T0259595

Screening and Prevention in Primary Care

Editors

MACK T. RUFFIN IV
CAMERON G. SHULTZ

PRIMARY CARE:
CLINICS IN OFFICE PRACTICE

www.primarycare.theclinics.com

Consulting Editor
JOEL J. HEIDELBAUGH

June 2014 • Volume 41 • Number 2

ELSEVIER

1600 John F. Kennedy Boulevard • Suite 1800 • Philadelphia, Pennsylvania, 19103-2899

http://www.theclinics.com

PRIMARY CARE: CLINICS IN OFFICE PRACTICE Volume 41, Number 2
June 2014 ISSN 0095-4543, ISBN-13: 978-0-323-29930-5

Editor: Jessica McCool
Developmental Editor: Yonah Korngold

© **2014 Elsevier Inc. All rights reserved.**

This periodical and the individual contributions contained in it are protected under copyright by Elsevier, and the following terms and conditions apply to their use:

Photocopying
Single photocopies of single articles may be made for personal use as allowed by national copyright laws. Permission of the Publisher and payment of a fee is required for all other photocopying, including multiple or systematic copying, copying for advertising or promotional purposes, resale, and all forms of document delivery. Special rates are available for educational institutions that wish to make photocopies for non-profit educational classroom use. For information on how to seek permission visit www.elsevier.com/permissions or call: (+44) 1865 843830 (UK)/(+1) 215 239 3804 (USA).

Derivative Works
Subscribers may reproduce tables of contents or prepare lists of articles including abstracts for internal circulation within their institutions. Permission of the Publisher is required for resale or distribution outside the institution. Permission of the Publisher is required for all other derivative works, including compilations and translations (please consult www.elsevier.com/permissions).

Electronic Storage or Usage
Permission of the Publisher is required to store or use electronically any material contained in this periodical, including any article or part of an article (please consult www.elsevier.com/permissions). Except as outlined above, no part of this publication may be reproduced, stored in a retrieval system or transmitted in any form or by any means, electronic, mechanical, photocopying, recording or otherwise, without prior written permission of the Publisher.

Notice
No responsibility is assumed by the Publisher for any injury and/or damage to persons or property as a matter of products liability, negligence or otherwise, or from any use or operation of any methods, products, instructions or ideas contained in the material herein. Because of rapid advances in the medical sciences, in particular, independent verification of diagnoses and drug dosages should be made.

Although all advertising material is expected to conform to ethical (medical) standards, inclusion in this publication does not constitute a guarantee or endorsement of the quality or value of such product or of the claims made of it by its manufacturer.

Primary Care: Clinics in Office Practice (ISSN: 0095–4543) is published quarterly by Elsevier Inc., 360 Park Avenue South, New York, NY 10010-1710. Months of issue are March, June, September, and December. Periodicals postage paid at New York, NY and additional mailing offices. Subscription prices are $225.00 per year (US individuals), $392.00 (US institutions), $115.00 (US students), $275.00 (Canadian individuals), $444.00 (Canadian institutions), $175.00 (Canadian students), $345.00 (international individuals), $444.00 (international institutions), and $175.00 (international students). Foreign air speed delivery is included in all *Clinics* subscription prices. All prices are subject to change without notice. POSTMASTER: Send address changes to *Primary Care: Clinics in Office Practice*, Elsevier Periodicals Customer Service, 11830 Westline Industrial Drive, St. Louis, MO 63146. Customer Service Health Sciences Division, Subscription Customer Service, 3251 Riverport Lane, Maryland Heights, MO 63043. **Customer Service: 1-800-654-2452 (U.S. and Canada); 314-447-8871 (outside U.S. and Canada). Fax: 314-447-8029. E-mail: journalscustomerservice-usa@elsevier.com (for print support); journalsonlinesupport-usa@elsevier.com (for online support).**

Reprints. For copies of 100 or more, of articles in this publication, please contact the Commercial Reprints Department, Elsevier Inc., 360 Park Avenue South, New York, NY 10010-1710. Tel. 212-633-3874; Fax: 212-633-3820; E-mail: reprints@elsevier.com.

Primary Care: Clinics in Office Practice is covered in *MEDLINE/PubMed (Index Medicus)* and *EMBASE/ Excerpta Medica, Current Contents/Clinical Medicine, and ISI/BIOMED.*

Contributors

CONSULTING EDITOR

JOEL J. HEIDELBAUGH, MD, FAAFP, FACG
Clinical Associate Professor, Departments of Family Medicine and Urology; Clerkship Director, Department of Family Medicine, University of Michigan Medical School, Ann Arbor, Michigan; Ypsilanti Health Center, Ypsilanti, Michigan

EDITORS

MACK T. RUFFIN IV, MD, MPH
Max and Buena Lichter Research Professor in Family Medicine, Department of Family Medicine, University of Michigan, Ann Arbor, Michigan

CAMERON G. SHULTZ, PhD, MSW
Director of Scholarly Projects, Department of Family Medicine, University of Michigan, Ann Arbor, Michigan

AUTHORS

LOUISE S. ACHESON, MD, MS
Professor of Family Medicine, Oncology, and Reproductive Biology, University Hospitals Case Medical Center, Case Western Reserve University, Cleveland, Ohio

BRUCE BARRETT, MD, PhD
Professor, Department of Family Medicine, University of Wisconsin, Madison, Wisconsin

EDITH BURBANK-SCHMITT, BA
Rutgers Robert Wood Johnson Medical School, New Brunswick, New Jersey

RALPH S. CARABALLO, PhD
Office of Smoking and Health, National Center for Chronic Disease Prevention and Health Promotion, Centers for Disease Control and Prevention, Atlanta, Georgia

JESSICA DALBY, MD
Assistant Professor, Department of Family Medicine, University of Wisconsin School of Medicine and Public Health, Madison, Wisconsin

MARIA SYL D. DE LA CRUZ, MD
Instructor, Department of Family and Community Medicine, Thomas Jefferson University, Philadelphia, Pennsylvania

D. EDWARD DENEKE, MD
Clinical Instructor, Department of Psychiatry, University of Michigan Health System, University of Michigan, Ann Arbor, Michigan

DOUGLAS H. FERNALD, MA
Senior Instructor, Department of Family Medicine, University of Colorado, Aurora, Colorado

THOMAS E. FLUENT, MD
Assistant Professor, Department of Psychiatry, University of Michigan Health System, University of Michigan, Ann Arbor, Michigan

BRIAN HALSTATER, MD
Physician, Department of Community and Family Medicine, Duke Family Medicine Center, Duke University, Durham, North Carolina

PAUL HUNTER, MD
Assistant Professor, Department of Family Medicine; Associate Medical Director, City of Milwaukee Health Department; Center Scientist, Center for Urban Population Health, University of Wisconsin School of Medicine and Public Health, Milwaukee, Wisconsin

KYLE E. KNIERIM, MD
Assistant Professor, Department of Family Medicine, University of Colorado, Aurora, Colorado

JAIME MARKS, MD
Assistant Professor, Department of Family Medicine, University of Wisconsin School of Medicine and Public Health, Augusta, Wisconsin

VIVIANA MARTINEZ-BIANCHI, MD, FAAFP
Physician, Department of Community and Family Medicine, Duke Family Medicine Center, Duke University, Durham, North Carolina

DONALD E. NEASE Jr, MD
Associate Professor and Vice Chair of Research, Department of Family Medicine, University of Colorado, Aurora, Colorado

KETTI PETERSEN, MD
Fellow, Hospice and Palliative Medicine; Department of Family Medicine, University of Michigan, Ann Arbor, Michigan; Department of Family Medicine, University of Michigan, Ypsilanti, Michigan

SARAH PICKLE, MD
Instructor, Department of Family Medicine and Community Health, Rutgers Robert Wood Johnson Medical School, New Brunswick, New Jersey

JOHN W. RAGSDALE III, MD
Physician, Department of Community and Family Medicine, Duke Family Medicine Center, Duke University, Durham, North Carolina

JASON A. RICCO, MD, MPH
Research Fellow, Department of Family Medicine, University of Wisconsin, Madison, Wisconsin

THOMAS B. RICHARDS, MD
Division of Cancer Prevention and Control, National Center for Chronic Disease Prevention and Health Promotion, Centers for Disease Control and Prevention, Atlanta, Georgia

MACK T. RUFFIN IV, MD, MPH
Max and Buena Lichter Research Professor in Family Medicine, Department of Family Medicine, University of Michigan, Ann Arbor, Michigan

MONA SARFATY, MD, MPH
Associate Professor, Department of Family and Community Medicine, Thomas Jefferson University, Philadelphia, Pennsylvania

SARINA SCHRAGER, MD, MS
Professor, Department of Family Medicine, University of Wisconsin School of Medicine and Public Health, Madison, Wisconsin

HEATHER SCHULTZ, MD, MPH
Chief Resident, Department of Psychiatry, University of Michigan Health System, University of Michigan, Ann Arbor, Michigan

SIMONE RAUSCHER SINGH, PhD, MA
Assistant Professor, Department of Health Management and Policy, School of Public Health, University of Michigan, Ann Arbor, Michigan

VIJAY SINGH, MD, MPH, MS
Clinical Lecturer, Department of Family Medicine, University of Michigan; Department of Emergency Medicine, Institute for Healthcare Policy and Innovation, University of Michigan Injury Center, Ann Arbor, Michigan

ELIZABETH W. STATON, MSTC
Instructor, Department of Family Medicine, University of Colorado, Aurora, Colorado

STEPHEN STROBBE, PhD, RN, PMHCNS-BC, CARN-AP
Clinical Associate Professor, Department of Psychiatry, University of Michigan School of Nursing, Ann Arbor, Michigan

GEOFFREY R. SWAIN, MD, MPH
Professor, Department of Family Medicine; Chief Medical Officer and Medical Director, City of Milwaukee Health Department; Center Scientist, Center for Urban Population Health, University of Wisconsin School of Medicine and Public Health, Milwaukee, Wisconsin

KATHRYN TENG, MD, FACP
Staff Physician, Internal Medicine; Director, Center for Personalized Healthcare, Cleveland Clinic, Cleveland, Ohio

D. KIM TURGEON, MD
Associate Professor, Division of Gastroenterology, Department of Internal Medicine, University of Michigan, Ann Arbor, Michigan

MARGARET L. WALLACE, PharmD, BCACP
Research Fellow, Department of Family Medicine, University of Wisconsin, Madison, Wisconsin

RICHARD C. WENDER, MD
Professor, Department of Family and Community Medicine, Thomas Jefferson University, Philadelphia, Pennsylvania; Chief Cancer Control Officer, American Cancer Society, Atlanta, Georgia

MARY C. WHITE, ScD
Division of Cancer Prevention and Control, National Center for Chronic Disease Prevention and Health Promotion, Centers for Disease Control and Prevention, Atlanta, Georgia

JUSTINE WU, MD, MPH
Associate Professor, Department of Family Medicine and Community Health, Rutgers Robert Wood Johnson Medical School, New Brunswick, New Jersey

Contents

Prevention plays an important role in achieving the triple aim of decreasing per capita health care costs, improving the health of populations, and bettering the patient experience. Primary care is uniquely positioned to provide preventive services. External forces are aligning to support the transition of primary care from traditional models focused on disease-specific, acute episodes of care to new ways of organizing that are more patient centered, team based, and quality driven. By aligning leadership, building change capacity, and selectively choosing relevant processes to change, those practicing primary care can successfully organize their practice environment to deliver preventive services.

Substance use and related disorders are among the leading causes of preventable injury and illness, chronic health conditions, medical complications, disability, increased suffering, and premature death. Primary care clinicians can help patients avoid, reduce, or eliminate high-risk behaviors and negative consequences associated with substance use by integrating prevention and screening, brief intervention, and referral to treatment into their clinical practices. This article provides the necessary information, evidence-based recommendations, and readily available resources to help address substance use and related disorders in primary care, with special emphasis on the use of tobacco, alcohol, cannabis, and nonmedical prescription opioid medications.

Sexually transmitted infections (STIs) are common and costly, in part because they are asymptomatic and result in serious complications. Primary care clinicians can easily diagnose and effectively treat most STIs. Clinicians should screen patients for STIs based on high-risk behaviors, and consult with local public health officials to adapt national screening guidelines to local epidemiology. Clinical encounters involving STI screening are opportunities to counsel patients on risk behaviors, and vaccinate against human papillomavirus and hepatitis B. Electronic health records and mobile phone apps show promise for improving the clinical care of STIs.

This article summarizes the literature regarding the epidemiology and prevention of unintended pregnancy in the United States. Because of the Affordable Care Act and its accompanying contraceptive provision, there is a need for more primary care clinicians to provide family planning services. Office-based interventions to incorporate family planning services in primary care are presented, including clinical tools and electronic health record use. Special attention is paid to long-acting reversible contraceptive methods (the subdermal implant and intrauterine devices); these highly effective and safe methods have the greatest potential to decrease the rate of unintended pregnancy, but have been underused.

In the United States, more than 1 out of 3 women experiences lifetime intimate partner violence (IPV) victimization. Short screening instruments such as HITS or the AAS can identify IPV victimization. Nonjudgmental statements that validate an IPV victim's experience should be followed by safety assessment and planning. Intervention includes referral to services, treatment of associated health conditions, mandatory reporting if required, and documentation. Counseling has been shown to reduce IPV victimization. Clinical guidelines recommend IPV screening for all or most women, and providing or referring victims to intervention. The Affordable Care Act will increase coverage of screening and counseling for IPV victims.

The goal of this article is to provide clinical guidance on breast cancer screening and prevention in primary care. The discussion highlights the importance of risk assessment, including screening options and risk-reduction strategies, for women at average and high risk. We review recommendations for breast cancer screening, evaluate current evidence on primary prevention, examine current practice patterns, and consider the impact of recent changes within health care.

This review provides an update on lung cancer screening with low-dose computed tomography (LDCT) and its implications for primary care providers. One of the unique features of lung cancer screening is the potential complexity in patient management if an LDCT scan reveals a small pulmonary nodule. Additional tests, consultation with multiple specialists, and follow-up evaluations may be needed to evaluate whether lung cancer is present. Primary care providers should know the resources available in their communities for lung cancer screening with LDCT and smoking cessation, and the key points to be addressed in informed and shared decision-making discussions with patients.

This article provides an update for the primary care community on the evidence and recommendations for colorectal cancer screening in the adult population without symptoms at average and increased risk, excluding patients with high-risk genetic syndromes. The current and possible new screening strategies are reviewed, along with clinical wisdom related to the implementation of each method.

Universal screening for prostate cancer (Pca) using prostate-specific antigen–based testing is not recommended, as the potential harms of screening (overdiagnosis and overtreatment) outweigh potential benefits. The case for Pca screening requires a paradigm shift, which emphasizes the risks of screening over the risks of undetected cancer. Physicians are encouraged to use shared decision making with patients who express an interest in Pca screening, taking into account both the patient's screening preferences and individual risk profile. New models of care informed by the Patient Protection and Affordable Care Act are intended to assist clinicians in providing recommended preventive services.

The purpose of this article is to update the primary care community on the evidence and guidelines for cardiovascular disease screening in a general-risk adult population, with the goal of assisting clinicians in developing an evidence-based approach toward screening. This article discusses global risk assessment and screening strategies, including blood pressure, lipids, C-reactive protein, homocysteine, coronary artery calcium score, carotid intima-media thickness, ultrasound of the abdominal aorta, and electrocardiography.

Despite strong efforts, the diagnosis and treatment of depression bring many challenges in the primary care setting. Screening for depression has been shown to be effective only if reliable systems of care are in place to ensure appropriate treatment by clinicians and adherence by patients. New evidence-based models of care for depression exist, but spread has been slow because of inadequate funding structures and conflicts within current clinical culture. The Affordable Care Act introduces potential opportunities to reorganize funding structures, conceivably leading to increased adoption of these collaborative care models. Suicide screening remains controversial.

This article discusses the clinical utility of genomic information for personalized preventive care of a healthy adult. Family health history is currently the most applicable genomic predictor for common, multifactorial diseases, and can also show patterns that suggest an inherited high susceptibility to a particular form of cancer or other disease. Both bloodline ancestry and shared environmental factors are important predictors for many disease states. DNA and family history analyses give information that is probabilistic, not deterministic. Therefore, family history can highlight behavioral, social, or cultural risk factors that can be modified to prevent diseases.

PRIMARY CARE:
CLINICS IN OFFICE PRACTICE

DOWNLOAD Free App!

Review Articles
THE CLINICS

NOW AVAILABLE FOR YOUR iPhone and iPad

Foreword

Preventive Medicine: Shared Responsibility

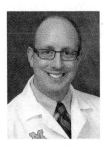

Joel J. Heidelbaugh, MD, FAAFP, FACG
Consulting Editor

The topic "preventive medicine" is defined by the American College of Preventive Medicine as the practice of medicine that *"focuses on the health of individuals, communities, and defined populations. Its goal is to protect, promote, and maintain health and well-being…and to prevent disease, disability, and death."*[1] Coupled with the provisions of the patient-centered medical home model, which seeks to improve the health of *"whole people, families, communities and populations, and on increasing the value of health care,"*[2] preventive medicine has a central tenet that aims to lower health care costs, maximize the overall patient–health care provider experience, and reduce morbidity and mortality.

As a family physician spending a substantial portion of my day performing health maintenance examinations, I'm always struck by what motivates patients to come to my office for "a physical," and I become quickly curious about what questions regarding preventive medicine services will arise during the visit. Perhaps dishearteningly, a very high percentage of such visits quickly center on "a form" that the patient brings to the visit, whereby they have been instructed by their insurance company to have me complete it. Some of these forms simply require me to sign them; some require vital signs such as body mass index and blood pressure, as well as fasting cholesterol and glucose measurements, while others may inquire about symptoms of depression and smoking status. None are complete in requesting preventive services, and none are risk-stratified based on age or gender. Most commonly, I find that patients with private insurances are "advised" to have these forms completed with a visible carrot at the end of the stick: do it or we may raise your rates. What happens for patients with Medicaid or Medicare? While many patients are inquisitive about screening tests and are proactive in prevention, we are missing significant opportunities to screen various populations of our patients appropriately within our communities.

Last week, a 51-year-old woman came to my office for a medication refill. She has a history of hypertension and had run out of hydrocholorothiazide in October 2010. (Yes,

Prim Care Clin Office Pract 41 (2014) xiii–xv
http://dx.doi.org/10.1016/j.pop.2014.03.001
0095-4543/14/$ – see front matter © 2014 Elsevier Inc. All rights reserved.

2010.) Fortunately, the positive light in the visit occurred when I told her that her blood pressure was 115/72; on repeat 10 minutes later it was 112/72, and I felt that she didn't need the medication at this point. In reviewing her chart, I noticed that she was due for a mammogram; a colonoscopy; a PAP smear; a renal panel (based on her previous diagnosis of hypertension); and influenza, pneumococcal, and tetanus/diphtheria/pertussis vaccinations. Always taking the opportunity to address preventive maintenance during office visits, I offered her these services, and she quickly became visibly infuriated with me. First, it was clear that she was offended that I offered her these preventive services. She likened my "offering of these services" to "bringing her car into the shop" to get "unnecessary tests done" when she didn't have any symptoms or in her opinion "didn't need them." She then asked me what "my kickback" was going to be from her insurance company for performing such tests. I apologized, reframed my offering of preventive services for her, and explained that I don't get direct financial incentives from anyone for her receiving such services. The reality is that the financial incentive portion may be only partially true (I don't get direct incentives, but my institution and employer might), and that failure to have this patient complete such services may likely negatively affect the quality metrics of my practice. As it would turn out, she complained to my checkout clerk that I wanted to give her a flu shot and was upset because she had "gotten the flu" from a flu shot previously...

As we have now embraced and employed the paradigm of population management in our practices, one which creates a level of accountability for health care providers and practices, the proverbial "bar has been raised" for us to more aggressively target appropriate interval preventive screening for our patients. So, what if they decline certain tests and screening provisions? How much responsibility do health care providers and practices assume for noncompliant patients and for those who decline screening and preventive services? To what degree will patients ultimately be responsible?

This issue of *Primary Care: Clinics in Office Practice* commences with an article dedicated to organizing our medical practices to enhance screening and secondary disease prevention practices in adults. It very deftly outlines key provisions of the Affordable Care Act relative to disease prevention and screening across populations of men and women throughout the life cycle. Additional articles outline current evidence-based guidelines for breast, lung, and colorectal cancer screening, as well as the highly controversial topic of prostate cancer screening. Articles dedicated to interpersonal violence screening and planned pregnancy provide profound insight into prevention within the family and in relationships. Screening for chronic diseases, including heart disease and depression, as well as sexually transmitted infections, is of paramount importance and is detailed through current literature reviews. While tobacco use in the United States has leveled off in recent years, rates of illicit substance abuse have dramatically increased, and this topic deserves and receives special attention. Finally, this volume concludes with an article dedicated to the use of genetic markers in disease and cancer screening, a topic that most primary care providers are not adequately taught at baseline, and a field of rapid advancement that may hold significant promise in future screening of terminal disease.

Drs Ruffin and Shultz, my colleagues in the Department of Family Medicine at the University of Michigan, have compiled and edited an exciting and detailed volume of articles from reputable experts across the country. This issue should serve as the template by which a reasonable approach to adult preventive services becomes based not only in theory but especially in practice. It is the responsibility of the health care provider to educate patients on appropriate preventive screening, and it is our collective responsibility to maximize the preventive health of our widely variable populations.

Joel J. Heidelbaugh, MD, FAAFP, FACG
Departments of Family Medicine and Urology
Department of Family Medicine
University of Michigan Medical School
Ann Arbor, MI, USA

Ypsilanti Health Center
200 Arnet Suite 200
Ypsilanti, MI 48198, USA

E-mail address:
jheidel@umich.edu

REFERENCES

1. The American College of Preventive Medicine. Available at: http://www.acpm.org/?page=WhatisPM. Accessed February 26, 2014.
2. Stange KC, Nutting PA, Miller WL, et al. Defining and measuring the patient-centered medical home. J Gen Intern Med 2010;25(6):601–2.

Preface

Screening and Prevention in Primary Care

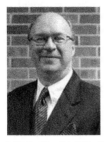   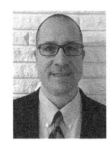

Mack T. Ruffin IV, MD, MPH   Cameron G. Shultz, PhD, MSW
Editors

Preventive services—both critical and essential to the foundation of primary care—are a unique feature of the primary care specialties. In this issue of *Primary Care: Clinics in Office Practice*, we selected a wide array of preventive service topics, including the commonly addressed issues of screening for breast cancer, heart disease, colorectal cancer, depression, and substance misuse (alcohol, tobacco, and other substances). Screening for sexually transmitted infections, intimate partner violence, prostate cancer, and lung cancer are also addressed, as well as the topics of preventing unintended pregnancy, genomics in primary care practice, and organizing primary care practice for screening and prevention. We challenged authors to summarize the evidence, review the service from the perspective of community-based primary care, and address the impact of recent changes in health care: the Patient Protection and Affordable Care Act, accountable care organizations, electronic health records, and the patient-centered medical home. To this end, authors have done an admirable job.

As discussed by the authors, primary care is on the cusp of revolutionary changes intended to improve the primary care clinicians' ability to effectively and efficiently deliver preventive services. While many of us in primary care have extolled the importance and priority of preventive services for years, data suggest only a modest percentage of eligible patients gets the preventive care they need. We have pointed to many barriers that keep us from doing better, including too little time or money, incomplete information or ineffective data management systems, and a lack of patient acceptance or access. Making the time to provide preventive services has in the past been one of the most challenging obstacles, as many of us practice within perverted systems that reward viewing patients as an output product, much like widgets on an assembly line.

The revolutionary changes to health care now on our doorstep could move us away from the sole focus of patient throughput to new models of care based on efficient, high-quality care that addresses the needs of individual patients and the health of

Prim Care Clin Office Pract 41 (2014) xvii–xviii
http://dx.doi.org/10.1016/j.pop.2014.02.013
0095-4543/14/$ – see front matter © 2014 Published by Elsevier Inc.

primarycare.theclinics.com

defined populations. Integral to these new models is the effective delivery of preventive services. However, an important challenge in transitioning one's practice comes from the duality of continuing to provide care within the existing primary care environment while at the same time (and with limited guidance and resources) transitioning to the new models of care. Despite this challenge, primary care clinicians need to step up and take leadership during this time of change. The first article of this issue is an essential primer on leadership and organizing primary care practice for health care in the twenty-first century. The last article, addressing the utility of genomic information for personalized preventive care, offers guidance for how the primary care clinician should—and should not—utilize this rapidly changing technology in everyday practice. The ten articles in-between offer guidance for setting priorities as they relate to each respective content area.

An analogy may help to communicate the urgency of our situation. If we gave you a Model T, most of you would not know how to start it. And even if you could start it, you could not make it down a modern superhighway. Our current practice models and information systems, in 20 years, will be seen like the Model T. To deal with our rapidly transforming health care system, primary care leaders must take a quantum leap equivalent to the gap between the Model T and the solar car. Whereas the Model T is cumbersome, ineffective, and ill-suited to meet the demands of the twenty-first century, the solar car is of the highest quality, incredibly efficient, and self-sustaining. While the transition to new models of primary care will not be easy, the future for primary care—and prevention—has never looked brighter.

Mack T. Ruffin IV, MD, MPH
Department of Family Medicine
University of Michigan
1018 Fuller Street
Ann Arbor, MI 48104-1213, USA

Cameron G. Shultz, PhD, MSW
Department of Family Medicine
University of Michigan
1018 Fuller Street
Ann Arbor, MI 48104-1213, USA

E-mail addresses:
mruffin@med.umich.edu (M.T. Ruffin)
cshultz@med.umich.edu (C.G. Shultz)

Organizing Your Practice for Screening and Secondary Prevention Among Adults

Kyle E. Knierim, MD*, Douglas H. Fernald, MA,
Elizabeth W. Staton, MSTC, Donald E. Nease Jr, MD

KEYWORDS

- Primary heath care • Practice transformation • Primary care organization
- Prevention

KEY POINTS

- Prevention is required to achieve the triple aim of lowering per capita health care costs, improving the health of populations, and bettering the patient experience.
- As the largest formal platform for health care delivery in the United States, primary care is uniquely positioned to provide preventive services.
- Recently passed health care legislation (the Affordable Care Act) and new models of organizing and delivering health care (accountable care organizations, patient-centered medical homes) compel those in primary care to abandon more traditional models of care and take up new models that are more patient centered, team based, and quality driven.
- By aligning leadership, building change capacity, and selectively choosing relevant processes to change, those practicing primary care can successfully organize to deliver preventive services.

INTRODUCTION

This issue of *Primary Care: Clinics in Office Practice* is devoted to prevention. The topic is timely not only because of the many new diagnostic and therapeutic techniques but also because of the broader goals to decrease costs, improve health, and improve the patient experience; goals that can be achieved, in part, by enhanced preventive services provided by better organized primary care. This article outlines several prevention shortfalls in the US health care system, the ability of

Conflict of Interest: None.
Department of Family Medicine, University of Colorado, Mail Stop F496, 12631 East 17th Avenue, Aurora, CO 80045, USA
* Corresponding author. 3055 Roslyn Street, Suite 100, Denver, CO 80238.
E-mail address: kyle.knierim@ucdenver.edu

prevention-oriented primary care to address these gaps, and how newly enacted legislation (the Patient Protection and Affordable Care Act [ACA]) and emerging models for organizing care (eg, accountable care organizations [ACOs], patient-centered medical homes [PCMHs]) are designed to help support the capacity of primary care to provide prevention-related services. This article offers guidance to the primary care practitioner for organizing one's practice to consistently deliver high-quality preventive services.

PRIMARY CARE: IMPORTANT TO PREVENTION

Primary care is the largest formal platform for health care delivery in the United States. Of the 1 billion outpatient visits in the United States in 2011, 55% were provided by primary care physicians.[1,2] The primary care workforce comprises nearly 295,000 providers, including physicians, nurse practitioners, and physician assistants.[3] Considering its substantial reach, primary care is considered the logical base to a sustainable US health care system.[4] The Institute of Medicine describes primary care as "the provision of integrated, accessible health care services by clinicians who are accountable for addressing a large majority of personal health care needs, developing a sustained partnership with patients, and practicing in the context of family and community."[5] As outlined in **Box 1**, more contemporary descriptions of primary care also include the tenets of person-centeredness, first-contact access, comprehensiveness, and coordination.[4] When implemented in a comprehensive manner and in accordance with these tenets, primary care leads to improved population health.[5–7]

Health care accounted for nearly 18% of US gross domestic product (GDP) in 2011. On its current trajectory, health care could account for 34% of GDP by 2040.[8] On average, the United States spent $8508 per person on health care in 2011 (2.5 times more than the average for developed countries) but achieved worse outcomes on nearly every health indicator.[9,10] Both primary care and preventive services are recognized as important components to slowing costs and improving the quality of US health care.

Box 1
Four key features of primary care

- It is person-focused rather than disease-focused. This focus entails sustained relationships between patients and providers in primary care practices over time, often referred to as continuity.

- It provides first contact for whatever people might consider a health or health care problem. In properly organized health care systems, primary care ensures access to needed services.

- It is comprehensive. By definition, it can encompass any problem. Many problems in primary care are ambiguous and defy precise diagnosis. Nonetheless, primary care meets most patients' needs without referral.

- It coordinates care. Primary care adopts mechanisms that facilitate the transfer of information about health care over time. Highly personalized solutions to patients' problems can be implemented when sustained relationships permit deeper knowledge and understanding of individuals' habits, preferences, and goals.

From Institute of Medicine. Primary care and public health: exploring integration to improve population health. Washington, DC: National Academies Press; 2012. Reprinted with permission from the National Academies Press, Copyright © 2012 National Academy of Sciences.

US populations with a greater supply of primary care providers have better health outcomes, including lower rates of all-cause mortality, and reduced mortality from heart disease, cancer, and stroke; likewise, populations in areas with a high ratio of primary care providers are more likely to have higher self-reported health. These positive correlations persist regardless of a person's age, income, or education, or the population's rurality, education levels, percentage of female-headed households, poverty rates, and minority status.[5–7,11,12] In addition to better health outcomes, access to primary care plays a key role in the provision of preventive services[13–20]; however, as outlined in **Table 1**, there remains room for improvement.

Improving the provision of preventive services within the primary care setting could make an important contribution toward reducing both excess morbidity and mortality. For example, evidence suggests that 1 in 10 hospitalizations could be prevented with comprehensive outpatient care,[27] and increasing the use of just 5 preventive services (daily aspirin, smoking cessation assistance, colorectal cancer screening, and immunization against influenza) in high-risk populations could save more than 100,000 lives in the United States each year.[19]

Many factors can restrict primary care providers from consistently performing high-value preventive interventions: lack of awareness, familiarity, or agreement with the recommended intervention; a belief that one cannot successfully deliver the intervention, or that the intervention will not bring about the desired outcome; practice inertia (ie, difficulty in changing the way things have previously been done); and external barriers (eg, too few resources).[28–30] One commonly cited external barrier is not having enough time, a complaint borne, in part, from the increasing number and complexity of recommended preventive services. In an effort to operationalize this complexity, Yarnall and colleagues[31] estimated that it would take a primary care provider with 2500 patients nearly 7.5 hours every working day to fully satisfy the recommendations (Yarnall and colleagues derived the time estimate based on services delineated in the 1996 US Preventive Services Task Force *Guide to Clinical Preventive Services*). Despite these challenges, recent policy changes and focused attention on providing better support to primary care providers represent a significant opportunity to reorganize primary care practice in ways that enable more effective delivery of preventive health care.

NATIONAL TRENDS SUPPORTING PREVENTION IN PRIMARY CARE

In the past, many primary care providers seeking to emphasize preventive services had to overcome multiple barriers, not the least of which was a payment system

Table 1
Actual versus healthy people 2020 target rates of preventive services

	Actual Rate (%)	Healthy People 2020 Target Rate (%)
Colon cancer screening[a]	59.2	70.5
Breast cancer screening[b]	72.4	81.1
Cervical cancer screening[c]	82.8	93
Annual influenza vaccination in adults aged 18–64 y[d]	38.6	90
Pneumococcal vaccination in adults aged ≥65 y[e]	60.1	90
Hypertension controlled[f]	45.9	61.2

[a–f] From the US Department of Health and Human Services.[21–26]

that, collectively, tended to create disincentives to providing preventive care. Several far-reaching policy efforts are under way to align incentives, emphasize prevention, and transform primary care to better deliver these services. These initiatives begin to address many of the long-standing barriers to providing preventive care in the primary care setting.

The ACA

The ACA is the most significant federal statute to affect the provision of health care in the United States in decades. Signed into law in 2010, the ACA expands health insurance coverage, requires insurers to provide recommended preventive services at no additional cost to patients (eg, no deductibles or copayments), and expands access to primary care.[32] Key components of the law are outlined in **Box 2**, including fully covered preventive care. For those in primary care practice, several provisions in the ACA specifically aim to support primary care providers' ability to serve more patients with better models of care (**Box 3**).

In addition to expanded insurance coverage and improved financing for primary care, the ACA supports the implementation of payment and organizational models that align with the objectives of delivering preventive care. One organizational model in particular has the potential to increase the provision of preventive services in primary care: the ACO.

ACOs are a network of providers and hospitals that share responsibility for providing coordinated care to a defined population. ACOs move away from purely fee-for-service (FFS) payments to a shared savings model. Participants receive financial

---

Box 2
Key components of the ACA that will expand insurance coverage

- Individual shared responsibility provision: starting in 2014, individuals of all ages (including children) must have minimum essential health coverage, qualify for an exemption, or make payment when filing a federal tax return.[a]

- Medicaid expansion: starting in 2014 in participating states, nearly all individuals younger than 65 years with income less than 133% of the federal poverty level (about $15,282 for an individual and $31,322 for a family of 4[b]) are eligible for Medicaid.[c] For state-specific policies, go to http://www.medicaid.gov/Medicaid-CHIP-Program-Information/By-State/By-State.html.

- Children's Health Insurance Program (CHIP): children currently covered by CHIP with family incomes between 100% and 133% of the federal poverty level will move to Medicaid, but states will keep their right to claim the enhanced CHIP matching rate, beginning in October 2015.[d] For state-specific policies go to http://insurekidsnow.gov/state/index.html.

- Children younger than 26 years: most health plans that cover children must make coverage available to children up to age 26 years.[e]

- Preexisting health conditions: starting in 2014, most health insurance plans cannot refuse coverage or charge higher premiums to those with preexisting health conditions.[f]

- Free preventive care: insurance plans must cover preventive services to patients with no out-of-pocket costs (eg, no deductible or copay) to the patient. This provision includes many immunizations, obesity counseling, and screening for important conditions like diabetes, human immunodeficiency virus, and alcohol misuse.[g]

[a] From the Internal Revenue Service.[33]

[b] From the US Department of Health and Human Services.[34]

[c–g] From the US Centers for Medicare and Medicaid Services.[35–39]

Box 3
ACA provisions that affect primary care

- Medicare 10% increase in primary care reimbursement rates, 2011 to 2016 ($3.5 billion)
- Medicaid reimbursement for primary care increased to at least Medicare levels, 2013 to 2014 ($8.3 billion)
- 32 million more people insured, with preventive and primary care coverage, leading to less uncompensated care
- Grants/contracts to support medical homes through:
  - Community health teams increasing access to coordinated care
  - Community-based collaborative care networks for low-income populations
  - Primary care extension center program providing technical assistance to primary care providers
- Scholarships, loan repayment, and training demonstration programs to invest in primary care physicians, midlevel providers, and community providers
- $11 billion for federally qualified health centers, 2011 to 2015, to serve 15 million to 20 million more patients by 2015

Data from Abrams M, Nuzum R, Mika S, et al. How the Affordable Care Act will strengthen primary care and benefit patients, providers, and payers. Issue Brief (Commonw Fund) 2011;1:1–28.

---

bonuses if they meet agreed performance benchmarks based on both quality and cost; ACOs can receive larger rewards if they accept financial risk if they fail to meet their benchmarks. The ACO model attempts to strike a balance between volume-based FFS payments and tightly controlled capitated budgets that place providers under full financial risk for all spending in their enrolled populations.[40]

ACOs can benefit primary care and prevention in at least 2 ways: they require a strong primary care foundation to achieve their value-based targets; and their quality markers include a focus on preventive health care. The ACO quality measures divide into 4 domains: patient and caregiver experience; care coordination and patient safety; at-risk populations (ie, patients with diabetes, hypertension, heart disease); and preventive health.[41] Primary care providers, with the proper resources, data, and leadership, can affect all of these domains.[42] **Table 2** details the preventive care measures that must be reported by ACOs to the Centers for Medicare and Medicaid Services (CMS). CMS initially rewards ACOs for complete and accurate reporting for all quality measures (including those related to prevention), then phases in additional performance standards over subsequent years.[43]

The partnership between ACOs and primary care practices can be synergistic: the ACOs provide financial support and collaboration across a network of providers and organizations, and primary care practices offer direct provision of services and efficient care coordination. The partnership fosters a new model of primary care practice that combines the traditional strengths of primary care (eg, continuity; accessible, coordinated, and comprehensive care) with modern advances in health information technology, population management, and team-based care.[44]

The PCMH and Primary Care Practice Transformation

As viewed through the lens of the ACA and ACOs, the model primary care practice is proactive, bundled, and shared: proactive, in that those providing care actively target

Table 2
CMS prevention-related reporting requirements for ACOs

Measure Title	Pay for Performance Phase in Reporting (R) and Performance (P)		
	Year 1	Year 2	Year 3
Influenza immunization	R	P	P
Pneumococcal vaccination	R	P	P
Tobacco use assessment and tobacco cessation intervention	R	P	P
Depression screening	R	P	P
Colorectal cancer screening	R	R	P
Mammography screening	R	R	P
Adults with blood pressure measured within the preceding 2 y	R	R	P

From CMS. Improving quality of care for Medicare patients: accountable care organizations. Available at: http://www.cms.gov/Medicare/Medicare-Fee-for-Service-Payment/sharedsavingsprogram/Downloads/ACO_Quality_Factsheet_ICN907407.pdf. Accessed March 13, 2014.

and prevent anticipated health problems; bundled, in that the focus is on providing comprehensive primary care over time rather than treating acute or episodic events; and shared, in that care is provided by a diverse multidisciplinary team, of which the informed, activated, and engaged patient is a member.[45,46] Because this vision represents a shift from more traditional forms of primary care practice in both its structures (ie, the physical environment and context of care) and processes (ie, the procedures associated with health care delivery and documentation), effective practice management requires a different administrative skill set. Successful administrators in this new model of primary care must not only possess the capacity to manage and understand complex data, they must have the know-how to leverage those data to improve efficiencies and outcomes.

The PCMH is the most widely recognized way of operationalizing the new model of primary care. The PCMH promotes patient-centered, comprehensive, team-based, coordinated, and accessible services focused on quality and safety.[47] First introduced in 1967 by the American Academy of Pediatrics, the concept of the medical home was updated in 2002 as part of the Future of Family Medicine project and presented as a way to transform primary care to better meet the needs of patients in a rapidly changing health care environment.[48] In 2007, the American Academy of Family Physicians, the American Academy of Pediatrics, the American College of Physicians, and the American Osteopathic Association jointly adopted a set of principles defining the PCMH as the foundation of a transformed health care delivery system positioned to meet patients' primary care needs. A contemporary interpretation of these principles (in which focus is placed on practice teams rather than individual providers) is outlined in **Box 4**.[47]

Although existing evidence is insufficient to establish the impact of PCMH on most clinical and economic outcomes, the model continues to hold promise for improving the quality of health care. A 2013 review of 19 comparative studies[49] showed that PCMH interventions had a small to moderate positive impact on the provision of preventive care, and a small positive effect on patient experience, provider satisfaction, and staff satisfaction. Researchers reported there was no evidence that PCMH led to cost savings, and a reduction in hospital admissions was not observed. However, evidence suggested reduced emergency department use among older adults, which may be related to the positive impact of PCMH on prevention and chronic disease

---

Box 4
Principles of the PCMH: team-based care and enhanced practice settings

- Personal provider: each patient has an ongoing relationship with a primary care provider (working within a practice team) who is trained to provide first-contact, continuous, and comprehensive care.

- Provider-directed medical practice: teams within the practice share responsibility for both the care of individual patients and the greater population they serve.

- Whole person orientation: the practice team provides care in all stages of life and across care settings or arranges such care with other professionals when necessary.

- Coordinated/integrated care: practice teams use information technology to ensure that patients are receiving the right care, at the right time, and in the right care settings.

- Focus on quality and safety: practice teams continuously strive to improve the tools of practice, such as clinical pathways that support evidence-based medicine, enhanced clinical decision support systems, and continuous quality improvement cycles, to ensure efficient and high-quality patient-centered outcomes.

- Enhanced access: practice teams adopt policies and procedures to improve patients' access to primary care, such as advanced access scheduling, extended hours, asynchronous communication (eg, e-mail, text messaging), and telemedicine (eg, 2-way video, wireless tools, smart phones).

- Payment reform: compensation for the wide range of services provided by practice teams within enhanced practice settings duly accounts for factors (eg, care coordination, enhanced communication, population management, case-mix complexity, practice efficiency) not typically recognized by FFS models based solely on face-to-face patient-provider encounters.

The 2007 Joint Principles of the PCMH identified the primary care provider as the principal locus of health care delivery; however, more contemporary PCMH models focus on primary care teams working within enhanced practice settings that optimize efficiency, quality, and the patient experience.

Adapted from American Academy of Family Physicians, American Academy of Pediatrics, American College of Physicians, America Osteopathic Association. Joint principles of the patient-centered medical home. 2007. Available at: http://www.aafp.org/dam/AAFP/documents/practice_management/pcmh/initiatives/PCMHJoint.pdf. Accessed December 7, 2011.

---

management in primary care settings. A 2012 summary released by the Patient-Centered Primary Care Collaborative rated PCMHs more positively, showing improvements in health outcomes, enhanced patient and provider experiences, and reductions in unnecessary emergency department use. Although it was not subjected to peer review, 1 strength of the summary is the diversity of PCMH models that it included, such as initiatives spearheaded by ACOs, health systems, insurance providers, public institutions, private institutions, and public-private partnerships.[42] Research investigating PCMHs has been limited by lack of consistent nomenclature, variation in model design and outcome measures, and unsatisfactory evaluation methods. Although future evaluations of PCMH need to address these issues, the PCMH model as whole is generally believed to hold promise for decreasing health care costs, improving health outcomes, and enhancing patients' experience of care.

More information on PCMH can be found by visiting the Web site of the Agency for Healthcare Research and Quality PCMH Resource Center (http://pcmh.ahrq.gov/), the American Academy of Family Physicians PCMH Overview (http://www.aafp.org/practice-management/pcmh/overview.html), and the Patient-Centered Primary Care Collaborative (http://www.pcpcc.org/).

ORGANIZING PRIMARY CARE PRACTICE TO PROVIDE PREVENTIVE SERVICES

Delivering preventive services is a core function of primary care. To fulfill this function, primary care providers in many practice settings have had to overcome several external barriers, including the increase of patient panels; increased demand (competition) for providers' time; insurance coverage that may deter prevention (eg, high patient deductibles and copays); inadequate compensation for some prevention-related tasks (eg, educating patients, shared decision making, using patient decision aids); and increased complexity of primary care practice generally, in which prevention is just one of an increasing list of responsibilities. New regulatory frameworks (the ACA) and emerging models for organizing care (ACOs and PCMHs) are designed to help reduce these external obstacles, replacing them with incentives that reward high-quality, low-cost, patient-centered care. For these new arrangements to be most effective, the structures and processes of the primary care practice setting must be appropriately organized.

Traditionally, FFS primary care practice settings have been managed to maximize the number of patient-provider face-to-face encounters. Under the new arrangements (in which costs, quality, and outcomes are aligned with reimbursement for an entire population), a team-based approach works more efficiently. In team-based primary care, a clinician (usually a physician) leads a team of professionals (eg, physician assistants and nurse practitioners, nurses, medical assistants, and support staff) who, collectively, share responsibility for the care of patients. Through planning and clear delineation of roles, the team draws on the respective strengths of each team member to best address a given patient's needs. For example, although a physician may be responsible for making complex diagnoses, a physician assistant meets patients' more routine needs (eg, ongoing chronic disease management), and the medical assistant performs necessary administrative or clinical tasks (eg, administering a vaccine following standing orders, drawing blood).[50] Team-based care has been associated with improvements in quality, including higher immunization rates[51,52]; improved chronic disease management[53–57]; improved screening processes for cancer, chronic disease, and tobacco use[52,58]; and higher patient and provider satisfaction.[59,60] To move to a team-based approach, significant changes are often required to the structures and processes of a clinic.[61]

Several strategies have been developed to help primary care providers improve the capacity of their clinic for change.[62–65] Solberg,[66] for example, developed a 3-pronged approach for practice improvement that includes aligning improvement priorities throughout the organization, building capacity for change, and carefully selecting the content of new processes. To effectively facilitate meaningful change, those coordinating the change process must ask themselves the following key questions: "Do[es] the practice...have sufficient priority for this change and will [the practice]...have enough capability for managing the process of change? Have the best and most feasible care process targets been chosen for improvement? Are there internal or external barriers that will prevent success no matter how well the other stars are aligned?"[66]

The following section describes how to use Solberg's model to enhance the provision of preventive services in the primary care setting. Using the Solberg model is not about following a step-by-step process; rather, it is about learning how to ask the right questions and find the right answers within the context of a given practice setting. Because no 2 settings are exactly alike, no 2 solutions are exactly alike. The following case example shows how the Solberg approach can be used to improve immunizations and cancer screening in a small, suburban primary care clinic. The questions posed under each heading are meant to stimulate thinking on the sort of issues leaders must consider when developing and implementing a practice improvement project.

Aligning Improvement Priorities

The task of implementing a practice improvement project within a given practice setting is analogous to a patient making a health behavior change: success emerges only after robust commitment and dedicated effort. To achieve the desired result, leaders must convey the importance of the proposed change by allocating sufficient resources (eg, time, money), minimizing competing demands, and communicating a consistent vision for why the change matters. If the clinic is affiliated with a larger institution (eg, a regional health center), it is also important that the parent institution be in support of the desired change process. Those carrying out the change must have not only explicit support from the clinic's leaders but support from all affected personnel.[67] For example, changing the workflow to improve immunization rates might require the involvement of several team members, such as the physician, nurse, medical assistant, and intake receptionist. If 1 team member is not on board, that person becomes the weak link and can undermine the entire change process. In general, staff are likely to get behind a change when they understand why it is needed and how it helps make things better.[67]

As the consumer of health care, patients can play an important role in identifying change priorities.[68,69] Patients can bring important insight to change efforts by helping providers select priority areas, understand the personal impact of change, and ensure that the change is carried out in a culturally sensitive manner. Despite these advantages, patients commonly remain underused as a strategic resource.[70] Several organizations, including the Agency for Healthcare Research and Quality (http://www.ahrq.gov/professionals/quality-patient-safety/patient-safety-resources/resources/patient-safety-advisory-council/), the Institute for Patient- and Family-Centered Care (http://www.ipfcc.org/advance/Advisory_Councils.pdf), and the Robert Wood Johnson Foundation (http://www.pcpcc.org/sites/default/files/resources/Engaging%20Patients%20in%20Improving%20Ambulatory%20Care%20-%20RWJF.pdf) offer guidance on how to effectively engage patients when undertaking a change-related initiative.

Box 5 presents several questions to consider when establishing improvement priorities.

Change Capacity

Before a change process can start (whether implementing new prevention practices or updating existing screening protocols), those engaged in the process must have the capacity to develop a sufficiently detailed plan, the means to execute the plan, and the resources to assess the impact of that execution over time. Each of these tasks (planning, execution, and assessment) requires effective leadership. In addition to ensuring that a change process has the resources it needs to be successful, effective leaders must be able to communicate a clear vision for the desired change, tailoring the message so it has relevance to all respective personnel within the change setting (from the intake receptionists to the administrators of the institution). Effective leaders must also build support among the myriad of potential stakeholders, who may in some cases have competing or conflicting interests. Similarly, leaders must also know how to overcome resistance among team members and bring energy and encouragement to the initiative when enthusiasm is lacking. Leaders must have the fortitude to stick with the change process through inevitable (and often multiple) setbacks.[67]

Leadership styles commonly fall into 2 camps: autocratic (or authoritative) and democratic (or participative). Autocratic leadership styles, in which a single leader issues

---

Box 5
Aligning improvement priorities

- What is the reason my practice needs to change? Is there a substantial issue (eg, safety, inequality, business) that needs attention?
- Do my colleagues think the issue is important?
- Do my patients find the issue meaningful?
- Compared with the other efforts already under way or about to start, how important is this issue?
- How will the larger organization react? Does the issue align with their current priorities?

Case example: Aligning Internal and External Priorities to Motivate Practice Change

A private, suburban primary care clinic with 3 clinicians opened about 2 years ago. At the start, the clinicians committed to a shared vision to treat the patient as a whole and to engage patients in their own health care. They quickly were caught up in the challenges of developing a new practice, but they dedicated time to participate in a regional quality improvement initiative that required them to share patient outcomes data with other clinics in the area. In return for their participation, the clinicians received technical support to achieve meaningful use stage 1 (MU). After a year of ups and downs, the operations of the clinic were stable, the data generated by the electronic health records (EHR) was accurate, and the MU requirements were satisfied. The clinicians and staff had put in a lot of hard work, but the patient outcomes were not turning out as they had hoped; many patients were not receiving recommended preventive care such as screening for colon and breast cancer and immunizations for flu and pneumonia, and markers of chronic disease control lagged behind other practices in the community. The clinic leaders decided it was time to refocus on their initial vision and become more proactive and patient centered.

Considering the case: are there any local or regional projects that your practice can join to support changes you want to do?

---

commands that the rest follow, can be effective when decisions need to be made quickly or when input from team members is unnecessary. However, because buy-in and feedback are essential for making changes within most primary care settings, an autocratic leadership style, in most cases, is neither helpful nor desirable. In contrast, a democratic leadership style, with its flatter organizational hierarchy and in which team members share decision-making responsibilities, is well suited for changing processes within primary care; it helps to keep team members engaged, it spurs creativity and enthusiasm, and can facilitate a sense of ownership over the change process itself.[71] An example of a democratic approach to change is to structure an improvement team with diverse membership (eg, physicians, nurses, medical assistants, front office staff), and adopt explicit ground rules that promote respect and unhindered disclosure of ideas, questions, and concerns. To optimize democratic principles, the meetings of the team should be scheduled at a time when all participants can attend, and in a setting in which interruptions are kept to a minimum. Although a democratic approach to change takes more effort to organize and sustain, evidence suggests that it is associated with improved performance on measures of quality in primary care.[72–74]

In addition to a democratic leadership style, effective leaders must have the expertise to identify and implement an appropriate change framework that fits the setting and improvement goal. Several change frameworks have proved useful in health care settings, including the Model for Improvement (http://www.ihi.org/knowledge/pages/howtoimprove/default.aspx), Lean (http://www.lean.org/whatslean/), and Six Sigma (http://www.innovations.ahrq.gov/content.aspx?id=2148).[75,76] Having a clearly identified and agreed framework supplies a common language, thus helping to improve communication, and provides a systematic process for implementing change. The most useful frameworks guide quality improvement teams through each of the tasks associated with the change process, including planning, execution, and assessment; effective frameworks also have a clear process for adjusting and reassessing, as needed, until improvement goals are met. With repetition, the steps associated with a given framework become routine, and, over time, change is no longer seen as a project to complete but a process to continue.

Table 3 expands on some of the key elements discussed in this section; **Box 6** presents several questions to consider.

Change Process Content

Quality improvement teams can find a seemingly endless number of areas needing improvement, and the volume of items requiring attention may be overwhelming. Not everything can be improved at once, and where to start is less important than the act of starting. The key is to start somewhere. Pick 1 thing that your team can agree on improving, get that working, and move on. Outlined in the following sections

Table 3 Key elements of change capacity	
Leadership	Skilled leadership can break down resistance among team members, allocate sufficient resources, and bring energy and encouragement, all of which can increase the likelihood of the team changing[77]
Teams	With appropriate accountability, trust, respect, safety, and inclusion, teams can effectively develop workflows, oversee projects, and spread change[77,78]
Time	Protected time for regular meetings and associated tasks is necessary to complete work, review changes, and decide on next steps. Reflecting on successes and failures during team meetings reinforces the sense of alignment and shared mission that is critical to sustaining the change process[67]
Improvement framework	Improvement frameworks give teams a common language and systematic process to approach change. Examples of models used in primary care settings include the Model for Improvement, Lean, and Six Sigma. A primer on continuous quality improvement developed by the National Learning Consortium can be found at http://www.healthit.gov/sites/default/files/tools/nlc_continuousqualityimprovementprimer.pdf
Measures	Measuring progress allows teams to better define goals, focus interventions, and show progress. To save time, consider using preexisting measures like those from the National Quality Forum: http://www.qualityforum.org/Measures_Reports_Tools.aspx
Information systems	Health information systems help collect, organize, and show data. EHRs are an obvious source of information, but many practice sites do not have EHRs, and others need to find solutions better suited to population management. The Agency for Healthcare Research and Quality provides a wealth of information on its Web site to help health care teams better understand how information systems can be used to improve quality and work flows: http://healthit.ahrq.gov/health-it-tools-and-resources/workflow-assessment-health-it-toolkit

---

Box 6
Building change capacity

- Who are the formal and informal leaders of our quality improvement teams?
- What framework for improvement does my practice use (or need)?
- Does our quality improvement team have dedicated time for meetings? Does the team meet often enough?
- Is the work being spread fairly? If not, are there other staff or providers who would like to get involved?
- What data do we have to support our change projects? Are there other data sources that we need?

Case Continued: Teams with Clear Goals, Enough Time, and Proper Resources Can Help Propel Clinic Reorganization Projects

The clinic leaders asked all the providers and staff to review the data generated by the EHR, reflect on the past year, and develop a plan to move forward. In a series of weekly lunchtime meetings, staff and providers were given time to discuss possible reasons for the lack of progress and to identify potential next steps. The team decided that improving mammography, colon cancer screening, and immunization rates needed the most atten-tion. They began to discuss interventions that involved patient outreach, developing self-management support resources, and creating point-of-care alerts. The plans were put on hold when everyone agreed that their days were already too busy to take on more responsibilities.

Recognizing the strain the new demands would put on their staff and providers, the clinic leaders proposed a solution: instead of the initial plan to divide the MU reward money among the team as a bonus, the money could be used to hire a new care manager to take on the new responsibilities. Thinking that some physicians and staff would want to keep the money for themselves, the leaders allowed each team member the choice to keep their bonus or to use it to fund the new position. To the leaders' surprise, all staff and providers agreed to fund the new plan.

Considering the case: what resources would your clinic need to have to start a quality improvement project related to prevention?

---

are several ideas that have improved the provision of preventive care in some health care systems.

Standing orders

Many recommendations for preventive services are purely algorithmic; hence, these tasks can be passed to nonphysician team members (eg, medical assistants, nursing staff) through standing orders (written policies and procedures for the provision of care in stipulated situations and for which sign-off from the physician is not required at the time of service). Standing orders have been shown to increase the use of many pre-ventive services,[79–82] and are a simple way to involve many staff in quality improve-ment. For some services, such as provision of immunizations, evidence suggests that standing orders may be more effective than provider-directed reminders.[79,83–85]

Outreach reminders

Outreach reminders directed toward patients can improve both patient attendance at scheduled visits and the provision of preventive services.[86–88] However, effective outreach requires a sufficiently organized and accessible data management system,

Box 7
Choosing what to change

- What gaps exist in our preventive care services?

- With the proper education and support, what tasks can our nurses, medical assistants, and administrative team members perform?

- Do we receive results from outside laboratories and clinics easily, consistently, and on time?

- How do our patients find out that they need a preventive service?

- How can we help our patients get more involved in their own health care?

- How can we improve our coordination and communication with specialists providing preventive care?

Case Conclusion: Implementing Focused Changes Can Help Practices Better Deliver Preventive Services and Organize for Future Improvements

After settling on the target outcomes and hiring the new care manager, team members began looking at what specific steps might improve their outcomes. Before deciding on the specific changes to implement, they first discussed how the improvement project may have unintended consequences or might disrupt the overall workflow of the clinic. The team discussed several questions: how would patients needing these services be identified and notified? Could any of the prevention-related activities happen outside the visit with the provider? And how would patients react to services being provided by the primary care team (as opposed by the primary care provider)?

After deliberating these questions, the team outlined the following tasks and responsibilities for each of the personnel involved:

Physicians

- *Develop standing orders for the care manager for ordering immunizations and completing mammography and colonoscopy referrals*

- *Share strategies for successful incorporation of preventive care into routine office visits*

Care manager

- *Work with EHR to develop lists of patients due for preventive services*

- *During team meetings, consult with providers about patients due for preventive services, identifying those patients who should be called in-person or mailed a customizable reminder letter*

- *Mail or call identified patients to remind them about preventive services, and schedule appointments as needed*

- *Track down outside study results and immunizations (eg, state registries, outstanding test results from laboratory tests, follow-up on referrals) and enter them into patients' EHR*

Medical assistants

- *Develop a method to draw attention to preventive care so that team members are properly prepared for the visit*

Receptionist

- *Develop a script to talk to patients about the outreach letters and phone calls*

- *Work with the care manager and staff to schedule immunization-only visits*

Clinic leadership

- *Submit, review, and present updated outcomes data to all practice personnel*

- *Gather patient feedback to refine the outreach process, and develop personalized preventive care tracking cards that the patients keep for their own records.*

All team members

- Set aside time for ongoing participation in team meetings (ie, at a time during which there are no clinic-related interruptions)
- Continue to remain open to team members or other clinic staff when feedback or constructive criticism is offered; continue to offer feedback or constructive criticism to team members or other clinic staff when lapses are observed

Testing the changes

Once the initial processes were in place, the team continued to watch how the implementation went and how patients reacted. Because there was some ongoing confusion among patients about the outreach calls and letters, the team looked for a script that they could use with patients. They had the receptionist and staff use the same script to send a consistent message to patients. Since then, they have tailored the script to suit their ongoing needs.

Because the practice also wanted to know what patients thought about the new outreach efforts, they surveyed a small sample of patients with a brief 1-page survey. They learned that most patients liked the calls more than the letters. They also held a focus group (during a time that the clinic was otherwise closed) to solicit input on creating a wallet card for patients to keep track of their preventive care services.

Planning for more change

From reviewing the EHR reports and the patient surveys, the team knew that the new processes were, for the most part, working well. They also recognized that they would have to revisit the process every month or 2 to identify gaps (ie, who was not up to date on preventive care) and make improvements. After a few cycles of outreach, they found that there were fewer and fewer patients needing calls, so they began planning for other areas needing improvement.

Considering the case: What new process has your practice introduced recently? Was it successful? Why or why not?

and the resources (eg, staff, time) to carry out the outreach tasks. Quality improvement teams must be able to define the population targeted for preventive services, identify patients in need of those services, and perform the outreach (eg, phone calls, e-mail, text messaging, postcards/letters). The anticipated costs (time, money) and benefits (improved delivery of preventive services) of a given outreach method should be thoughtfully considered before initiating the outreach effort. Although live phone calls may be more effective than mail, they can also be more expensive.[88,89] Automated phone calls seem to add no additional benefit to reminder letters alone.[86] Patient navigators (using high-intensity outreach methods tailored to specific patients) have proved effective at improving cancer screening among some historically underserved populations.[90] Reaching out to patients via targeted reminders can be an important step toward reorganizing one's practice and improving the delivery of preventive services.

Engaging patients
Because even the sickest patients spend only a little of their time in the primary care setting, it is essential to activate patients to engage in the care of their own health. Patients activated with the knowledge, skills, and confidence to manage their own health tend to have improved health, better experience of care, and fewer unhealthy

behaviors and costly emergency room visits.[91–93] Several strategies can effectively improve patient engagement, including written materials (eg, brochures) to improve health literacy,[94] online and paper-based decision aids to promote shared decision making,[95] online portals to provide patients with direct access to their personal health information,[96,97] and group visits to foster improved self-management of chronic diseases.[98]

Coordinated care

The coordination of care can occur on many different levels, such as referral tracking, data sharing agreements, monitoring follow-up, and linking patients to community resources. In some settings, care coordination is supported by health coaches or care managers who review action plans with patients, assist with follow-up activities after appointments or between office visits, and help ensure that preventive care is completed.[58] Providing care within a well-integrated PCMH can improve communication between primary care providers, specialists, and laboratories, thereby reducing fragmentation and inefficiencies with care.[73,99,100] Several provisions of the ACA are intended to improve the coordination of care between primary care providers and specialists, which could help streamline care for several preventive services, including colorectal, lung, and breast cancer screening. Specifically, the ACA creates incentives for improved coordination of services within PCMHs and ACOs; supports workforce development to increase the number of caregivers trained in care transition services; and calls for coordinated, comprehensive case management and transitional care.[101,102] These far-reaching provisions have the potential to improve primary care providers' capacity to effectively manage patients receiving care from multiple providers, including specialists providing preventive care.

Box 7 outlines several questions to help quality improvement teams identify care coordination processes that may warrant change.

SUMMARY

Prevention is an important component to achieving the triple aim of decreasing per capita costs, improving the health of populations, and bettering the patient experience. Primary care providers are instrumental in providing preventive services but may need to adopt new models of care that are patient centered, team based, and quality driven. Although the ACA is anticipated to help facilitate this process, it is too early to measure its success. By aligning leadership, building change capacity, and selectively choosing relevant processes to change, providers can successfully organize their practice to effectively deliver preventive services.

REFERENCES

1. Centers for Disease Control and Prevention, National Center for Health Statistics. Ambulatory care use and physician visits. 2013. Available at: http://www.cdc.gov/nchs/fastats/docvisit.htm. Accessed August 29, 2013.
2. Centers for Disease Control and Prevention. National ambulatory medical care survey: 2010 summary tables. 2010. Available at: http://www.cdc.gov/nchs/data/ahcd/namcs_summary/2010_namcs_web_tables.pdf. Accessed August 29, 2013.
3. Agency for Healthcare Research and Quality. Primary care workforce facts and stats No. 3. 2012. Available at: http://www.ahrq.gov/research/findings/factsheets/primary/pcwork3/index.html. Accessed August 29, 2013.

4. National Research Council. Primary Care and Public Health: Exploring Integration to Improve Population Health. Washington, DC: The National Academies Press; 2012.

5. Donaldson MS, Yordy KD, Lohr KN, et al. Primary care: America's health in a new era. Washington, DC: National Academy Press; 1996.

6. Macinko J, Starfield B, Shi L. Quantifying the health benefits of primary care physician supply in the United States. Int J Health Serv 2007;37(1):111–26.

7. Starfield B, Shi L, Macinko J. Contribution of primary care to health systems and health. Milbank Q 2005;83(3):457–502.

8. Council of Economic Advisors. The economic case for health care reform. 2009. Available at: http://www.whitehouse.gov/administration/eop/cea/TheEconomic CaseforHealthCareReform.

9. Organization for Economic Co-operation and Development. Health at a glance 2013: OECD indicators. 2013. Available at: http://www.oecd.org/els/health-systems/Health-at-a-Glance-2013.pdf. Accessed December 22, 2013.

10. National Research Council. US Health in International Perspective: Shorter Lives, Poorer Health. Washington, DC: The National Academies Press; 2013.

11. Institute of Medicine. Primary care and public health: exploring integration to improve population health. Washington, DC: The National Academies Press; 2012.

12. Starfield B, Horder J. Interpersonal continuity: old and new perspectives. Br J Gen Pract 2007;57(540):527–9.

13. Centers for Disease Control and Prevention (CDC). Cancer screening–United States, 2010. MMWR Morb Mortal Wkly Rep 2012;61(3):41–5.

14. Centers for Disease Control and Prevention (CDC). National, state, and local area vaccination coverage among children aged 19-35 months–United States, 2012. MMWR Morb Mortal Wkly Rep 2013;62(36):733–40.

15. Bindman AB, Grumbach K, Osmond D, et al. Primary care and receipt of preventive services. J Gen Intern Med 1996;11(5):269–76.

16. Dietrich AJ, Goldberg H. Preventive content of adult primary care: do generalists and subspecialists differ? Am J Public Health 1984;74(3):223–7.

17. Ferrante JM, Balasubramanian BA, Hudson SV, et al. Principles of the patient-centered medical home and preventive services delivery. Ann Fam Med 2010; 8(2):108–16.

18. Pandhi N, DeVoe JE, Schumacher JR, et al. Preventive service gains from first contact access in the primary care home. J Am Board Fam Med 2011;24(4): 351–9.

19. National Commission on Prevention Priorities. Preventive Care: A National Profile on Use, Disparities, and Health Benefits. Washington, DC: Partnership for Prevention; 2007.

20. Rosenthal TC. The medical home: growing evidence to support a new approach to primary care. J Am Board Fam Med 2008;21(5):427–40.

21. US Department of Health and Human Services, Office of Disease Prevention and Health Promotion, Healthy People 2020. Increase the proportion of women who receive a breast cancer screening based on the most recent guidelines. Available at: http://www.healthypeople.gov/2020/Data/SearchResult.aspx? topicid=5&topic=Cancer&objective=C-17&anchor=355. Accessed December 15, 2013.

22. US Department of Health and Human Services, Office of Disease Prevention and Health Promotion, Healthy People 2020. Increase the proportion of adults who receive a colorectal cancer screening based on the most recent guidelines.

Available at: http://healthypeople.gov/2020/Data/SearchResult.aspx?topicid=5&topic=Cancer&objective=C-16&anchor=354. Accessed December 15, 2013.

23. US Department of Health and Human Services. Office of Disease Prevention and Health Promotion. Healthy People 2020. Washington DC. Increase the proportion of women who receive a cervical cancer screening based on the most recent guidelines. Available at: http://healthypeople.gov/2020/Data/SearchResult.aspx?topicid=5&topic=Cancer&objective=C-15&anchor=353. Accessed December 15, 2013.

24. US Department of Health and Human Services. Office of Disease Prevention and Health Promotion. Healthy people 2020. Washington DC. Increase the percentage of noninstitutionalized high-risk adults aged 18 to 64 years who are vaccinated annually against seasonal influenza. Available at: http://healthypeople.gov/2020/Data/SearchResult.aspx?topicid=23&topic=Immunization and Infectious Diseases&objective=IID-12.6&anchor=578822. Accessed December 15, 2013.

25. US Department of Health and Human Services. Office of Disease Prevention and Health Promotion. Healthy People 2020. Washington DC. Increase the percentage of noninstitutionalized adults aged 65 years and older who are vaccinated against pneumococcal disease. Available at: http://www.healthypeople.gov/2020/Data/SearchResult.aspx?topicid=23&topic=Immunization and Infectious Diseases&objective=IID-13.1&anchor=569814. Accessed December 15, 2013.

26. US Department of Health and Human Services. Office of Disease Prevention and Health Promotion. Healthy People 2020. Washington DC. Increase the proportion of adults with hypertension whose blood pressure is under control. Available at: http://healthypeople.gov/2020/Data/SearchResult.aspx?topicid=21&topic=Heart Disease and Stroke&objective=HDS-12&anchor=526. Accessed December 15, 2013.

27. Stranges E, Stocks C. Potentially preventable hospitalizations for acute and chronic conditions, 2008: statistical brief #99. Rockville (MD): Healthcare Cost and Utilization Project (HCUP) Statistical Briefs; 2006.

28. Cabana MD, Rand CS, Powe NR, et al. Why don't physicians follow clinical practice guidelines? A framework for improvement. JAMA 1999;282(15):1458–65.

29. Cornuz J, Ghali WA, Di Carlantonio D, et al. Physicians' attitudes towards prevention: importance of intervention-specific barriers and physicians' health habits. Fam Pract 2000;17(6):535–40.

30. Burack RC. Barriers to clinical preventive medicine. Prim Care 1989;16(1):245–50.

31. Yarnall KS, Pollak KI, Ostbye T, et al. Primary care: is there enough time for prevention? Am J Public Health 2003;93(4):635–41.

32. Library of Congress. Patient Protection and Affordable Care Act: bill summary and status 111th congress (2009-2010) H.R. 3590. 2010.

33. Internal Revenue Service. Questions and answers on the individual shared responsibility provision. 2013. Available at: http://www.irs.gov/uac/Questions-and-Answers-on-the-Individual-Shared-Responsibility-Provision. Accessed December 16, 2013.

34. US Department of Health and Human Services. 2013 poverty guidelines. Available at: http://aspe.hhs.gov/poverty/13poverty.cfm. Accessed December 16, 2013.

35. US Centers for Medicare and Medicaid Services. Assuring access to affordable coverage: Medicaid and the Children's Health Insurance Program final rule.

2012. Available at: http://www.medicaid.gov/AffordableCareAct/Provisions/Downloads/MedicaidCHIP-Eligibility-Final-Rule-Fact-Sheet-Final-3-16-12.pdf. Accessed March 13, 2014.

36. US Centers for Medicare and Medicaid Services. Eligibility. Available at: http://www.medicaid.gov/Medicaid-CHIP-Program-Information/By-Topics/Eligibility/Eligibility.html. Accessed December 16, 2013.

37. US Centers for Medicare and Medicaid Services. Young adult coverage. Available at: http://www.hhs.gov/healthcare/rights/youngadults/. Accessed December 16, 2013.

38. US Centers for Medicare and Medicaid Services. What if I have a pre-existing health condition? Available at: https://http://www.healthcare.gov/what-if-i-have-a-pre-existing-health-condition/. Accessed December 16, 2013.

39. US Centers for Medicare and Medicaid Services. What are my preventive care benefits? Available at: https://http://www.healthcare.gov/what-are-my-preventive-care-benefits/. Accessed December 16, 2013.

40. Berenson RA, Burton RA. Health policy brief: next steps for ACOs. Health Aff (Millwood) 2012.

41. US Centers for Medicare and Medicaid Services. Accountable care organization 2013 program analysis. 2012. Available at: http://www.cms.gov/Medicare/Medicare-Fee-for-Service-Payment/sharedsavingsprogram/Downloads/ACO-NarrativeMeasures-Specs.pdf. Accessed March 13, 2014.

42. Nielsen M, Langner B, Zema C, et al. Benefits of implementing the primary care patient-centered medical home: a review of cost and quality results. 2012. Available at: http://www.pcpcc.org/sites/default/files/media/benefits_of_implementing_the_primary_care_pcmh.pdf. Accessed January 29, 2014.

43. Department of Health and Human Services, US Centers for Medicare and Medicaid Services. Improving quality of care for Medicare patients: accountable care organizations. 2012. Available at: http://www.cms.gov/Medicare/Medicare-Fee-for-Service-Payment/sharedsavingsprogram/Downloads/ACO_Quality_Factsheet_ICN907407.pdf. Accessed March 13, 2014.

44. Rittenhouse DR, Shortell SM, Fisher ES. Primary care and accountable care—two essential elements of delivery-system reform. N Engl J Med 2009;361(24):2301–3.

45. Bohmer RM. Managing the new primary care: the new skills that will be needed. Health Aff (Millwood) 2010;29(5):1010–4.

46. Patient-Centered Primary Care Collaborative. Defining the medical home: a patient-centered philosophy that drives primary care excellence. 2013. Available at: http://www.pcpcc.org/about/medical-home. Accessed September 10, 2013.

47. American Academy of Family Physicians, American Academy of Pediatrics, American College of Physicians, American Osteopathic Association. Joint principles of the patient-centered medical home. 2007. Available at: http://www.aafp.org/dam/AAFP/documents/practice_management/pcmh/initiatives/PCMHJoint.pdf. Accessed December 7, 2011.

48. Future of Family Medicine Project Leadership Committee. The future of family medicine: a collaborative project of the family medicine community. Ann Fam Med 2004;2(Suppl 1):S3–32.

49. Jackson GL, Powers BJ, Chatterjee R, et al. The patient-centered medical home: a systematic review. Ann Intern Med 2013;158(3):169–78.

50. American Academy of Family Physicians. Primary care for the 21st century: ensuring a quality, physician-led team for every patient. 2012. Available at:

http://www.aafp.org/dam/AAFP/documents/about_us/initiatives/AAFP-PCMHWhite
Paper.pdf. Accessed December 31, 2013.

51. Sokos DR, Skledar SJ, Ervin KA, et al. Designing and implementing a hospital-based vaccine standing orders program. Am J Health Syst Pharm 2007;64(10): 1096–102.

52. Kanter M, Martinez O, Lindsay G, et al. Proactive office encounter: a systematic approach to preventive and chronic care at every patient encounter. Perm J 2010;14(3):38–43.

53. Carter BL, Bosworth HB, Green BB. The hypertension team: the role of the pharmacist, nurse, and teamwork in hypertension therapy. J Clin Hypertens (Greenwich) 2012;14(1):51–65.

54. Carter BL, Rogers M, Daly J, et al. The potency of team-based care interventions for hypertension: a meta-analysis. Arch Intern Med 2009;169(19): 1748–55.

55. McLean DL, McAlister FA, Johnson JA, et al. A randomized trial of the effect of community pharmacist and nurse care on improving blood pressure management in patients with diabetes mellitus: study of cardiovascular risk intervention by pharmacists-hypertension (SCRIP-HTN). Arch Intern Med 2008;168(21): 2355–61.

56. Wubben DP, Vivian EM. Effects of pharmacist outpatient interventions on adults with diabetes mellitus: a systematic review. Pharmacotherapy 2008;28(4): 421–36.

57. Holland R, Battersby J, Harvey I, et al. Systematic review of multidisciplinary interventions in heart failure. Heart 2005;91(7):899–906.

58. Chen EH, Thom DH, Hessler DM, et al. Using the Teamlet Model to improve chronic care in an academic primary care practice. J Gen Intern Med 2010; 25(Suppl 4):S610–4.

59. Reid RJ, Coleman K, Johnson EA, et al. The Group Health medical home at year two: cost savings, higher patient satisfaction, and less burnout for providers. Health Aff (Millwood) 2010;29(5):835–43.

60. Sinsky CA, Willard-Grace R, Schutzbank AM, et al. In search of joy in practice: a report of 23 high-functioning primary care practices. Ann Fam Med 2013;11(3): 272–8.

61. Saba GW, Villela TJ, Chen E, et al. The myth of the lone physician: toward a collaborative alternative. Ann Fam Med 2012;10(2):169–73.

62. Taylor EF, Genevro J, Peikes D, et al. Building quality improvement capacity in primary care: supports and resources. 2013. Available at: http://www.ahrq.gov/professionals/prevention-chronic-care/improve/capacity-building/pcmhqi2.html. Accessed December 31, 2013.

63. Cohen D, McDaniel RR Jr, Crabtree BF, et al. A practice change model for quality improvement in primary care practice. J Healthc Manag 2004;49(3):155–68 [discussion: 169–70].

64. Institute for Healthcare Improvement. How to improve. 2012. Available at: http://www.ihi.org/knowledge/Pages/HowtoImprove/default.aspx. Accessed December 31, 2013.

65. McNellis RJ, Genevro JL, Meyers DS. Lessons learned from the study of primary care transformation. Ann Fam Med 2013;11(Suppl 1):S1–5.

66. Solberg LI. Improving medical practice: a conceptual framework. Ann Fam Med 2007;5(3):251–6.

67. Fernald DH, Deaner N, O'Neill C, et al. Overcoming early barriers to PCMH practice improvement in family medicine residencies. Fam Med 2011;43(7):503.

68. American Academy of Pediatrics. Patient- and family-centered care and the pediatrician's role. Pediatrics 2012;129(2):394–404.

69. Jim Conway BJ, Edgman-Levitan S, Schlucter J, et al. Partnering with patients and families to design a patient- and family-centered health care system. A roadmap for the future, a work in progress. Bethesda (MD): Institute for Family-Centered Care; 2006.

70. Han E, Scholle SH, Morton S, et al. Survey shows that fewer than a third of patient-centered medical home practices engage patients in quality improvement. Health Aff (Millwood) 2013;32(2):368–75.

71. Rajan RG, Wulf J. The flattening firm: evidence from panel data on the changing nature of corporate hierarchies. Rev Econ Stat 2006;88(4):759–73.

72. Friedberg MW, Coltin KL, Safran DG, et al. Associations between structural capabilities of primary care practices and performance on selected quality measures. Ann Intern Med 2009;151(7):456–63.

73. Nutting PA, Crabtree BF, Miller WL, et al. Transforming physician practices to patient-centered medical homes: lessons from the national demonstration project. Health Aff (Millwood) 2011;30(3):439–45.

74. Nease DE, Nutting PA, Dickinson WP, et al. Inducing sustainable improvement in depression care in primary care practices. Jt Comm J Qual Patient Saf 2008; 34(5):247–55.

75. Kaplan GS. Advanced lean thinking: proven methods to reduce waste and improve quality in health care. Oak Brook (IL): Joint Commission Resources; 2008.

76. Meyer H. Life in the 'lean' lane: performance improvement at Denver Health. Health Aff (Millwood) 2010;29(11):2054–60.

77. Hroscikoski MC, Solberg LI, Sperl-Hillen JM, et al. Challenges of change: a qualitative study of chronic care model implementation. Ann Fam Med 2006; 4(4):317–26.

78. Stevenson K, Baker R, Farooqi A, et al. Features of primary health care teams associated with successful quality improvement of diabetes care: a qualitative study. Fam Pract 2001;18(1):21–6.

79. Dexter PR, Perkins SM, Maharry KS, et al. Inpatient computer-based standing orders vs physician reminders to increase influenza and pneumococcal vaccination rates: a randomized trial. JAMA 2004;292(19):2366–71.

80. Nemeth LS, Ornstein SM, Jenkins RG, et al. Implementing and evaluating electronic standing orders in primary care practice: a PPRNet study. J Am Board Fam Med 2012;25(5):594–604.

81. Potter MB, Walsh JM, Yu TM, et al. The effectiveness of the FLU-FOBT program in primary care a randomized trial. Am J Prev Med 2011;41(1):9–16.

82. Braun RA, Provost JM. Bridging the gap: using school-based health services to improve Chlamydia screening among young women. Am J Public Health 2010; 100(9):1624–9.

83. Zimmerman RK, Nowalk MP, Tabbarah M, et al. Understanding adult vaccination in urban, lower-socioeconomic settings: influence of physician and prevention systems. Ann Fam Med 2009;7(6):534–41.

84. Trick WE, Das K, Gerard MN, et al. Clinical trial of standing-orders strategies to increase the inpatient influenza vaccination rate. Infect Control Hosp Epidemiol 2009;30(1):86–8.

85. Coyle CM, Currie BP. Improving the rates of inpatient pneumococcal vaccination: impact of standing orders versus computerized reminders to physicians. Infect Control Hosp Epidemiol 2004;25(11):904–7.

86. Fortuna RJ, Idris A, Winters P, et al. Get screened: a randomized trial of the incremental benefits of reminders, recall, and outreach on cancer screening. J Gen Intern Med 2014;29(1):90–7.

87. Guy R, Hocking J, Wand H, et al. How effective are short message service reminders at increasing clinic attendance? A meta-analysis and systematic review. Health Serv Res 2012;47(2):614–32.

88. Jacobson Vann JC, Szilagyi P. Patient reminder and patient recall systems to improve immunization rates. Cochrane Database Syst Rev 2005;(3):CD003941.

89. Jones Cooper SN, Walton-Moss B. Using reminder/recall systems to improve influenza immunization rates in children with asthma. J Pediatr Health Care 2013;27(5):327–33.

90. Phillips CE, Rothstein JD, Beaver K, et al. Patient navigation to increase mammography screening among inner city women. J Gen Intern Med 2011; 26(2):123–9.

91. Greene J, Hibbard JH. Why does patient activation matter? An examination of the relationships between patient activation and health-related outcomes. J Gen Intern Med 2012;27(5):520–6.

92. Greene J, Hibbard JH, Sacks R, et al. When seeing the same physician, highly activated patients have better care experiences than less activated patients. Health Aff (Millwood) 2013;32(7):1299–305.

93. Coulter A, Ellins J. Effectiveness of strategies for informing, educating, and involving patients. BMJ 2007;335(7609):24–7.

94. McPherson CJ, Higginson IJ, Hearn J. Effective methods of giving information in cancer: a systematic literature review of randomized controlled trials. J Public Health Med 2001;23(3):227–34.

95. Stacey D, Bennett CL, Barry MJ, et al. Decision aids for people facing health treatment or screening decisions. Cochrane Database Syst Rev 2011;(10):CD001431.

96. Nagykaldi Z, Aspy CB, Chou A, et al. Impact of a wellness portal on the delivery of patient-centered preventive care. J Am Board Fam Med 2012;25(2):158–67.

97. Brown H, Smith H. Giving women their own case notes to carry during pregnancy. Cochrane Database Syst Rev 2004;(2):CD002856.

98. Deakin T, McShane CE, Cade JE, et al. Group based training for self-management strategies in people with type 2 diabetes mellitus. Cochrane Database Syst Rev 2005;(2):CD003417.

99. Fisher ES. Building a medical neighborhood for the medical home. N Engl J Med 2008;359(12):1202–5.

100. Maeng DD, Graham J, Graf TR, et al. Reducing long-term cost by transforming primary care: evidence from Geisinger's medical home model. Am J Manag Care 2012;18(3):149–55.

101. Moreo K, Moreo N, Urbano FL, et al. Are we prepared for affordable care act provisions of care coordination? Case managers' self-assessments and views on physicians' roles. Prof Case Manag 2014;19(1):18–26.

102. Burton R. Health policy brief: improving care transitions. Health Aff (Millwood) 2012.

Prevention and Screening, Brief Intervention, and Referral to Treatment for Substance Use in Primary Care

Stephen Strobbe, PhD, RN, PMHCNS-BC, CARN-AP

KEYWORDS

- Prevention • Screening • Brief intervention • SBIRT • Substance use • Primary care

KEY POINTS

- Substance use and related disorders are a major public health concern in the United States, adding to increased health care costs and needless human suffering.
- Effective prevention and screening, brief intervention, and referral to treatment (SBIRT) can reduce the burdens of injury, illness, and premature death.
- The US Preventive Services Task Force periodically issues evidence-based recommendations for prevention and screening across a broad array of health conditions, including substance use and related disorders.
- Primary care clinicians are in prime positions to integrate prevention and SBIRT into their respective practices, thereby contributing to the improved health of patients, families, and communities.

INTRODUCTION

More than a decade ago, a monograph prepared for the Robert Wood Johnson Foundation called the problematic use of alcohol, tobacco, and illicit substances "the nation's number one health problem," contributing to "the death and ill health of millions of Americans every year and to the high cost of health care."[1] More recently, the National Center on Addiction and Substance Abuse (CASA) at Columbia University reported the total annual cost of substance use to federal, state, and local governments, based on data from 2005, was approaching half a trillion dollars.[2] In its landmark 2011 report titled "Adolescent Substance Use: America's #1 Public Health Problem," CASA reported that three-quarters of high school students (75.6%) in the

Conflicts of Interest: None.
Department of Psychiatry, University of Michigan School of Nursing, 400 North Ingalls Street, Ann Arbor, MI 48109-5482, USA
E-mail address: strobbe@umich.edu

0095-4543/14/$ – see front matter © 2014 Elsevier Inc. All rights reserved.

United States have smoked cigarettes or used alcohol or another drug, and just less than half (46.1%) have smoked or used within the past 30 days.[3]

Historically, substance use disorders were treated almost exclusively from a tertiary care perspective, often among only the most acutely and chronically ill, long after serious negative consequences had accrued across physical, biopsychosocial, and spiritual domains. Now, in response to clinical research, evidence-based practices, and recommendations from professional organizations and governmental agencies, increased emphasis has been placed on prevention, screening, and early intervention. With this gradual shift in focus, primary care clinicians (including physicians, physician assistants, and nurse practitioners) are in prime positions to further contribute to the improved health of patients, families, and communities.

The purpose of this article is to provide primary care clinicians with the necessary information, recommendations, and resources to successfully integrate prevention and screening, brief intervention, and referral to treatment (SBIRT) for substance use and related disorders into clinical practice. Although the main focus of this issue of *Primary Care: Clinics in Office Practice* is on prevention and screening for various health concerns among adults, many of the formal recommendations specific to substance use also include brief intervention and referral to treatment, approaches consistent with the delivery of primary care. In addition, because risk factors and initial signs of substance use often emerge during childhood or adolescence, specific measures for these special populations are discussed. Although many of the prevention and SBRIT strategies may apply across multiple categories of substances, particular attention is paid here to tobacco, alcohol, cannabis, and the nonmedical use of prescription opioid medications.

DSM-5: NOMENCLATURE, CLASSES OF SUBSTANCES, AND DIAGNOSTIC CRITERIA

Effective prevention and screening for substance use requires at least some familiarity with diagnostic criteria. The release of the *Diagnostic and Statistical Manual for Mental Disorders*, 5th Edition (DSM-5) in May 2013 brought changes to preferred nomenclature, classes of substances, and diagnostic criteria.[4] To begin, both the previous terms and formal diagnoses of substance abuse and substance dependence were eliminated in favor of the broader conceptualization of Substance Use Disorders.

Classes of substances have also been modified (**Box 1**), with amphetamine-like substances and cocaine now being listed under the broader category of Stimulants. Former diagnoses of nicotine abuse and nicotine dependence are now referred to as Tobacco Use Disorders, and include cigarettes and other forms of smoking tobacco, as well as smokeless tobacco.

Criteria from the 2 previous DSM-IV diagnostic sets of abuse and dependence were combined, with 2 notable changes: (1) the abuse criterion for recurrent substance-related legal problems was deleted, and (2) a new criterion was added to include the physiologic phenomenon of craving, or a strong desire or urge to use a specific substance (**Box 2**). Diagnoses remain substance specific, such as alcohol use disorder. However, for certain classes greater specificity is requested when known, such as alprazolam use disorder, rather than the previous and more generic sedative, hypnotic, or anxiolytic use disorder. In addition, any individual who has previously qualified for a diagnosis of a substance use disorder, now rated in severity as mild, moderate, or severe, must be free from any of these criteria, with the possible exception of craving, for a minimum of 3 months (rather than the previous 1 month) before the condition is considered to be in early remission. The required period to establish sustained remission remains 1 year, again with the caveat of possible craving.

Box 1
Classes of substances

- Alcohol
- Caffeine
- Cannabis
- Hallucinogens
  - Phencyclidine
  - Other hallucinogens
- Inhalants
- Opioids
- Sedatives, hypnotics, or anxiolytics
- Stimulants
  - Amphetamine-type substances
  - Cocaine
  - Other or unspecified stimulants
- Tobacco
- Other (or unknown)

Adapted from American Psychiatric Association (APA). Diagnostic and statistical manual for mental disorders. 5th edition. Arlington (VA): APA; 2013.

Box 2
Abbreviated diagnostic criteria for substance use disorders

A problematic pattern of substance use leading to clinically significant impairment or distress, manifested by at least 2 of the following in a 12-month period:

1. Taken in larger amounts or over a longer period than intended
2. Persistent desire or unsuccessful efforts to cut down or control use
3. Great deal of time spent obtaining, using, or recovering from effects
4. Craving, or strong desire or urge to use the substance
5. Recurrent use resulting in failure to fulfill major role obligations
6. Continued use despite related personal or interpersonal problems
7. Important activities given up or reduced because of use
8. Recurrent use in situations in which it is physically hazardous
9. Continued use despite related physiologic or psychological problems
10. Tolerance
11. Withdrawal

Severity: Mild (2–3 symptoms); Moderate (4–5 symptoms); Severe (6 or more symptoms).

Early remission: Criteria no longer met ≥3 months and <12 months, except possible craving.

Sustained remission: Criteria no longer met ≥12 months, except possible craving.

Adapted from American Psychiatric Association (APA). Diagnostic and statistical manual for mental disorders. 5th edition. Arlington (VA): APA; 2013.

RISK FACTORS, PREVALENCE, AND CONSEQUENCES

Although an exhaustive review of risk factors, prevalence, and consequences related to substance use across each of the respective classes is beyond the scope of this offering, there are a few general principles with practical implications for primary practice that do apply. First, one of the most consistent predictors for substance use is family history. Addictions, in particular, are considered to be moderately to highly heritable, with genetics accounting for approximately half of the explained variance for such disorders, although rates differ across various classes of substances.[5] Second, earlier onset of substance use is associated with an increased risk for the development of a frank substance use disorder and related negative consequences. Third, personal history, or the presence of any current substance use disorder in a given individual, increases the risk for another substance use disorder.[6] Fourth, the presence of a mental health disorder, such as anxiety, bipolar disorder, depression, a personality disorder, or a trauma-related disorder, also increases the risk for a substance use disorder.[7]

Prevalence rates and representative consequences associated with the use of tobacco, alcohol, cannabis, and the nonmedical use of prescription opioid medications provide important information to support efforts toward prevention and SBIRT. According to the National Comorbidity Survey replication, lifetime prevalence for substance use disorders other than tobacco and alcohol was 10.9%, or approximately 1 in 9 individuals in the United States aged 18 years and older.[8] In addition to identified intrinsic factors (family history, earlier onset, personal history, presence of another mental health disorder), extrinsic factors play a role, including environmental considerations such as culture, social and family attitudes, and access to various substances.

In terms of serious consequences that cut across different classes of substances, it must be noted that DSM-5 specifically and repeatedly speaks to an increased risk for attempted and completed suicides in the context of substance use, intoxication, withdrawal, and certain substance use disorders. These substances include alcohol (intoxication, alcohol use disorder), hallucinogens (intoxication), inhalants (use, inhalant use disorder), opioids (intoxication, withdrawal, opioid use disorder), sedatives, hypnotics, or anxiolytics (intoxication), and stimulants (withdrawal).[4]

Tobacco Use

Tobacco use, specifically cigarette smoking, remains the single greatest cause of preventable morbidity and mortality in the United States, resulting in more than 440,000 premature deaths annually from cardiovascular disease, respiratory disease, and cancer[9]; this includes the death of some 49,000 individuals from exposure to secondhand smoke.[10] Despite significant reductions in overall smoking rates in the United States over the past 5 decades, due in part to vigorous public health campaigns, 19.0% of adults were current cigarette smokers in 2011. Rates were higher among men (21.6%), those living below the federal poverty level (29.0%), American Indians and Alaskan Natives (31.5%), and those with a General Education Development diploma (45.3%).[11]

Unfortunately the ranks of cigarette smokers continue to be filled by youth, and tobacco use has now been termed a pediatric epidemic.[12] Each day nearly 4000 individuals under the age of 18 smoke their first cigarettes.[12] Among high school seniors in the United States, approximately 1 in 4 is a regular cigarette smoker,[13] and about 80% of these young people will continue to smoke into adulthood. Tobacco use among United States youth is not limited to cigarette smoking, as 1 in 5 white adolescent males (aged 12–17 years) reportedly uses smokeless tobacco, which has also been linked to oral cancers.[12]

It was recently reported that smoking rates during pregnancy among women aged 15 to 44 years in the United States were 21.8% among whites, 14.2% among blacks, and 7.4% among Hispanics.[14] Smoking during pregnancy has been associated with several adverse outcomes, including spontaneous abortions, stillbirth, preterm birth, and fetal growth restriction.[15] Although most women may cease smoking early in pregnancy, many relapse following delivery.[16] Children who are subsequently exposed to secondhand smoke are also more likely to suffer from several health conditions, including increased rates of ear infections, asthma, and other respiratory illnesses.[17]

Alcohol Use

More than 85,000 deaths per year are attributable to alcohol consumption, making it the third leading cause of preventable death in the United States after tobacco use and the combination of poor diet and physical inactivity.[18] In one epidemiologic study, lifetime prevalence of any alcohol use disorder in the United States was more than 30%.[19] Another survey, conducted across multiple primary care practices, revealed risky or hazardous alcohol use among 22.3% of adult patients during the previous 30 days.[20] Risky or hazardous drinking, that is, consuming alcohol in excess of established guidelines set forth by the National Institute on Alcohol Abuse and Alcoholism (NIAAA) (**Box 3**), has been associated with negative physical, emotional, and social consequences.[21]

Many adults who eventually develop alcohol use disorders establish patterns of problematic drinking during adolescence. In 2011, based on Monitoring the Future (MTF) data, a total of 70% of United States high school seniors reported some lifetime alcohol use, 51% reported having been drunk at least once, and 22% reported binge drinking (defined as ≥ 5 drinks in a row) during the last 2 weeks.[22]

More recently, the phenomenon of extreme binge drinking has been described, during which high school seniors reported episodes of alcohol consumption that

---

Box 3
National Institute on Alcohol Abuse and Alcoholism guidelines for alcohol use

- Healthy men younger than 65: consume no more than...
  - Fourteen standard drinks per week or
  - Four drinks per drinking occasion.
- Healthy, nonpregnant women and healthy adults older than 65: consume no more than...
  - Seven standard drinks per week or
  - Three drinks per drinking occasion.
- A standard drink is defined as
  - A 12-ounce glass of beer,
  - A 5-ounce glass of table wine, or
  - 1.5 ounces of 80-proof spirits.

Adapted from National Institute on Alcohol Abuse and Alcoholism (NIAAA). Helping patients who drink too much: a clinician's guide (NIH Publication No. 05-3769). Rockville (MD): NIAAA; 2005. Available at: http://pubs.niaaa.nih.gov/publications/Practitioner/CliniciansGuide2005/clinicians_guide.htm. Accessed October 29, 2013.

surpassed traditional definitions of binge drinking. Between 2005 and 2011, a total of 20.2% of high school seniors reported drinking 5 or more standard drinks, 10.5% reported drinking 10 or more drinks, and 5.6% reported drinking 15 or more drinks in a row during the past 2 weeks. Extreme binge drinking, with subsequently elevated blood alcohol levels, places young people at still greater risk for accidents and injuries, including alcohol poisoning, respiratory depression, coma, and death. Consistent with most other categories of alcohol use, binge drinkers were more likely to be male. Other predictors for binge drinking included more days of skipping school, perceiving that more friends got drunk, spending more evenings out with friends, and use of cigarettes or marijuana during the last month.[23]

Concerns related to excessive alcohol use are not limited to boys or men. While overall rates of alcohol use may be lower among girls and women, the impact of associated consequences is not. Binge drinking is a risk factor for several health and social problems among women, including unintended pregnancy, sexually transmitted diseases, and breast cancer.[24] In 2004, NIAAA reduced criteria for what constituted risky or hazardous drinking for women (from >14 to >7 drinks per week), as well as binge drinking (from >4 to >3 drinks per drinking occasion), to better reflect physiologic differences between men and women that affect the absorption of alcohol.[25]

According to the 2011 national Youth Risk Behavior Survey, 45.4% of senior high school girls reported current (past month) alcohol use, and 27.0% reported current binge drinking (in this survey, ≥ 5 drinks). By comparison, based on results from the 2011 Behavioral Risk Factor Surveillance System (BRFSS) survey, binge drinking among women aged 18 to 44 years was most prevalent among those aged 18 to 24 years (24.2%), non-Hispanic whites (13.3%), and those with annual household incomes of US $75,000 or more (16.0%).[24]

Heavy alcohol use during pregnancy is associated with adverse outcomes, including fetal alcohol syndrome and other fetal alcohol spectrum disorders (FASDs), and can result in neurodevelopmental deficits and lifelong disability.[26] FASDs are estimated to affect at least 1% of all births in the United States,[27] and have been associated with patterns of alcohol consumption that result in high blood alcohol concentrations, such as those seen in binge drinking.[28]

Based on BRFSS data from 2006 to 2010, an estimated 51.5% of nonpregnant women used alcohol and 15.0% engaged in binge drinking. Women who binge drink in the preconception period are also more likely than non–binge drinkers to continue using alcohol, even after becoming pregnant.[25] Among pregnant women, 7.6% used alcohol and 1.4% engaged in binge drinking. Prevalence rates for drinking during pregnancy were highest among women aged 35 to 44 years (14.3%), white (8.3%), college graduates (10.0%), and employed (9.6%).[24] In 2005, the Surgeon General issued an advisory urging women who are pregnant, or who may become pregnant, to abstain from alcohol.[29]

Cannabis Use

Cannabis use continues to increase among residents of the United States aged 12 years and older. According the 2012 National Survey on Drug Use and Health (NSDUH), an estimated 31.5 million individuals reported having used marijuana in the past year, up from approximately 25 million each year from 2002 to 2008.[30]

Marijuana also remains the most widely used illicit substance among youth. Data from MTF 2012 indicated that among high school seniors, 36% had used marijuana during the past year and 23% during the past month, and 6.5% said they smoked daily, up from 5.1% in 2007. One explanation for increased use is a corresponding decrease in perceived risk. Contrary to this perception, a systematic review published in the *Lancet* linked early cannabis use to an increased risk for the development of psychotic illness later in life.[31]

Continued controversy surrounding the use of cannabis has created a compelling clinical conundrum. On one extreme, federal law continues to classify cannabis as a Schedule I drug, "with no currently accepted medical use and a high potential for abuse. Schedule I drugs are the most dangerous drugs of all the drug schedules with potentially severe psychological or physical dependence."[32] Other substances in this class include heroin, lysergic acid diethylamide (LSD), 3,4-methylenedioxyme-thamphetamine (ecstasy), methaqualone (Quaalude), and peyote.[32]

By contrast, and potential conflict, several local and state referenda have produced an inconsistent patchwork of varied legislation and law-enforcement efforts. Some of the more controversial initiatives include the wholesale legalization or decriminalization of cannabis, whereas others advocate for the use of "medical marijuana." As a result, primary care clinicians may find themselves in the position of being asked to prescribe cannabis, or to provide documentation for the procurement of a medical marijuana card, and to care for individuals with chronic cannabis use. These eventualities may prompt the clinician to engage in clarification of personal and professional values, and to set and communicate practice parameters accordingly.

Nonmedical Use of Prescription Opioid Medications

In a report released by the Executive Office of the President of the United States, nonmedical use of prescription medications was called "the nation's fastest-growing drug problem."[33] Although more specific typologies exist,[34] for the purposes of this article nonmedical use of prescription medications includes (1) taking a medication that has been prescribed for somebody else, (2) taking a drug in a higher quantity or in another manner than prescribed, or (3) taking a drug for another purpose than prescribed,[35] for example, changing one's mood or getting high. Although this broader category of nonmedical prescription drug use also includes prescription stimulants, as well as sedatives, hypnotics, or anxiolytics, most attention thus far has focused on the misuse of prescription opioid medications.

Recent years have seen dramatic increases in the prescribing and nonmedical use of opioid pain relievers across the life span, with serious consequences from a public health perspective. From 1997 to 2007, the milligram-per-person use of prescription opioids in the United States escalated from 74 to 369 mg, an increase of 402%.[36] From 2000 to 2009, the number of prescriptions dispensed by retail pharmacies increased from 174 million to 257 million, or 48%.[33] Across multiple studies and regions, it has been noted that approximately 20% of all prescribers are responsible for 80% of the prescriptions written for opioid pain relievers.[37]

According to data from the 2010 NSDUH, in the United States 13.8% of residents aged 12 years and older, or 34.8 million people, reported lifetime nonmedical use of prescription opioid analgesics, such as hydrocodone (9.5%), codeine or propoxyphene (7.8%), and/or oxycodone (6.1%).[38] That same year, 5.1 million people reported current (past month) use, with the majority (60.1%) indicating they had obtained these medications from a friend or relative for free.[39] In 2011 more than 420,000 emergency department visits involved the nonmedical use of opioid analgesics.[40] In addition, a nationally representative study recently found a strong association between prior nonmedical use of opioid pain relievers and initiation of heroin use in the past year.[41] Of note, in addition to having devastating psychosocial consequences, heroin use is a contributing factor in other serious medical illnesses including hepatitis B and C, human immunodeficiency virus, and AIDS.

In 2008, opioid pain relievers were involved in 14,800 overdose deaths, or 73.8% of all overdose deaths involving prescription drugs.[42] While men remain more likely to die from drug overdoses, there has been an alarming increase in the number of opioid overdose deaths among women. Between 1999 and 2010, nearly 48,000 women died of such overdoses, representing an increase of more than 500% over the 12-year period. Women at greatest risk of dying from a prescription opioid overdose, including unintentional, suicide, and other deaths, were those aged 45 to 54 years, as well as non-Hispanic whites, American Indians, and Alaskan Natives.[43]

Among pregnant women, opioid use disorders also place infants at risk. Between 2000 and 2009, the number of neonates who experienced neonatal abstinence syndrome in the United States increased by nearly 300%.[43] At the other end of the life span, with the aging of the baby-boomer generation, it has been estimated that nonmedical use of prescription medications will increase dramatically among older adults.[44,45] With increasing age, a reduced physiologic capacity to metabolize medications places seniors at greater risk for injuries and potentially fatal drug-drug interactions including, most notably, combinations of central nervous system depressants such as alcohol; sedatives, hypnotics, or anxiolytics; and opioid analgesics.

EVIDENCE THAT PREVENTION AND SBIRT WORK
Prevention

Prevention, in the context of substance use and related disorders, includes abstinence from potentially harmful substances or engaging in other behaviors, such as limited alcohol consumption, to reduce the risks of substance-related injury or illness. Earlier use of tobacco, alcohol, or other drugs is a predictor for the development of substance use disorders across virtually all classes of substances. Among youth aged 12 to 17, cigarette smoking before the age of 12 years has been associated with higher rates of alcohol (12.0% vs 9.6%), cannabis (4.8% vs 2.2%), and other illicit drug (5.8% vs 1.9%) use compared with those who began smoking at age 16 years or older.[46] Conversely, avoiding or delaying the use of substances during childhood, adolescence, and young adulthood—critical phases of neurodevelopment—has been associated with continued abstinence or nonproblematic use. For example, in one study adults who initiated alcohol use at age 21 years or older were 6 times less likely (2.5%) to have developed an alcohol use disorder later in life than those who had started drinking at age 14 years or younger (16.5%).[47]

The effectiveness of preventive measures extends beyond the individual to families, schools, and society at large. In one frequently cited study, teens who had dinner with their families 5 times a week or more were less likely to use tobacco, alcohol, or other drugs than those who had dinner with their families fewer than 3 times a week.[48] Youth aged 12 to 17 years who attended drug-free and gang-free schools were less likely to have ever tried tobacco, alcohol, or marijuana.[49] Increases in cigarette taxes at state and federal levels have been linked to reduced rates of youth smoking.[50,51] Each of these examples serves as a reminder of the potential benefits that can be realized by implementing an array of preventive strategies, across a variety of settings, and targeting children at younger ages. Specific to clinical practice and prevention, particularly in light of the relationship between cigarette smoking and other substance-related behaviors, the US Preventive Services Task Force (USPSTF) "found adequate evidence that behavioral counseling interventions, such as face-to-face or phone interaction with a health care provider, print materials, and computer applications, can reduce the risk of smoking initiation of school-aged children and adolescents."[52]

SBIRT as Defined by the Substance Abuse and Mental Health Services Administration (SAMHSA)

SBIRT is a comprehensive, integrated public health approach to the delivery of early intervention and treatment services for people with substance use disorders as well as those who are at risk for developing these disorders. Primary care centers,... office-based practices, and other community settings provide opportunities for early intervention with at-risk substance users before more serious consequences occur.

- Screening quickly assesses the severity of substance use and identifies the appropriate level of treatment.
- Brief intervention focuses on increasing insight and awareness regarding substance use and motivation toward behavioral change.
- Referral to treatment provides those identified as needing more extensive treatment with access to specialty care.[53]

SBIRT has its roots in the transtheoretical stages of change model[54] and motivational interviewing techniques[55] which, together, identify a patient's readiness to change and assist in continued movement toward healthy, adaptive responses related to substance use. A seminal review article published in 2007 described research on the components of SBIRT, including the development of screening tests, clinical trials of brief interventions, and implementation research. Evidence from this review clearly showed that SBIRT can improve individuals' health over the short term. Reviewers noted, however, that the long-term impact of SBIRT on population health has yet to be shown. Despite this limitation, reviewers cited optimism, as simulation models suggest the long-term benefits of SBRIT could be substantial.[56]

In an earlier review evaluating 32 controlled studies with a combined total of more than 6000 patients, Bien and colleagues[57] concluded that brief interventions directed toward alcohol use had a positive impact on outcomes when compared with no counseling, and were frequently as positive as more extensive treatments. In general, these brief interventions appeared to be equally effective when directed toward adolescents, adults, older adults, and pregnant women.[56] When provided by primary care clinicians, brief interventions have been found to lessen alcohol consumption,[56] reduce hospital days and health care costs,[58] and decrease mortality.[59]

Although initial research efforts were meant to provide an evidence base for alcohol screening and brief intervention in primary health care settings, they were followed by trials for other substances, including tobacco, illicit drugs, and the nonmedical use of prescription medications. Although results from the brief intervention portion of SBIRT have sometimes varied when applied to substances other than alcohol, universal screening still plays a role in helping to identify substance-related problems, and a successful referral to specialized treatment can be viewed as a positive outcome.

USPSTF AND OTHER RECOMMENDATIONS RELATED TO SUBSTANCE USE
USPSTF Recommendations

The USPSTF is an independent panel of nonfederal experts in prevention and evidence-based medicine and is composed of primary care clinicians. It conducts scientific reviews of a broad range of clinical preventive health care services, and develops recommendations for primary care clinicians and health systems.[60] Recommendations are based and graded on current available evidence; it is suggested that clinicians offer or provide services that receive a letter grade of A or B.[61] Current USPSTF recommendations specific to substance use and related disorders are provided in **Box 4**.

Box 4
United States Preventive Services Task Force (USPSTF) recommendations pertaining to substance use and related disorders

Tobacco

The USPSTF recommends...

- Primary care clinicians provide interventions, including education or brief counseling, to prevent initiation of tobacco use in school-aged children and adolescents (Grade B Recommendation).[52]

- Clinicians ask all adults about tobacco use and provide tobacco cessation interventions for those who use tobacco products (Grade A Recommendation).[62]

- Clinicians ask all pregnant women about tobacco use and provide augmented, pregnancy-tailored counseling for those who smoke (Grade A Recommendation).[62]

Alcohol

The USPSTF recommends...

- Clinicians screen adults aged 18 years or older for alcohol misuse, and provide persons engaged in risky or hazardous drinking with brief behavioral counseling interventions to reduce alcohol misuse (Grade B Recommendation).[63]

Screening for Hepatitis C Virus Infection in Adults

The USPSTF recommends...

Screening for hepatitis C virus (HCV) infections in persons at high risk for infection (Grade B Recommendation). Note: "The most important risk factor for HCV infection is past or current injection drug use."[64]

Grade A Recommendation: High certainty that the net benefit is substantial; Grade B Recommendation: High certainty that the net benefit is moderate, or moderate certainty that the net benefit is moderate to substantial.[61]

In addition to graded recommendations, the USPSTF may also issue an I Statement, indicating that current evidence is insufficient to formulate recommendations either for or against a particular service. I statements indicate that evidence on the topic is lacking, of poor quality, or conflicting, and that additional research is needed to formulate a recommendation.[61] At the time of writing, such statements had been issued for the following 2 services: (1) screening and behavioral counseling interventions in primary care settings to reduce alcohol misuse in adolescents,[63] and (2) screening adolescents, adults, and pregnant women for illicit drug use.[65]

Other Recommendations

Whereas substance use recommendations from the American Academy of Family Physicians (AAFP) mirrored those of the USPSTF,[66] recommendations from other professional entities expand prevention and screening efforts. For example, the American Academy of Pediatrics recommends that pediatricians incorporate substance use prevention into daily practice, acquire the necessary skills to identify young people at risk for substance use, and provide or facilitate assessment, intervention, and treatment as necessary.[67] The American College of Obstetrics and Gynecology recommends direct questioning by clinicians of all patients about their use of drugs (in addition to tobacco and alcohol) as part of periodic assessments.[68] The American Lung Association's Lung Cancer Screening Committee issued interim recommendations for low-dose computed tomography screening for lung cancer among current smokers aged 55 to 74 years with a smoking history of at least 30 pack-years and no history of lung cancer.[69]

PREVENTION AND SBIRT: PUTTING IT INTO PRACTICE

One of the single most important things a primary care clinician can do to help promote healthy lifestyle patterns among patients and their families is to demonstrate a consistent willingness to raise and discuss issues pertaining to substance use in a clear, supportive, matter-of-fact, and nonjudgmental fashion.[70] The goal is to establish and sustain a positive professional relationship over time that will allow and encourage patients to raise and address inherently difficult topics related to substance use. Much of this work is educational and supportive in nature. From an SBIRT perspective, prevention of substance use and related disorders is an ongoing process that continues across the life span, and is integrated into the delivery of routine clinical care, including wellness visits. **Box 5** lists suggested topics for patient and family education in the prevention of substance use and related disorders.

A simple graphic model of the SBIRT process[71] is provided in **Fig. 1**. The essential elements of SBIRT also align with the 5 As approach to behavioral counseling as adopted by USPSTF. The 5 As stand for Assess, Advise, Agree, Assist, and Arrange (**Table 1**). These elements also serve as the basis for reimbursement for behavioral counseling, such as SBIRT, from the Centers for Medicare and Medicaid Services (CMS).[72]

Screening

The first step of SBIRT is the implementation of universal screening to help identify patients who may be at risk for, or are currently experiencing, problematic substance use. Many primary care clinicians ask about cigarette smoking and other tobacco use in the context of the patient's health, but fewer inquire about alcohol and other substance use. Examples of validated 1-item and 2-item screening tests for alcohol and/or other drug misuse are provided in **Box 6**.[73–75]

Screening negative on the 1- or 2-item screening test (ie, no alcohol or other drug misuse), in the absence of any evidence to the contrary, indicates that screening is complete; this affords the clinician an opportunity to provide positive verbal reinforcement to the patient for healthy behaviors related to substance use. It is generally recommended that screening be repeated on a routine basis at least annually, or earlier as changes in behavior, health status, or other personal circumstances warrant.

Screening positive for either alcohol or other drug misuse on the 1- or 2-item screening test leads to further screening using a valid and reliable scale. Perhaps foremost among these for alcohol use is the AUDIT-C (Alcohol Use Disorders Identification Test—Consumption).[76] See **Table 2** for the AUDIT-C questionnaire, and **Table 3** for this and other selected screening instruments for substance use.[76–82] Alternatively, clinicians could use the newly structured DSM-5 diagnostic criteria (see **Box 2**) as a checklist for potentially problematic substances, which would also provide an indication of severity.

Brief Intervention

Brief intervention is the cornerstone of SBIRT. The object of brief intervention is to help patients move along a continuum of cognitive and behavioral health, recognizing that progress is seldom linear, and that setbacks may occur. Brief interventions are short (5–15 minutes) semistructured discussions intended to raise awareness and increase motivation to avoid, reduce, or discontinue potentially problematic use of alcohol or other substances. Six elements critical to brief interventions are captured in the

Box 5
Suggested topics for patient and family education in the prevention of substance use and related disorders across the life span

Children

- Decide now to be tobacco-free
- Avoid secondhand smoke
- Choose friends who do not use tobacco, alcohol, or other drugs
- Learn and use appropriate refusal skills for tobacco, alcohol, and other drugs
- Do not ride with drivers who have been drinking or using other drugs
- Only use medicines that are meant for you, and use them in accordance with the label or prescription

Adolescents

- Continue to be tobacco-free and alcohol-free
- Understand and avoid the risks of cannabis and other substance use
- Spend time with peers who have similar goals and interests
- Only ride in cars with people who have not been drinking or getting high
- Do not take prescription medications that were not prescribed for you
- If prescribed a medication, take only as directed
- Do not give, lend, trade, or sell prescription medications

Young Adults

- Continue to avoid tobacco in all forms, or obtain help to quit now
- If you have a strong family history of substance use, consider abstinence
- If you choose to use alcohol, observe recommended levels, avoid binge drinking (see **Box 3**)
- Know the continued risks of cannabis and other substance use during young adulthood
- Use prescription medications only as directed
- Do not give, lend, trade, or sell prescription medications

Women Who Are Pregnant, or Who May Become Pregnant

- Abstain from tobacco, alcohol, and other substances
- Seek professional help to quit smoking, drinking, or using other substances if needed

Parents of Children, Adolescents, or Young Adults

- Model and encourage substance-free lifestyles for your children
- Teach and reinforce refusal skills for tobacco, alcohol, and other drugs
- If you choose to use alcohol, adhere to NIAAA guidelines (see **Box 3**)
- Do not administer prescription medications to children other than as prescribed
- Always secure and dispose of prescription medications properly

Older Adults

- Recognize a decreased capacity to metabolize alcohol and medications with age
- If you choose to use alcohol, adhere to NIAAA guidelines (see **Box 3**)
- Avoid the use of alcohol with any medication, whether over-the-counter or prescription
- Always secure and dispose of prescription medications properly

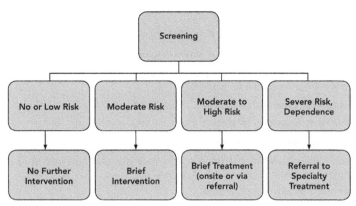

Fig. 1. Graphic model of the screening, brief intervention, and referral to treatment (SBIRT) process. (*From* Substance Abuse and Mental Health Services Administration (SAMHSA). Systems-level implementation of screening, brief intervention and referral to treatment. Technical Assistance Publication (TAP) Series 33. HHS Publication No. (SMA) 13-4741. Rockville (MD): SAMHSA; 2013. Available at: http://www.integration.samhsa.gov/sbirt/TAP33.pdf. Accessed November 22, 2013.)

acronym FRAMES, which provides both a philosophic stance and a practical structure for the delivery of care:

- *Feedback* is given to the individual about personal risk or impairment.
- *Responsibility* for change is placed on the patient.
- *Advice* to change is given by the provider.
- *Menu* of options is offered for behavioral change, supports, and/or treatment options.
- *Empathic style* is used in counseling.
- *Self-efficacy* or optimistic empowerment is engendered in the patient.[83]

Table 1	
The 5 As of behavioral counseling	
Assess	Ask about/assess behavioral health risk(s) and factors affecting choice of behavior change goals/methods
Advise	Give clear, specific, and personalized behavior-change advice, including information about personal health harms and benefits
Agree	Collaboratively select appropriate treatment goals and methods based on the patient's interest in and willingness to change behavior
Assist	Using behavior-change techniques (self-help and/or counseling), aid the patient in achieving agreed-upon goals by acquiring the skills, confidence, and social/environmental supports for behavior change, supplemented with adjunctive medical treatments when appropriate
Arrange	Schedule follow-up contacts (in person or by telephone) to provide ongoing assistance/support and to adjust the treatment plan as needed, including referral to more intensive or specialized treatment

From Centers for Medicare & Medicaid Services (CMS), Department of Health and Human Services (DHHS). Screening and behavioral counseling interventions in primary care to reduce alcohol misuse. Publication ICN 907798. CMS; 2013. Available at: http://www.cms.gov/Outreach-and-Education/Medicare-Learning-Network-MLN/MLNProducts/downloads/Reduce-Alcohol-Misuse-ICN907798.pdf. Accessed November 22, 2013.

Box 6
One-item and 2-item screening tests for alcohol and/or other drug misuse

- Single-question screening test for unhealthy alcohol use
  - Question: "How many times in the past year have you had X or more drinks in a day?" (where X is 5 for men and 4 for women)
  - Response: A response of >1 is positive
  - Sensitivity 82%, specificity 79%[73]
- Single-question screening test for drug use
  - Question: "How many times in the past year have you used an illegal drug or used a prescription medication for nonmedical reasons?"
  - Response: A response of ≥1 is positive
  - Sensitivity 100%, specificity 73.5%[74]
- Two-item conjoint screen for alcohol and other drug problems
  - Questions:
    - "In the last year, have you ever drunk or used drugs more than you meant to?"
    - "Have you felt you wanted or needed to cut down on your drinking or drug use in the last year?"
  - Response: A response of ≥1 is positive for a current substance use disorder
  - Sensitivity 79%, specificity 78%[75]

Table 2
AUDIT-C questionnaire

Questions	Scoring					Score
	0	1	2	3	4	
How often do you have a drink containing alcohol?	Never	Monthly or less	2 to 4 times a month	2 to 3 times a week	4 or more times a week	
If score to first question is zero, Stop screening here						
How many drinks containing alcohol do you have on a typical day when you are drinking?	1 to 2 drinks	3 to 4 drinks	5 to 6 drinks	7 to 9 drinks	10 or more drinks	
How often do you have 5 or more drinks on one occasion?	Never	Less than monthly	Monthly	Weekly	Daily or almost daily	
Total score						

The AUDIT-C is scored on a scale of 0–12 (scores of 0 reflect no alcohol use). In men, a score of 4 or more is considered positive; in women, a score of 3 or more is considered positive.

In general, the higher the AUDIT-C score, the more likely it is that the patient's drinking is affecting his or her health and safety.

From Babor TF, Higgins-Biddle JC, Saunders JB, et al. AUDIT: the alcohol use disorders identification test guidelines for use in primary care, second edition. Department of Mental Health and Substance Dependence, World Health Organization; 2011.

Table 3
Selected screening instruments for tobacco, alcohol, and/or other substance use

Substance	Instrument	Target Population	Description
Tobacco	Fagerström Test for Nicotine Dependence (FTND)	Adults	6-item screen measuring intensity of physical addiction to nicotine (cigarettes); level of severity assists in treatment planning[77]
Alcohol	Youth Guide	Children, adolescents	2-item screening tool for students in elementary school (aged 9–11 y), middle school (aged 11–14 y), and high school (aged 14–18 y); identifies risk factors for alcohol use[78]
	Alcohol Use Disorders Identification Test (AUDIT)	Adults	10-item screening tool, developed by the World Health Organization, to identify risky or hazardous alcohol use[79]
	Alcohol Use Disorders Identification Test—Consumption (AUDIT-C)	Adults	First 3 questions of AUDIT, focusing on alcohol consumption[76]
	TWEAK (Tolerance, Worried, Eye-opener, Amnesia, K/cut down)	Adults, pregnant women	5-item screening tool for risky drinking, with questions related to tolerance, worried, eye-opener, amnesia, and attempts to k/cut down[80]
Alcohol and other drugs	CRAFFT (Car, Relax, Alone, Forget, Family or Friends, Trouble)	Adolescents	6-item screening tool for alcohol and other drugs; targets situations relevant to adolescents: Car, Relax, Alone, Forget, Family or Friends, Trouble[81]
Other drugs	Drug Abuse Screening Test-20	Adolescents, adults	20-item screening tool to detect consequences related to drug use; includes prescribed or over-the-counter drugs, and any nonmedical use of drugs[82]

One set of resources, in particular, may be especially valuable to the primary care clinician striving to learn and integrate screening and brief intervention into their practice: the NIAAA publication *Helping Patients Who Drink Too Much: Clinician's Guide*,[21] which is available in both hardcopy and electronic versions (**Box 7**). An online training program has also been developed that includes step-by-step instructions for clinicians, handouts for patients, information regarding pharmacotherapy for alcohol use disorders, and video case presentations.[84] In addition, free continuing education credits are available for physicians and nurses when this course is taken through Medscape (see **Box 7**).

The number of sessions for screening and brief intervention may vary based on several factors, including (1) the patient's level of risk or severity related to substance use, (2) current medical conditions and/or other complicating factors, and (3) his or her response to screening and brief intervention. As one guideline states, "Medicare covers annual alcohol misuse screenings and, for those who screen positive, up to 4 brief face-to-face behavioral interventions in a 12-month period...for Medicare

---

Box 7
Clinical resources for primary care clinicians

National Institute on Alcohol Abuse and Alcoholism (NIAAA)

- Alcohol Screening and Brief Interventions for Youth: A Practitioner's Guide

  www.niaaa.nih.gov/YouthGuide

- Helping Patients Who Drink Too Much: A Clinician's Guide

  http://pubs.niaaa.nih.gov/publications/Practitioner/CliniciansGuide2005/clinicians_guide.htm.

- Clinician's Guide Online Video

  www.niaaa.nih.gov/publications/clinical-guides-and-manuals/niaaa-clinicians-guide-online-training

National Institute on Drug Abuse (NIDA)

- NIDA Drug Use Screening Tool: Clinician's Screening Tool for Drug Use in General Medical Settings

  www.drugabuse.gov/medical-health-professionals

- Safe Prescribing for Pain CME/CE (Medscape online)

  http://www.medscape.org/viewarticle/770687

- Managing Pain Patients Who Abuse Prescription Drugs CME/CE (Medscape online)

  http://www.medscape.org/viewarticle/770440

Substance Abuse and Mental Health Services Administration (SAMHSA)

- Brief Interventions and Brief Therapies for Substance Abuse (TIP 34)

  http://store.samhsa.gov/product/TIP-34-Brief-Interventions-and-Brief-Therapies-for-Substance-Abuse/SMA12-3952

- A Guide to Substance Abuse Services for Primary Care Clinicians (TIP 24)

  http://store.samhsa.gov/product/TIP-24-Guide-to-Substance-Abuse-Services-for-Primary-Care-Clinicians/SMA08-4075

- Incorporating Alcohol Pharmacotherapies into Medical Practice (TIP 49)

  http://store.samhsa.gov/product/TIP-49-Incorporating-Alcohol-Pharmacotherapies-Into-Medical-Practice/SMA13-4380

- Substance Abuse Treatment Services Locator

  www.findtreatment.samhsa.gov

- SBIRT: Screening, Brief Intervention, and Referral to Treatment

  http://www.integration.samhsa.gov/clinical-practice/sbirt

US Department of Justice, Drug Enforcement Agency (DEA)

- State Prescription Drug Monitoring Programs, Frequently Asked Questions (FAQs)

  http://www.deadiversion.usdoj.gov/faq/rx_monitor.htm

---

beneficiaries, including pregnant women."[72] Some SBIRT models (see **Fig. 1**) describe brief treatment as an intermediate step between brief intervention and referral to treatment. This approach may involve more intensive counseling sessions, delivered by clinicians with additional qualifications or experience in counseling, addictions medicine, addictions nursing, or other addictions specialist. The level of intervention should match the potential risk or severity of use (**Fig. 2**).

Referral to Treatment

Patients identified as needing more help than brief interventions can successfully provide are referred to specialty treatment. In preparation for this eventuality, primary care clinicians are encouraged to identify, establish, and maintain collaborative relationships with clinicians and facilities that specialize in the treatment of substance use disorders. This approach may include consulting with colleagues, or contacting and visiting local treatment centers.

The SAMHSA Substance Abuse Treatment Services Locator lists and provides pertinent information about state-licensed substance use treatment facilities throughout the United States, which currently number more than 11,000. This information can be accessed electronically (see **Box 7**).[85]

Because most treatment for substance use disorders occurs on an outpatient basis, the primary care clinician will likely continue to provide routine medical care while the patient participates in substance use treatment, as well as after discharge. This interaction presents a unique opportunity to create a culture of collaboration between primary care clinicians and addiction treatment services, and to provide true continuity of care.

Other Considerations

Mutual help groups
An essential part of treatment and recovery for many individuals with substance use disorders includes regular meeting attendance and affiliation with a mutual help group such as Alcoholics Anonymous (www.aa.org), Women for Sobriety (www.womenforsobriety.org), Narcotics Anonymous (www.na.org), or SMART Recovery

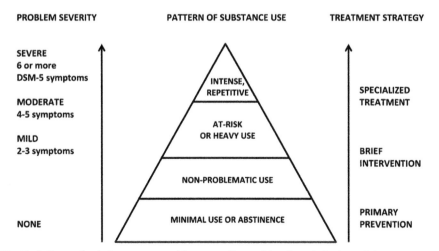

Fig. 2. Pattern of substance use, problem severity, and treatment strategy. Primary prevention is advised for those who are abstinent, or with minimal or nonproblematic use. Brief intervention is appropriate for at-risk or heavy-drinking individuals. For moderate to severe use, refer the patient to specialized addictions treatment. The use of illegal substances is inherently problematic. (*From* Strobbe S. Addressing substance use in primary care. Nurse Pract 2013;38(10):45–54.)

(www.smartrecovery.org). Family members and friends of those with substance use disorders can also seek and obtain support in several parallel organizations such as Al-Anon (www.al-anon.alateen.org) or Nar-Anon (www.nar-anon.org). Because mutual help group meetings play such a vital role in the treatment and recovery of individuals across the country and around the world, health care professionals, including primary care clinicians, are encouraged to familiarize themselves with these societies by attending 1 or more open meetings (ie, meetings open to the general public).[86]

Medications for substance use disorders

Several medications have been approved by the US Food and Drug Administration for the treatment of substance use disorders (**Box 8**). These medications can assist some patients in the transition from physiologic dependence to abstinence, or with replacement therapy. It is generally recommended that pharmacotherapy for addictions be provided in conjunction with psychosocial rehabilitation, which could include mutual help group meeting attendance and/or formal substance use treatment. The SAMHSA

Box 8
Pharmacotherapy for substance use disorders

Tobacco
- Nicotine replacement therapy
  - Nicotine gum
  - Nicotine lozenges
  - Nicotine nasal spray
  - Nicotine transdermal patches
  - Nicotine inhalers
- Medications
  - Bupropion (Zyban)
  - Varenicline (Chantix)

Alcohol
- Acamprosate (Campral)
- Disulfiram (Antabuse)
- Naltrexone
  - Oral (ReVia)
  - Injectable (Vivitrol)

Opioids
- Antagonist therapy
  - Naltrexone
    - Oral (ReVia)
    - Injectable (Vivitrol)
- Replacement/maintenance therapy
  - Buprenorphine (Suboxone, Subutex)
  - Methadone

publication *Incorporating Alcohol Pharmacotherapies into Medical Practice (TIP 49)* (see **Box 7**) has more information on medications for substance use disorders.[87]

Prescribing practices

When prescribing medications to patients with a history of problematic use of alcohol or other substances, clinicians are encouraged to avoid the use of agents that may place the patient at increased risk for misuse or relapse, particularly benzodiazepines or opioid medications. For specific procedures that require the use of such agents on a limited basis, additional education, monitoring, and support may be necessary. If questions arise regarding the possibility that a patient may be "doctor shopping" (eg, obtaining controlled substances from multiple prescribers), most states now have prescription drug monitoring programs (PDMPs) in place.[88] More information about PDMPs can be found through accessing the Web site of the US Department of Justice Drug Enforcement Administration's Office of Diversion Control (http://www.deadiversion.usdoj.gov/faq/rx_monitor.htm).

Pain management

In 2012, the National Institute of Drug Abuse (NIDA) and the Office of National Drug Control Policy (ONDCP) launched a new online learning tool to provide training to health care professionals on proper prescribing and patient management practices for patients receiving opioid analgesics. Continuing Medical Education/Continuing Education (CME/CE) credits are available when these offerings are accessed through Medscape (see **Box 7** under the National Institute on Drug Abuse for *Safe Prescribing for Pain CME/CE*[89] and *Managing Pain Patients Who Abuse Prescription Drugs*[90]).

Principles and strategies related to pain management are also addressed in detail in a position statement issued by the American Society of Pain Management Nurses. In this position statement, clinical recommendations are delineated for patients at low, moderate, and high risk for addiction. Ethical tenets are discussed, including the notion that all patients have the proper high-quality assessment and pain management, including those with substance use disorders. Adherence monitoring procedures are also considered, including urine toxicology studies. Although such studies are not yet regarded as part of universal screening, they can in some situations play a constructive role.[91]

CURRENT PRACTICE PATTERNS
Current Practice

Despite compelling evidence that prevention and SBIRT can be efficacious and cost-effective in addressing substance use and related disorders, primary care clinicians have been slow to adopt these practices.[92] Alcohol problems, in particular, are commonly not identified during the course of routine health care services.[93]

In a national sample of individuals aged 18 to 39 years, slightly fewer than half (49%) of those who had seen a doctor during the past year recalled having been asked about their alcohol consumption. Among those who exceeded NIAAA guidelines for per-day or per-week limits, only 14% recalled being advised about these limits, and fewer still (7%) were advised to cut down. Proportions were somewhat higher among those who exceeded both daily and weekly limits, with 24% having been advised about safe limits, and 21% advised to cut down.[94]

Barriers to Delivery

Commonly identified barriers for implementing screening and preventive services include: (1) a concern that the tools do not reflect the realities of practice (eg, they take too much time, they are not tailored to the setting's demographics); (2) worry that screening will identify patients whose needs exceed available resources; (3) the clinician lacks the requisite expertise to successfully carry out the screening (or subsequent intervention); (4) a general lack of comfort in asking patients about their alcohol use (eg, fear of offending the patient, the clinician is him/herself an at-risk alcohol user); and (5) inadequate reimbursement from some insurance providers (and in some cases, no reimbursement at all).[92,95] Certain of these concerns may be reduced, if not eliminated, in the context of SBIRT and other recent developments in health care. As time remains a precious commodity in clinical services, brief interventions are intended to be just that, and the potential return on investment in relation to patient outcomes can be significant.

Until fairly recently, inadequate insurance reimbursement had the potential to negatively affect both primary care clinicians and addiction treatment facilities, ultimately leaving many patients without access to essential care. There was little incentive for clinicians in primary care to screen patients for substance use if there was insufficient payment for the services (screening, brief intervention, brief treatment) they provided, or inadequate coverage to facilitate a referral to treatment (if indicated).

Reimbursement for screening and brief intervention is now available through commercial insurance Current Procedural Terminology (CPT) codes, Medicare G codes, and Medicaid Healthcare Common Procedure Coding System (HCPCS) codes.[96] In addition, on January 1, 2010 the Mental Health Parity and Addiction Equity Act of 2008 went into effect, stipulating that group health plans that provided both medical and surgical benefits and mental health or substance use disorder benefits be similarly structured in terms of benefits and restrictions.[97]

Health care professionals continue to receive limited education on substance use and related disorders, particularly in comparison with the prevalence and impact that these conditions can have on individual and public health.[98,99] In response to a pressing sense of urgency to offset this deficiency, several high-quality educational and training opportunities have been developed and offered, often with CME/CE credits available free of charge, several of which have been described here.

Characteristics of Organizations that Facilitate Best Practice

One group of researchers examined the Chronic Care Model as a framework for the prevention of risk behaviors, including tobacco use and risky drinking. These investigators found that primary care practices were more likely to offer recommended services such as health risk assessment, behavioral counseling, and referral to community-based programs if they were owned by a hospital health system that exhibited a culture of quality improvement, had a multispecialty staff, received support for decision making through point-of-care reminders and clinical staff meetings, and benefited from information systems such as an electronic health record (EHR).[100]

A team-based approach to SBIRT may also help to improve screening and related services (brief intervention, brief treatment, referral) within the primary care setting. A team-based approach to primary care capitalizes on the respective strengths of each team member in the provision of patient care. Through planning and clear delineation of roles, nonclinician team members can carry out some aspects of SBIRT, thus enabling clinicians to attend most closely to those patients with the highest severity. For example, nurses or social workers (and in some cases medical assistants) can administer screening instruments, provide patient education, answer patients' question, and triage patients with a positive screen to the clinician or dedicated SBIRT provider. The clinician or dedicated SBIRT provider can then carry out SBIRT in accordance with the 6 elements as delineated by the FRAMES model. Leaders within the primary care setting can champion SBIRT by establishing a culture that takes substance misuse seriously, and support staff and clinician training in SBIRT methods. Because team-based models for SBIRT remain on the cutting edge of care, there are insufficient data to assess its efficacy; however, emerging evidence suggests that this approach shows promise.[101]

IMPACT OF CHANGES WITHIN HEALTH CARE
Electronic Health Records

Although transitions to EHRs can be costly, disruptive, and stressful in the short term, the potential benefits of coordinated clinical care for patients with substance use and related disorders could prove to be transformative. Historically, because of stigma, shame, and discrimination, substance use and mental health disorders were frequently treated in isolation and secrecy, resulting in a predictable fragmentation and discontinuity of services, often to the detriment of the very patients whom these practices were presumably meant to protect.

While misunderstandings and prejudice persist, increasing numbers of professionals in the health care field have come to view addictions as chronic medical illnesses,[102] rooted in genetics and neurobiology,[103] with possibilities for full and sustained recovery. Some of the potential benefits of an EHR in the prevention and treatment of substance use disorders could include, but are not limited to:

- A single, comprehensive medical record, accessible across sites, providers, and services, over time
- The creation of mandatory fields for information related to tobacco, alcohol, and other substance use
- Ready access to patient-specific educational materials
- The potential to generate automated charges for provided services, such as prevention, screening, and brief intervention
- Prompts for follow-up care during subsequent visits
- The ability to track and graph laboratory values and other clinical activities
- Improved monitoring of prescription medications, including controlled substances

Affordable Care Act

The Affordable Care Act (ACA) promises to enhance and expand efforts toward the prevention and treatment of substance use disorders. First, the ACA requires most health insurance plans to cover preventive services recommended by USPSTF,[104] including current measures related to tobacco (children and adolescents, adults, and pregnant women) and alcohol (adults), as well as persons at high risk for HCV infections, most notably those with past or current injection drug use (see **Box 4**). Second, the ACA "includes substance use disorders as one of the ten elements of essential health benefits," meaning that "more health care providers can offer and be reimbursed for these services, resulting in more individuals having access to treatment."[105] Third, benefits for substance use disorders are now more closely aligned with those for other chronic health conditions, with related prospects for more continual, rather than episodic, care.[106]

Patient-Centered Medical Homes

The patient-centered medical home (PCMH) is described as a transformative model for primary care that encompasses 5 functions and attributes: comprehensive care, patient-centered care, coordinated care, accessible services, and quality and safety.[107] Interestingly these are many of the same holistic values that have defined quality addictions treatment for decades. The Minnesota Model, which became the prevailing approach to abstinence-based 12-step treatment and recovery, embraces individualized treatment plans with active family involvement; an interprofessional collaborative team focused on comprehensive care; and integrated health in mind, body, and spirit.[108] The prospect of a true partnership with the medical community in the form of PCMHs bodes well for the future prevention and treatment of addictive disorders, and recovery from such disorders.

SUMMARY

Alcohol and substance use disorders are a major public health concern, contributing to increased health care costs and needless human suffering. SBIRT can help to reduce these burdens by improving the health and well-being not only of individuals but also of families and communities. Primary care clinicians, including physicians, physician assistants, and nurse practitioners, are on the leading edge of transformative changes to the nation's health care system, including unprecedented access to alcohol and substance use screening and care. Although the full benefit of the ACA and the Mental Health Parity and Addiction Equity Act have yet to be realized, the outlook for a more humane, effective, and holistic future for alcohol and substance use prevention, screening, and treatment is hopeful.

ACKNOWLEDGMENTS

This article is dedicated to the memory of Dr Patrick W. Gibbons (1954–2014), a tireless clinician, teacher, and advocate for those in need of addictions treatment.

REFERENCES

1. Horgan C, Skwara KC, Strickler G. Substance abuse: the nation's number one health problem. Princeton (NJ): Robert Wood Johnson Foundation; 2001.
2. National Center on Addictions and Substance Abuse (CASA). Shoveling it up II: the impact of substance abuse on federal, state and local budgets. New York: CASA; 2009. Available at: http://www.casacolumbia.org/templates/publications_reports.aspx. Accessed July 15, 2013.
3. National Center on Addiction and Substance Abuse at Columbia University (CASA). Adolescent substance use: America's #1 public health problem. New York: CASA; 2011. Available at: http://www.casacolumbia.org/upload/2011/20110629adolescentsubstanceuse.pdf. Accessed July 15, 2013.
4. American Psychiatric Association (APA). Diagnostic and statistical manual for mental disorders. 5th edition. Arlington (VA): APA; 2013.
5. Goldman D, Oroszi G, Ducci F. The genetics of addictions: uncovering the genes. Nat Rev Genet 2005;6:521–32.
6. Kessler RC, Crum RM, Warner LA, et al. Lifetime co-occurrence of DSM-III-R alcohol abuse and dependence with other psychiatric disorders in the national comorbidity survey. Arch Gen Psychiatry 1997;54:313–21.
7. Kessler RC. The epidemiology of dual diagnosis. Biol Psychiatry 2004;56:730–7.
8. Kessler RC, Berlund P, Demler O, et al. Lifetime prevalence of age-of-onset distributions of DSM-IV disorders in the National Comorbidity Survey Replication. Arch Gen Psychiatry 2005;62(6):593–602.
9. Centers for Disease Control and Prevention (CDC). Smoking attributable mortality, years of potential life lost, and productivity losses—United States,

2000-2004. MMWR Morb Mortal Wkly Rep 2008;57:1226–8. Available at: http://www.cdc.gov/mmwr/preview/mmwrhtml/mm5745a3.htm. Accessed October 29, 2013.

10. US Department of Health and Human Services (USDHHS). How tobacco smoke causes disease: the biology and behavioral basis for smoking-attributable disease. Atlanta (GA): USDHHS, Centers for Disease Control and Prevention, National Center for Chronic Disease Prevention and Health Promotion, Office on Smoking and Health; 2010. Available at: http://www.surgeongeneral.gov/library/reports/tobaccosmoke/. Accessed October 29, 2013.

11. Centers for Disease Control and Prevention (CDC). Current cigarette smoking among adults—United States, 2011. MMWR Morb Mortal Wkly Rep 2012; 61(44):889–94. Available at: http://www.cdc.gov/mmwr/preview/mmwrhtml/mm6144a2.htm. Accessed October 29, 2013.

12. US Department of Health and Human Services (USDHHS). Preventing tobacco use among youth and young adults: a report of the Surgeon General. Atlanta (GA): USDHHS, CDC, National Center for Chronic Disease Prevention and Health Promotion, Office on Smoking and Health; 2012. Available at: http://www.cdc.gov/tobacco/data_statistics/sgr/2012/consumer_booklet/pdfs/consumer.pdf. Accessed October 29, 2013.

13. Centers for Disease Control and Prevention (CDC). Youth risk behavior surveillance—United States, 2009. Surveillance Summaries, June 4, 2010. MMWR Morb Mortal Wkly Rep 2010;59(No. SS05). Available at: http://www.cdc.gov/mmwr/preview/mmwrhtml/ss5905a1.htm. Accessed October 29, 2013.

14. Substance Abuse and Mental Health Services Administration (SAMHSA). Substance use during pregnancy varies by race and ethnicity. Center for Behavioral Health Statistics and Quality; 2012. Available at: http://www.samhsa.gov/data/spotlight/Spot062PregnantRaceEthnicity2012.pdf. Accessed October 29, 2013.

15. US Department of Health and Human Services (USDHHS). Health consequences of tobacco use among women. In: Ernster VL, Lloyd G, Norman LA, et al, editors. Women and smoking: a report of the Surgeon General. Rockville (MD): USDHHS, Centers for Disease Control and Prevention, National Center for Chronic Disease Prevention and Health Promotion, Office of Smoking and Health; 2001. p. 177–450. Available at: http://www.cdc.gov/tobacco/data_statistics/sgr/2001/complete_report/. Accessed October 29, 2013.

16. Bittoun R. Smoking cessation in pregnancy. Obstet Med 2010;3(3):90–3. http://dx.doi.org/10.1258/om.2010.090059.

17. Ober M, Jaakkola MS, Woodward A, et al. Worldwide burden of disease from exposure to second-hand smoke: a retrospective analysis of data from 192 countries. Lancet 2011;377:139–46. http://dx.doi.org/10.1016/S0140-6736(10)61388-8.

18. Mokdad AH, Marks JS, Stroup DF, et al. Actual causes of death in the United States, 2000. JAMA 2004;291(10):1238–45.

19. Hasin DS, Stinson FS, Ogburn E, et al. Prevalence, correlates, disability, and comorbidity of DSM-IV alcohol abuse and dependence in the United States: results from the National Epidemiologic Survey on Alcohol and Related Conditions. Arch Gen Psychiatry 2007;64(7):830–42.

20. Jonas DE, Garbutt JC, Amick HR, et al. Behavioral counseling after screening for alcohol misuse in primary care: a systematic review and meta-analysis for the U.S. Preventative Services Task Force. Ann Intern Med 2012;157(9):645–54.

21. National Institute on Alcohol Abuse and Alcoholism (NIAAA). Helping patients who drink too much: a clinician's guide (NIH Publication No. 05–3769). Rockville

(MD): NIAAA; 2005. Available at: http://pubs.niaaa.nih.gov/publications/Prac titioner/CliniciansGuide2005/clinicians_guide.htm. Accessed October 29, 2013.

22. Johnson LD, O'Malley PM, Bachman JG, et al. Monitoring the future: national survey results on drug use, 1975-2011: volume I: secondary school students. 2012. Available at: http://monitoringthefuture.org/pubs/monographs/mtf-vol1_ 2011.pdf. Accessed November 9, 2013.

23. Patrick ME, Schulenberg JE, Martz ME, et al. Extreme binge drinking among 12th-grade students in the United States: prevalence and predictors. JAMA Pediatr 2013;167(11):1019–25. http://dx.doi.org/10.1001/jamapediatrics.2013. 2392.

24. Centers for Disease Control and Prevention (CDC). Vital signs: binge drinking among women and high school girls—United States, 2011. MMWR Morb Mortal Wkly Rep 2013;62(1):9–13. Available at: http://www.cdc.gov/mmwr/preview/ mmwrhtml/mm6201a3.htm. Accessed November 9, 2013.

25. Centers for Disease Control and Prevention (CDC). Alcohol use and binge drinking among women of childbearing age—United States, 2006-2010. MMWR Morb Mortal Wkly Rep 2012;61(28):534–8. Available at: http://www.cdc.gov/ mmwr/preview/mmwrhtml/mm6128a4.htm. Accessed November 9, 2013.

26. Naimi TS, Libscomb LE, Brewer RD, et al. Binge drinking in the preconception period and the risk of unintended pregnancy: implications for women and their children. Pediatrics 2003;111:1136–41.

27. May PA, Gossage PA. Estimating the prevalence of fetal alcohol syndrome: a summary. Alcohol Res Health 2001;25:159–67.

28. Maier SE, West JR. Drinking patterns and alcohol-related birth defects. Alcohol Res Health 2001;25:168–74.

29. US Department of Health and Human Services (USDHHS). US Surgeon General releases advisory on alcohol use in pregnancy. Washington, DC: USDHHS; 2005. Available at: http://www.surgeongeneral.gov/pressreleases/sg02222005. html. Accessed November 9, 2013.

30. CESAR. Recently released drug survey shows marijuana use among U.S. residents continues to increase; no change in heroin use. Cesar Fax 2013;22(36):1. Available at: http://www.cesar.umd.edu/cesar/cesarfax/vol22/22-36.pdf. Accessed November 10, 2013.

31. Moore TH, Zammit S, Lingford-Hughes A, et al. Cannabis use and risk of psychotic or affective mental health outcomes: a systematic review. Lancet 2007; 370(9584):319–28.

32. US Drug Enforcement Administration (DEA), US Department of Justice. Drug scheduling. Available at: http://www.justice.gov/dea/druginfo/ds.shtml. Accessed November 10, 2013.

33. Office of National Drug Control Policy (ONDCP), US Executive Office of the President of the United States. Epidemic: responding to America's prescription drug abuse crisis. Rockville (MD): ONDCP; 2011. Available at: http://www.whitehouse. gov/sites/default/files/ondcp/policy-and-research/rx_abuse_plan.pdf. Accessed November 10, 2013.

34. Boyd CJ, McCabe SE. Commentary: coming to terms with the nonmedical use of prescription medications. Subst Abuse Treat Prev Policy 2008;3(1):22–3. http://dx.doi.org/10.1186/1747-597X-3-22.

35. National Institute on Drug Abuse (NIDA). Drug facts: prescription and over-the-counter medications [revised]. NIDA; 2013. Available at: http://www.drugabuse. gov/publications/drugfacts/prescription-over-counter-medications. Accessed November 10, 2013.

36. Manchikanti L, Fellow B, Ailinani H, et al. Therapeutic use, abuse, and nonmedical use of opioids: a ten-year perspective. Pain Physician 2010;13: 401–35.
37. Centers for Disease Control and Prevention (CDC). Policy impact: prescription painkiller overdoses. CDC; 2013. Available at: http://www.cdc.gov/Homeand RecreationalSafety/pdf/PolicyImpact-PrescriptionPainkillerOD.pdf.   Accessed November 10, 2013.
38. CESAR. Nearly 14% of U.S. residents report lifetime nonmedical use of prescription pain relievers; hydrocodone, codeine/propoxyphene, and oxycodone most commonly used. Cesar Fax 2011;20(44):1. Available at: http://www.cesar.umd.edu/cesar/cesarfax/vol20/20-44.pdf.   Accessed   November   10, 2013.
39. CESAR. Majority of nonmedical users of prescription pain relievers get the drugs from friends/relatives or doctors. Cesar Fax 2011;20(41):1. Available at: http://www.cesar.umd.edu/cesar/cesarfax/vol20/20-41.pdf. Accessed November 10, 2013.
40. Substance Abuse and Mental Health Services Administration (SAMHSA). Highlights of the 2011 Drug Abuse Warning Network (DAWN) findings on drug-related emergency department visits. The DAWN Report. Rockville (MD): US Department of Health and Human Services (USDHHS), SAMHSA; 2013. Available at: http://www.samhsa.gov/data/2k13/DAWN127/sr127-DAWN-highlights. htm. Accessed November 10, 2013.
41. Muhuri PD, Gfroerer JC, Davies MC. CBHSQ data review: associations of nonmedical pain reliever use and initiation of heroin use in the United States. Substance Abuse and Mental Health Services Administration (SAMHSA), Center for Behavioral Health Statistics and Quality (CBHSQ); 2013. Available at: http://www.samhsa.gov/data/2k13/DataReview/DR006/nonmedical-pain-reliever-use-2013.pdf. Accessed November 11, 2013.
42. Centers for Disease Control and Prevention (CDC). Vital signs: overdoses of prescription opioid pain relievers—United States, 1999-2008. MMWR Morb Mortal Wkly Rep 2011;60(43):1487–92. Available at: http://www.cdc.gov/mmwr/preview/mmwrhtml/mm6043a4.htm?s_cid=mm6043a4_w. Accessed November 10, 2013.
43. Centers for Disease Control and Prevention (CDC). Vital signs: prescription painkiller overdoses: a growing epidemic, especially among women. CDC; 2013. Available at: http://www.cdc.gov/vitalsigns/PrescriptionPainkillerOverdoses/. Accessed November 10, 2013.
44. Colliver JD, Compton WM, Gfroerer JC, et al. Projecting drug use among again baby boomers in 2020. Ann Epidemiol 2006;16(4):257–65.
45. Martin CM. Prescription drug abuse in the elderly. Consult Pharm 2008;23(12): 930–4, 936, 941–2.
46. CESAR. Smoking by age 12 related to alcohol and drug use/dependence. Cesar Fax 2007;16(47):1. Available at: http://www.cesar.umd.edu/cesar/cesarfax/vol16/16-47.pdf. Accessed November 10, 2013.
47. CESAR. Adults who initiate alcohol use before age 21 more likely to abuse or become dependent on alcohol. Cesar Fax 2010;19(40):1. Available at: http://www.cesar.umd.edu/cesar/cesarfax/vol19/19-40.pdf. Accessed November 10, 2013.
48. CESAR. Teens who frequently have family dinners less likely to drink, smoke, or use drugs. Cesar Fax 2006;15(39):1. Available at: http://www.cesar.umd.edu/cesar/cesarfax/vol15/15-39.pdf. Accessed November 10, 2013.

49. CESAR. Youth attending drug-free and gang-free schools least likely to have ever tried tobacco, alcohol, or marijuana. Cesar Fax 2010;19(34):1. Available at: http://www.cesar.umd.edu/cesar/cesarfax/vol19/19-34.pdf. Accessed November 10, 2013.

50. CESAR. Smoking among high school students decreases as cigarette prices increase. Cesar Fax 2010;19(7):1. Available at: http://www.cesar.umd.edu/cesar/cesarfax/vol19/19-07.pdf. Accessed November 10, 2013.

51. CESAR. Federal tobacco tax to increase by 62¢ per pack; increases in tobacco tax have been shown to reduce youth smoking. Cesar Fax 2009;18(6):1. Available at: http://www.cesar.umd.edu/cesar/cesarfax/vol18/18-06.pdf. Accessed November 10, 2013.

52. US Preventive Services Task Force (USPSTF). Primary care interventions to prevent tobacco use in children and adolescents. USPSTF; 2013. Available at: http://www.uspreventiveservicestaskforce.org/uspstf12/tobacco/tbacfinalrs.htm. Accessed October 29, 2013.

53. Substance Abuse and Mental Health Services Administration (SAMHSA). Screening, brief intervention, and referral to treatment (SBIRT). Available at: http://www.samhsa.gov/prevention/sbirt. Accessed November 17, 2013.

54. Prochaska JO, DiClemente CC, Norcross JC. In search of how people change: applications to addictive behaviors. Am Psychol 1992;47(9):1102–14.

55. Miller WR, Rollnick S. Motivational interviewing: preparing people for change. 2nd edition. New York: Guilford Press; 2002.

56. Babor TF, McRee BG, Kassesaum PA, et al. Screening, brief intervention, and referral to treatment (SBIRT): toward a public health approach to the management of substance abuse. Subst Abus 2007;28(3):7–30.

57. Bien T, Miller WR, Tonigan JS. Brief interventions for alcohol problems: a review. Addiction 1992;88:315–36.

58. Fleming MF, Mundt MP, French MT, et al. Brief physician advice for problem drinkers: long-term efficacy and benefit-cost analysis. Alcohol Clin Exp Res 2002;26(1):36–43.

59. Cuijpers R, Riper H, Lemmers L. The effects on mortality of brief interventions for problem drinking: a meta-analysis. Addiction 2004;99(7):839–45.

60. US Preventive Services Task Force (USPSTF). USPFTF. 2013. Available at: http://www.uspreventiveservicestaskforce.org/. Accessed October 29, 2013.

61. US Preventive Services Task Force (USPSTF). Grade definitions. USPSTF. 2008. Available at: http://www.uspreventiveservicestaskforce.org/uspstf/grades.htm. Accessed October 29, 2013.

62. US Preventive Services Task Force (USPSTF). Counseling and interventions to prevent tobacco use and tobacco-caused disease in adults and pregnant women, Topic Page. USPSTF; 2013. Available at: http://www.uspreventiveservicestaskforce.org/uspstf/uspstbac2.htm. Accessed October 29, 2013.

63. US Preventive Services Task Force (USPSTF). Screening and behavioral counseling interventions in primary care to reduce alcohol misuse, Topic Page. USPSTF; 2013. Available at: http://www.uspreventiveservicestaskforce.org/uspstf/uspsdrin.htm. Accessed October 29, 2013.

64. US Preventive Services Task Force (USPSTF). Screening for hepatitis C virus infection in adults, Topic Page. USPSTF; 2013. Available at: http://www.uspreventiveservicestaskforce.org/uspstf/uspshepc.htm. Accessed November 17, 2013.

65. US Preventive Services Task Force (USPSTF). Screening for illicit drug use, Topic Page. USPSTF; 2008. Available at: http://www.uspreventiveservicestaskforce.org/uspstf/uspsdrug.htm. Accessed October 29, 2013.

66. American Academy of Family Physicians (AAFP). Summary of recommendations for clinical preventive services. AAPF; 2013. Available at: http://www.aafp.org/dam/AAFP/documents/patient_care/clinical_recommendations/cps-recommendations.pdf. Accessed October 29, 2013.

67. Kulig JW, Committee on Substance Abuse. Tobacco, alcohol and other drugs: the role of the pediatrician in prevention, identification and management of substance abuse. Pediatrics 2005;115(3):816–21.

68. American College of Obstetrics and Gynecology (ACOG). Guidelines for women's health care. 2nd edition. Washington, DC: ACOG; 2002.

69. American Lung Association (ALA). Providing guidance on lung cancer screening to patients and physicians. ALA; 2012. Available at: http://www.lung.org/lung-disease/lung-cancer/lung-cancer-screening-guidelines/lung-cancer-screening.pdf. Accessed October 29, 2013.

70. Strobbe S. Addressing substance use in primary care. Nurse Pract 2013;38(10): 45–54. http://dx.doi.org/10.1097/01.NPR.0000433078.14775.15.

71. Substance Abuse and Mental Health Services Administration (SAMHSA). Systems-level implementation of screening, brief intervention and referral to treatment. Technical Assistance Publication (TAP) Series 33. HHS Publication No. (SMA) 13–4741. Rockville (MD): SAMHSA; 2013. Available at: http://www.integration.samhsa.gov/sbirt/TAP33.pdf. Accessed November 22, 2013.

72. Centers for Medicare & Medicaid Services (CMS), Department of Health and Human Services (DHHS). Screening and behavioral counseling interventions in primary care to reduce alcohol misuse. Publication ICN 907798. CMS; 2013. Available at: http://www.cms.gov/Outreach-and-Education/Medicare-Learning-Network-MLN/MLNProducts/downloads/Reduce-Alcohol-Misuse-ICN907798.pdf. Accessed November 22, 2013.

73. Smith PC, Schmidt SM, Allensworth-Davies D, et al. Primary care validation of a single-question alcohol screening test. J Gen Intern Med 2009;24(7): 783–8.

74. Smith PC, Schmidt SM, Allensworth-Davies D, et al. A single-question screening test for drug use in primary care. Arch Intern Med 2010;170(13): 1155–60.

75. Brown RL, Leonard T, Saunders LA, et al. A two-item conjoint screen for alcohol and other drug problems. J Am Board Fam Pract 2001;14(2):95–106.

76. Bush K, Kivlahan DR, McDonnell MB, et al. The AUDIT alcohol consumption questions (AUDIT-C): an effective brief screening test for problem drinking. Arch Intern Med 1998;158:1789–95.

77. Heatherton TF, Kozlowki LT, Frecker RC, et al. The Fagerström Test for Nicotine Dependence: a revision of the Fagerström Tolerance Questionnaire. Br J Addict 1991;86:1119–27.

78. National Institute on Alcohol Abuse and Alcoholism (NIAAA). Alcohol screening and brief intervention for youth: a practitioner's guide. Bethesda (MD): NIAAA; 2011. Available at: http://pubs.niaaa.nih.gov/publications/Practitioner/YouthGuide/YouthGuide.pdf. Accessed November 22, 2013.

79. Babor TF, Higgings-Biddle JC, Saunders JB, et al. AUDIT: the Alcohol Use Disorders Identification Test, guidelines for use in primary care. 2nd edition. Geneva (Switzerland): World Health Organization; 2001. Available at: http://apps.who.int/iris/bitstream/10665/67205/1/WHO_MSD_MSB_01.6a.pdf. Accessed November 22, 2013.

80. Russell M. New assessment tools for risk drinking during pregnancy: T-ACE, TWEAK, and others. Alcohol Health Res World 1994;18(1):55–61.

81. Knight JR, Sherritt L, Shrier LA, et al. Validity of the CRAFFT substance abuse screening test among adolescent clinic patients. Arch Pediatr Adolesc Med 1992;156:607–14.

82. Yudko E, Lozhkina O, Fouts A. A comprehensive review of the psychometric properties of the Drug Abuse Screening Test. J Subst Abuse Treat 2007;32: 189–98.

83. Miller WR, Sanchez VC. Motivating young adults for treatment and lifestyle change. In: Howard GS, Nathan PE, editors. Alcohol use and misuse by young adults. Notre Dame (IN): University of Notre Dame Press; 1994. p. 55–82.

84. National Institute on Alcohol Abuse and Alcoholism (NIAAA). NIAAA online clinician's guide online training. Available at: http://www.niaaa.nih.gov/publications/clinical-guides-and-manuals/niaaa-clinicians-guide-online-training. Accessed November 22, 2013.

85. Substance Abuse and Mental Health Services Administration (SAMHSA). Behavioral health treatment services locator, substance abuse treatment services locator. Available at: www.findtreatment.samhsa.gov. Accessed November 22, 2013.

86. Strobbe S, Thompson SM, Zucker RA. Teaching students about Alcoholics Anonymous an experiential approach. J Addict Nurs 2013;24(1):51–7. http://dx.doi.org/10.1097/JAN.Ob013e31828768e4.

87. Substance Abuse and Mental Health Services Administration (SAMHSA). Incorporating alcohol pharmacotherapies into medical practice. HHS Publication No. (SMA) 09–4380. Rockville (MD): SAMHSA; 2009.

88. US Department of Justice, Drug Enforcement Agency (DEA). State prescription drug monitoring programs. Available at: http://www.deadiversion.usdoj.gov/faq/rx_monitor.htm. Accessed November 23, 2013.

89. Dowling G, Denisco RA. Safe prescribing for pain (Medscape CME/CE). Available at: http://www.medscape.org/viewarticle/770687. Accessed November 22, 2013.

90. Dowling GJ, Denisco RA. Managing pain patients who abuse prescription drugs (Medscape CME/CE). Available at: http://www.medscape.org/viewarticle/770440. Accessed November 22, 2013.

91. Oliver J, Coggins C, Compton P, et al. American Society of Pain Management Nursing position statement: pain management in patients with substance use disorders [Dual publication]. Pain Manag Nurs 2012;13(3):169–83. http://dx.doi.org/10.1016/j.pmn.2012.07.001, J Addict Nurs 2012;23(3):210–22. http://dx.doi.org/10.1097/JAN.Ob013e31827c123.

92. Kuehn BM. Despite benefit, physicians slow to offer brief advice on harmful use. JAMA 2008;299(7):751–3.

93. Vinson DC, Turner BJ, Manning BK, et al. Clinician suspicion of an alcohol problem: an observational study from the AAFP National Research Network. Ann Fam Med 2013;11(1):53–9. http://dx.doi.org/10.1370/afm.1464.

94. Hingson R, Heeren T, Edwards E, et al. Young adults at risk for excess alcohol consumption are often not asked or counseled about drinking alcohol. J Gen Intern Med 2012;27(2):179–84. http://dx.doi.org/10.1007/s11606-011-1851-1.

95. Yarnall KS, Pollak KI, Ostbye T, et al. Primary care: is there enough time for prevention? Am J Public Health 2003;93(4):635–41.

96. Substance Abuse and Mental Health Services Administration (SAMHSA). Coding for SBI reimbursement. Available at: http://www.samhsa.gov/prevention/sbirt/coding.aspx. Accessed November 22, 2013.

97. H.R. 1424-117. Subtitle B—Paul Wellstone and Pete Domenici Mental Health Parity and Addiction Equity Act of 2008. Available at: http://www.cms.gov/Regulations-and-Guidance/Health-InsuranceReform/HealthInsReformforConsume/downloads/MHPAEA.pdf. Accessed November 22, 2013.

98. Boodman SG. Few doctors know how to treat addiction. A new program aims to change that. Washington Post 2012. Available at: http://www.washingtonpost.com/national/health-science/few-doctors-know-how-to-treat-addiction-a-new-program-aims-to-change-that/2012/08/31/d43f85bc-db27-11e1-bd1f-8f2b57de6d94_print.html. Accessed November 22, 2013.

99. Campbell-Heider NC, Finnell DS, Feigenbaum JC, et al. Survey on addictions: towards curricular change for family nurse practitioners. Int J Nurs Educ Scholarsh 2009;6:1–17.

100. Hung DY, Rundall TG, Tallia AF, et al. Rethinking prevention in primary care: applying the Chronic Care Model to address health risk behaviors. Milbank Q 2007;85(1):69–91.

101. Muench J, Jarvis K, Gray M, et al. Implementing a team-based SBIRT model in primary care clinics. J Subst Use 2013. http://dx.doi.org/10.3109/14659891.2013.866176.

102. McLellan TA, Lewis DC, O'Brien CP, et al. Drug dependence, a chronic medical illness: implications for treatment, insurance, and outcomes evaluation. JAMA 2000;284(13):1689–95.

103. Volkow ND, Li TK. Drug addiction: the neurobiology of behavior gone awry. Nat Rev Neurosci 2004;5(12):963–70.

104. Patient Protection and Affordable Care Act (Public Law 111-148). 2010. Available at: http://www.healthcare.gov/where-can-i-read-the-affordable-care-act/. Accessed November 22, 2013.

105. Office of National Drug Control Policy (ONDCP). Substance abuse and the Affordable Care Act. ONDCP. 2013. Available at: http://www.whitehouse.gov/ondcp/healthcare. Accessed November 22, 2013.

106. McLellan TA. Healthcare reform and substance use disorders: how will it affect opportunities for nurses? International Nurses Society on Addictions (IntNSA) 37th Annual Educational Conference, Keynote Address. Washington, DC, October 10, 2013.

107. Agency for Healthcare Research and Quality (AHRQ), Patient Centered Medical Home (PCMH) Resource Center. Defining the PCMH. Available at: http://pcmh.ahrq.gov/page/defining-pcmh. Accessed December 23, 2013.

108. Anderson DJ, McGovern JP, DuPont RL. The origins of the Minnesota Model of addiction treatment—a first person account. J Addict Dis 1999;18(1):107–14.

Screening and Prevention of Sexually Transmitted Infections

Paul Hunter, MD[a], Jessica Dalby, MD[b], Jaime Marks, MD[c],
Geoffrey R. Swain, MD, MPH[a], Sarina Schrager, MD, MS[b,*]

KEYWORDS

- Sexually transmitted infections • Screening • Prevention • *Chlamydia* • Gonorrhea
- Syphilis • Human immunodeficiency virus • United States

KEY POINTS

- Primary care clinicians should follow established guidelines for screening for sexually transmitted infection (STIs).
- The US Preventive Services Task Force, Centers for Disease Control and Prevention, American Academy of Family Physicians, American College of Obstetricians and Gynecologists, and American Academy of Pediatrics have all agreed on STI screening recommendations.
- Screening for an STI can also include counseling about risk-reduction behavior, and may be an opportune time to provide vaccinations to prevent other STIs.
- Each state has a list of different reportable STIs, so clinicians should be familiar with their state's legally mandated reporting requirements.
- High-risk behaviors put people at risk of STIs.
- Guidelines are based on national norms; clinicians should know the local prevalence of STIs and local recommendations, if any, to make more patient-centered decisions about screening.

INTRODUCTION

Sexually transmitted infections (STIs) are among the most frequently reported and prevalent medical conditions in the United States (**Table 1**). In total, nearly 20 million new cases of STIs occur in the United States each year, contributing to more than

Conflict of Interest: None.

[a] Department of Family Medicine, University of Wisconsin School of Medicine and Public Health, Center for Urban Population Health, City of Milwaukee Health Department, 841 North Broadway Street, 3rd Floor, Milwaukee, WI 53202, USA; [b] Department of Family Medicine, University of Wisconsin School of Medicine and Public Health, 1100 Delaplaine Court, Madison, WI 53715-1896, USA; [c] Department of Family Medicine, University of Wisconsin School of Medicine and Public Health, 207 West Lincoln Street, Suite 1, Augusta, WI 54722, USA
* Corresponding author.
E-mail address: sbschrag@wisc.edu

Table 1
Causes, complications, and burden[a] of selected sexually transmitted infections (STI) in the United States

STI	Description	Incidence Estimates (New Cases)	Incidence Rate (per 100,000)	Prevalence Estimates (Total Cases)	Prevalence Rate (per 100,000)
Chlamydia	An obligate intracellular bacterium, *Chlamydia trachomatis* causes urethritis and cervicitis, as well as pharyngeal and anal infections. Complications include pelvic inflammatory disease (and subsequent risk for infertility, pelvic pain, tubal ectopic pregnancy) as well as neonatal conjunctivitis and pneumonia	2,860,000	926.2	1,570,000	508.4
Gonorrhea	*Neisseria gonorrhoeae*, also known as gonococcus, is a gram-negative diplococcus that causes urethritis and cervicitis, as well as pharyngeal and anal infections. Complications are essentially identical to those of *Chlamydia*	820,000	265.5	270,000	87.4
Syphilis (primary, secondary, and early latent)	The spiral bacterium *Treponema pallidum* manifests itself in several stages, including primary (typically a painless chancre), early latent (asymptomatic), secondary (typically a rash), and late latent (asymptomatic). Tertiary syphilis includes neurosyphilis (eg, dorsalis tabes and dementia), gummas, and cardiovascular syphilis (eg, aortitis, aneurysm, and rupture). Vertical transmission to newborns is common, resulting in congenital syphilis	55,400	17.9	117,000	—
Hepatitis B	This chronic viral infection is transmitted through sharing of blood and body fluids (including saliva) as well as vertically from mother to newborn. Sequelae include hepatocellular carcinoma and hepatic failure	19,000	6.2	442,000	143.1

	Description				
HIV[b] (ages 13 and up)	This chronic retroviral infection, if not treated, creates immune-system dysfunction, resulting in AIDS and its hallmark opportunistic infections (eg, *Pneumocystis carinii*, Kaposi sarcoma). It can be transmitted sexually or through other blood and body fluid exposure (eg, needle sharing), and vertically from mother to newborn (eg, through breastfeeding). About 75% of case reports are in men	50,000	19.7	1,148,200	453.4
Genital herpes[c]	Caused by herpes simplex viruses 1 and 2, genital herpes is a chronic viral infection that causes painful recurrent herpetic outbreaks at the original site of infection	776,000	251.3	24,100,000	7804.4
Trichomoniasis	Trichomoniasis is a flagellate parasitic infection of the urethra or vagina that can persist for months. Testing is insensitive, and complications of its associated mucosal irritation include urinary tract infections and increased risk for HIV infection	1,090,000	353.0	3,710,000	1201.4
Human papillomavirus (HPV)[d]	This viral infection of the penis or cervix is nearly ubiquitous after 2 or more lifetime sexual partners. There are nearly 100 viral subtypes, and while some infections are transient, infection with high-risk subtypes leads to cervical intraepithelial neoplasia. Chronic infection with types 16 and 18 cause about 70% of cervical cancers. HPV-related anal, penile, and especially oropharyngeal cancers are rising. Infections with other subtypes (eg, 6 and 11) cause visible genital warts	14,100,000	4566.1	79,100,000	25,615.3 (25.6%)

[a] Except for human immunodeficiency virus (HIV), all incidence case and prevalence case estimates are for 2008, include both reported cases and estimates of unreported cases, use a 2008 US population denominator of 308,800,000, and are derived from the Centers for Disease Control and Prevention (CDC).[50]
[b] For HIV, incidence case and prevalence case estimates are for 2009, include both reported cases and estimates of unreported cases, use a 2009 US population denominator of the US population ages 13 years and older, and are derived from the CDC.[51]
[c] Incidence and prevalence estimates of herpes simplex virus are for type 2 only, even though genital herpes is also caused by type 1.
[d] HPV prevalence may be more than 40% according to the American Sexual Health Association.[52]

US$17 billion in health care costs.[1] Most costs are due to human immunodeficiency virus (HIV), cervical cancer, and complications of pelvic inflammatory disease, such as infertility, chronic pelvic pain, and tubal ectopic pregnancy. Because of their high incidence, high prevalence, serious complications, lack of symptoms, ease of diagnosis, and availability of effective treatment, STIs are of great importance to primary care clinicians. Furthermore, primary care clinicians are in unique positions to prevent future infections by identifying and treating existing infections, by treating exposed partners, and by serving as effective change agents to help reduce patients' risk behaviors.

Although sexual images and themes are nearly inescapable in American popular culture, there can often be social, psychological, and political awkwardness surrounding frank and open discussions of sexuality in general and STIs specifically; this is in contrast to western European countries, where sexuality is often seen as part of a healthy life and is discussed more openly. Perhaps not coincidentally, Europe has *Chlamydia* and gonorrhea rates that are 60% to 90% lower than American rates.[2]

RISK GROUPS AND RISK BEHAVIORS

Behaviors that put patients at higher risk for STIs include multiple sexual partners; unprotected oral, anal, or vaginal sex; exchanging money, housing, or drugs for sex; engaging in commercial, survival (prostitution to earn money), or coerced sex; and using mind-altering drugs or alcohol during sex. Certain demographic groups also have higher rates of STIs; however, race and ethnicity are of much less relevance than risk behaviors in clinical encounters.[3]

Adolescents and Young Adults

Sexually active adolescents and young adults (ages 15–24 years) have particularly high rates of *Chlamydia* and gonorrhea. The risk for STI is even higher among young people who engage in high-risk behaviors, initiate sexual activity earlier in adolescence, are in detention facilities, have multiple sexual partners concurrently, or have multiple sequential sexual partnerships of limited duration. In addition, adolescents have increased biological susceptibility to infection (eg, immature cervical epithelium) and multiple obstacles to accessing health care.

Clinicians treating adolescents frequently fail to inquire about sexual behaviors, assess STI risks, provide risk-reduction counseling, and screen for asymptomatic infections. Sexual health discussions should be appropriate for the patient's developmental level and should be aimed at identifying high-risk behaviors. Careful, nonjudgmental, and thorough counseling is particularly vital for adolescents who might not feel comfortable acknowledging high-risk behaviors.

Pregnant Women

Although pregnant women usually have been participating in unprotected sexual activity, many have no behavioral risks that increase the risk for STI. However, untreated STIs can result in serious, preventable complications for newborns. Therefore, recommendations to screen pregnant women for STIs are based on disease severity and sequelae, risk to the newborn, prevalence in the population, costs, medicolegal considerations (eg, state laws), and other factors.

Men Who Have Sex with Men

Since the mid-1990s, men who have sex with men (MSM) have had increasing rates of early syphilis (primary, secondary, or early latent), gonorrhea, and *Chlamydia*. Unsafe sexual behaviors, including the use of mind-altering drugs during sex (eg, methamphetamine and volatile nitrites or "poppers") have also increased. These trends have in turn led to increased rates of HIV, especially in some urban centers, and particularly among racial and ethnic minority groups.

The recent increases in HIV rates likely reflect the changing attitudes concerning HIV infection that have accompanied advances in HIV therapy. Because persons with HIV have improved quality of life and survival, fear of disease is no longer sufficient to motivate safe sexual practices. More MSM live longer while infectious, owing to medical management of HIV. New venues for partner acquisition (eg, Internet and smartphone apps) and increases in substance abuse have led to increased high-risk sexual behavior. This combination of factors has resulted in increased rates of STIs and HIV among MSM.

Clinicians should assess STI and HIV-related risks for all male patients, including the sex of their sexual partners.[4] MSM, including those with HIV infection, should receive nonjudgmental STI/HIV risk assessment and client-centered prevention counseling to reduce the likelihood of acquiring or transmitting HIV or other STIs. Clinicians should be familiar with the local community resources available to assist high-risk MSM in facilitating behavioral change and to enable partner notification activities. Clinicians should routinely ask sexually active MSM about the following: (1) symptoms consistent with common STIs, including urethral discharge, dysuria, genital and perianal ulcers, regional lymphadenopathy, and rash; and (2) anorectal symptoms consistent with proctitis, including discharge and pain on defecation or during anal intercourse.

Injection Drug Users

Injection drug users (IDUs) are at particularly high risk for HIV and hepatitis B; they are also at risk for other STIs if they exchange money or drugs for sex, or if they have sex while drunk or high.[5]

Racial and Ethnic Groups

In aggregate, black and Hispanic persons have significantly higher rates of *Chlamydia*, gonorrhea, and syphilis; however, race and ethnicity serve as surrogate markers for the underlying social factors that increase STI risk[6] among large populations. In addition to reduced access to health care, racial discrimination may also lead to elevated rates of STIs in blacks via intermediary factors[7] such as poverty, chronic unemployment, drug and alcohol marketing tactics, social disorganization, and male incarceration.

Therefore, it is important for clinicians to focus on individual risk behaviors when managing individual patients, rather than assuming that skin color of an individual provides causal information regarding that individual's pretest likelihood of having an STI.[8]

SCREENING RECOMMENDATIONS

Screening means testing asymptomatic individuals. When a disease is prevalent and has serious complications, screening may be appropriate. Screening requires accurate tests and effective treatments that are available and affordable (**Box 1**).

PROFESSIONAL GROUP RECOMMENDATIONS

Screening recommendations from various expert panels and authoritative institutions sometimes diverge because of differences in organizational mission and target audience; emphases on the harms of screening; methodology for evidence reviews; experts with vested interests (professional or economic); and demands by clinicians

---

Box 1
Developing local screening criteria from national guidelines

1. The US Preventive Services Task Force uses national epidemiologic data and the prevalence of risk behaviors to provide clinical guidance about what age to begin screening and what age to stop screening.[9]

2. Clinicians should consult with local public health officials and use available local epidemiologic data to tailor screening programs based on the community and populations served.[10]

3. Communities with STI rates higher than the national averages should have local screening criteria, usually formulated by that jurisdiction's local health department.

4. An example of evidence-based local screening criteria for a high-prevalence community is available at http://city.milwaukee.gov/ImageLibrary/Groups/healthAuthors/DCP/PDFs/STD_Screen_Tx_Guide_updated_20080121.pdf.[9]

---

for guidance despite limited evidence or resources. In 2008, there was agreement on STI screening among the US Preventive Services Task Force (USPSTF), Centers for Disease Control and Prevention (CDC), American Academy of Family Physicians (AAFP), American Academy of Pediatrics (AAP), and American College of Obstetricians and Gynecologists (ACOG).[10] The current guidelines from the USPSTF, CDC, AAFP, and ACOG were reviewed to develop the recommendations as outlined in **Tables 2** and **3**. These tables represent national guidance; however, local practice needs to be tailored to local conditions and prevalence of disease.

Known Contacts

Known contacts of patients with STIs should receive screening for STIs to which they have been exposed.[11] In addition, the following populations meet national criteria for routine screening for certain STIs.[12]

Sexually Active Adolescents and Young Adults

Nationally, *Chlamydia* screening is recommended annually for females aged 25 years and younger, but local prevalence sometimes warrants raising or lowering this age. Depending on local conditions, young men in high-prevalence settings such as adolescent clinics, correctional facilities, and STI clinics should also be considered for annual *Chlamydia* screening, despite national recommendations not including screening men.

The CDC recommends targeted gonorrhea screening for women meeting 1 of more of the following criteria: younger than 25 years; previous gonorrhea infection; other STIs; new or multiple sex partners; inconsistent condom use; or involved in commercial sex work or illicit drug use. Young women living in high-prevalence communities should also be screened.

HIV screening should be discussed with all adolescents, and encouraged for those who are sexually active or who use injection drugs.

No screening of adolescents is recommended nationally for syphilis, trichomoniasis, herpes simplex virus (HSV), human papillomavirus (HPV), or hepatitis B virus (HBV), except for MSM and pregnant women.

Pregnant Women

Chlamydia

Screening for *Chlamydia* should occur at the first prenatal visit. Rescreening in the third trimester is recommended for women aged 25 years or younger, who tested

Table 2
Screening and testing recommendations for STIs in the United States

Recommended Screening by Disease[a,b]		Testing Method	Strength of Recommendation (USPSTF Evidence Grade[c])
Chlamydia	Annually for all sexually active women <25 y of age	Cervical, vaginal, or urethral fluid by NAAT; pharyngeal and anorectal swabs for NAATs are available in some laboratories	A
	All women aged ≥25 y who are at increased risk[d]		A
	Insufficient evidence to recommend screening in asymptomatic men		I
Gonorrhea	Annually for all sexually active women <25 y of age	Cervical, vaginal, or urethral fluid by NAAT; pharyngeal and anorectal swabs for NAATs are available in some laboratories	B
	All women aged ≥25 y who are at increased risk[d]		B
	Insufficient evidence to recommend screening in asymptomatic men		I
Hepatitis B	No screening in asymptomatic individuals	Blood for HBsAg	D
Hepatitis C	All patients at increased risk, including those with past or current injection drug use, those who have had sex with intravenous drug users, and those having a blood transfusion before 1992	Blood for hepatitis C antibody	B
	One-time screening for all patients born between 1945 and 1965		B
Herpes	No screening in asymptomatic individuals	Viral culture of lesion or blood for HSV 1/2 PCR	D
HIV	All patients aged 13–65 y unless the prevalence of undiagnosed HIV infection in the population is proven to be <0.1%	Blood EIA with third-/fourth-generation antigen and antibody testing with no Western blot	A
	All patients initiating treatment for tuberculosis		A
	All patients seeking treatment for STIs		A
	All pregnant patients, including those presenting to labor and delivery if their status is unknown		A
HPV	Routine screening not recommended	Cervical swab for HPV DNA high risk or with supernatant from liquid-based Pap testing for cervical cancer	I
	Screening may be done in combination with Pap smear for women between 30 and 65 y of age as part of a cervical cancer screening program		A

(continued on next page)

Table 2 (continued)			
Recommended Screening by Disease[a,b]		Testing Method	Strength of Recommendation (USPSTF Evidence Grade[c])
Syphilis	Screen all persons at increased risk[d]	Blood for RPR or VDRL[e]	A
	Screen all pregnant women		A
Trichomonas	No screening in asymptomatic individuals	Wet mount (low sensitivity); Culture improves sensitivity; PCR testing, available in some laboratories, is more accurate, but currently is expensive	D

Abbreviations: EIA, enzyme immunoassay; HBsAg, hepatitis B surface antigen; HIV, human immunodeficiency virus; HPV, human papillomavirus; NAAT, nucleic acid amplification test; Pap, Papanicolaou; PCR, polymerase chain reaction; RPR, rapid plasma reagin; USPSTF, US Preventive Services Task Force; VDRL, Venereal Disease Research Laboratory.

[a] This table represents national guidance. Local practice needs to be tailored to local conditions and prevalence of disease. See Box 1 for suggestions of how clinicians can consult with local public health officials to develop local screening criteria.

[b] Data were derived from USPSTF recommendation statements.[10,53–62]

[c] Grade A: The USPSTF recommends the service. There is high certainty that the net benefit is substantial. Grade B: The USPSTF recommends the service. There is high certainty that the net benefit is moderate, or there is moderate certainty that the net benefit is moderate to substantial. Grade D: The USPSTF recommends selectively offering or providing this service to individual patients based on professional judgment and patient preferences. There is at least moderate certainty that the net benefit is small. I Statement: The USPSTF concludes that the current evidence is insufficient to assess the balance of benefits and harms of the service. Evidence is lacking, of poor quality, or conflicting, and the balance of benefits and harms cannot be determined.

[d] Increased risk includes areas of high disease prevalence, men who have sex with men, persons engaging in high-risk sexual behavior, commercial sex workers, persons who exchange sex for drugs, and persons in adult correctional facilities.

[e] Some health systems default to the more rapid, less expensive, treponemal EIA test for syphilis with a reflex, nontreponemal RPR or VDRL.

positive for Chlamydia or gonorrhea earlier in pregnancy, or who have new or multiple sex partners.

Gonorrhea

Gonorrhea screening should be done at the first prenatal visit for women aged 25 years or younger, living in high-prevalence areas, with a previous STI, with new or multiple sex partners, or involved in commercial sex work or illicit drug use. Rescreening in the third trimester should be done for women who still have one of the aforementioned risks.

HBV

HBV screening with hepatitis B surface antigen (HBsAg) should occur in the first trimester, even if women were previously vaccinated or tested. Rescreening at delivery should be done for women who were not screened prenatally; had multiple sex partners in the previous 6 months; acquired another STI; have recent or current injection drug use; have an HBsAg-positive sex partner; and/or have clinical hepatitis.

Table 3
Recommended screening by population[a]

Pregnant women	*Chlamydia*	All pregnant women
		Rescreen in third trimester if aged <25 y or at increased risk[b]
	Gonorrhea	All pregnant women aged <25 y or at increased risk[b]
		Rescreen in third trimester if aged <25 y or at increased risk[b]
	Hepatitis B	All pregnant women
		Rescreen at delivery if at increased risk[b]
	HIV	All pregnant women
		Rescreen in third trimester, preferably before 36 wk gestation, if at increased risk[b]
	Syphilis	All pregnant women
		Rescreen in third trimester and at delivery if at increased risk[b]
Nonpregnant women	*Chlamydia*	All women aged <25 y or at increased risk[b]
	Gonorrhea	All women aged <25 y or at increased risk[b]
	HIV	All women aged 13–65 y unless the prevalence of undiagnosed HIV infection in the population is proven to be <0.1%
	Syphilis	All women at increased risk[b]
Men who have sex with men	*Chlamydia*	Urine DNA or urethral or rectal swab in men who have had insertive or receptive anal intercourse within the last year
		Routine screening for oropharyngeal *Chlamydia* infection is not recommended
	Gonorrhea	Urine DNA or urethral or rectal swab in men who have had insertive or receptive anal intercourse within the last year
		DNA swab or culture for pharyngeal infection in men who have had receptive oral intercourse within the last year
	HIV	All men
	Syphilis	All men
Men	HIV	All men at increased risk[b]
	Syphilis	All men at increased risk[b]

[a] Data were derived from USPSTF recommendation statements.[10,53–62]
[b] Increased risk includes areas of high disease prevalence, men who have sex with men, persons engaging in high-risk sexual behavior, commercial sex workers, persons who exchange sex for drugs, and persons in adult correctional facilities.

Syphilis

Syphilis screening should be done at the first prenatal visit. Rescreening should be done at the beginning of the third trimester and again at delivery for women diagnosed with another STI during pregnancy or living in high-prevalence areas. To prevent congenital syphilis, infants should not be discharged from the hospital unless the syphilis serologic status of the mother has been determined at least one time during pregnancy and preferably again at delivery. Women who deliver stillborn infants should be tested for syphilis.

HIV

HIV screening should occur as early in pregnancy as possible.[13] Rescreening is recommended in the third trimester (preferably before 36 weeks' gestation) in women with illicit drug use, STIs during pregnancy, multiple sex partners during pregnancy, residence in areas with high HIV prevalence, or HIV-infected partners.

Other Populations

Individuals with active tuberculosis, MSM, IDU, and those with a new diagnosis of any other STI should be screened for HIV and syphilis. Foreign-born individuals, especially those born in Asia, should be screened once for HBV. To detect reinfection, patients diagnosed with *Chlamydia* or gonorrhea should be retested in 3 months; if not retested at 3 months, such patients should be retested at any visit up to 12 months after diagnosis. Incarcerated individuals are often at significantly higher risk for STIs. More aggressive screening for STIs among incarcerated individuals is recommended, although the details are beyond the scope of this article.

TESTING METHODS
Chlamydia and Gonorrhea

Chlamydia and gonorrhea can be detected by urethral, cervical, pharyngeal, and anorectal swabs for culture, polymerase chain reaction (PCR), or point-of-care tests. Urine PCR can also be used for screening.

HIV

HIV testing performed using blood for third-generation fourth-generation enzyme immunoassays (EIAs) does not require Western blot for confirmation (**Box 2**).

Syphilis

Syphilis testing has traditionally been performed using blood for nontreponemal rapid plasma reagin (RPR) and Venereal Disease Research Laboratory (VDRL) tests, and confirmed with treponemal fluorescent treponemal antibody and *Treponema pallidum* particle agglutination tests. However, some health systems screen prenatal patients with newer EIA treponemal tests and confirm these with nontreponemal (RPR and VDRL) tests.

HBV

HBV testing is performed using blood for antigen/antibody testing.

HPV

High-risk HPV types can be detected in the supernatant from cervical brushings collected for Papanicolaou testing.

Box 2
Anonymous versus confidential HIV testing

- Primary care clinicians should disclose to patients that HIV testing in the primary care setting is confidential, whereas testing done at some STI clinics and health departments is anonymous.

- Patients can find HIV-testing sites that may have anonymous testing by searching by ZIP code at http://hivtest.cdc.gov/, contacting their local health department, or calling 1-800-CDC-INFO (800-232-4636). Not all HIV test sites offer anonymous testing.

- Confidential testing means that the patient's name and other identifying information will be attached to the test results. The results will go in the medical record and may be shared with health care providers and the insurance company.

- Anonymous testing means that nothing ties the test results to the patient. The patient receives a unique identifier that allows the patient to obtain personal test results.

Adapted from U.S. Department of Health & Human Services (DHHS). HIV/AIDS basics/prevention: HIV testing: confidential & anonymous testing. DHHS. Available at: http://aids.gov/hiv-aids-basics/prevention/hiv-testing/confidential-anonymous-testing/. Accessed December 18, 2013.

HSV

Testing for HSV is done using viral cultures of lesions. Blood testing for HSV using PCR has limited clinical value.

Trichomoniasis

Wet-mount microscopy of vaginal discharges is only 51% to 65% sensitive for trichomoniasis. The nucleic acid amplification test for *Trichomonas* is 95% to 100% sensitive, but not currently widely available.[14]

REPORTING REQUIREMENTS

The accurate and timely reporting of STIs is integral to assessing morbidity trends, allocating limited resources, and assisting local health authorities in partner identification, notification, and treatment. STI/HIV and AIDS cases should be reported in accordance with state and local statutory requirements. Syphilis, gonorrhea, *Chlamydia*, chancroid, HIV infection, and AIDS are reportable diseases in every state (**Box 3**).

OPTIMIZING SCREENING OPPORTUNITIES
Shared Decision Making and Decision Aids

Primary care clinicians can optimize screening opportunities by using shared decision making.[15] The shared-decision model includes introducing choice, describing options, and helping patients explore preferences and make decisions. Clinicians offer options and describe risks and benefits; patients express preferences and values. Each participant is thus armed with a better understanding of the relevant factors, and shares responsibility in the decision about how to proceed.[16]

When more than 1 viable treatment or screening option exists, clinicians can facilitate shared decision making by encouraging patients to let clinicians know what they care about, and by providing decision aids that raise the patient's awareness and understanding of treatment options and possible outcomes. For example, shared decision making may be helpful when deciding on self-collected versus clinician-collected vaginal swabs for *Chlamydia* testing, and in-person partner follow-up versus expedited or patient-delivered therapy.

HPV and HBV Vaccines

Screening encounters are also excellent opportunities for preventing HPV and HBV with vaccinations. **Table 4** outlines the vaccination schedule for HPV and HBV.

HPV

There are 2 types of HPV vaccines available in the United States. The first, HPV2, is a bivalent vaccine covering HPV subtypes 16 and 18 that cause 70% of cervical cancer. The second, HPV4, covers subtypes 16 and 18 as well as the wart-causing subtypes 6 and 11 (**Box 4**).

Box 3
Reporting STIs in different states

1. The requirements for reporting other STIs differ by state

2. Clinicians must be familiar with and follow the reporting requirements for their jurisdictions

3. Detailed information on reporting requirements can be accessed through state health departments and this Web site: http://www.cdc.gov/mmwr/international/relres.html

Table 4
Recommended vaccines to prevent STIs[a]

STI	Recommended Schedule	Catch-Up Schedule
HPV	3 dose series at age 11–12 y (intervals 0, 2, 6 mo)	Same as recommended but at ages 9–26 y[b]
HBV	Birth, 1–2 mo of age, 6–18 mo of age	3 dose series (intervals 0, 1, 4 mo) All persons ≤18 y old High-risk persons aged ≥19 y[c]

[a] Data derived from Advisory Committee on Immunization Practices.[17–20]
[b] HPV vaccination is optional for men aged 22–26 years who are not HIV infected or men who have sex with men (MSM).
[c] High-risk persons include seeking STI evaluation or treatment; persons with multiple sex partners in the past 6 months; sex partners and household contacts of HBsAg-positive persons; MSM; injection drug users; health care and public safety personnel with potential exposure to blood; and persons with diabetes, HIV, renal failure on dialysis, and liver disease.

At present, the Advisory Committee on Immunization Practices recommends 3 doses of HPV vaccination for all children at age 11 or 12 years. The vaccine works best if given before exposure to the HPV virus, but is still effective after exposure to 1 or more of the subtypes. Vaccination can also begin as young as age 9 years and proceed up to age 26.[17,18]

HBV

HBV vaccination is recommended for persons without HBV who are seeking STI evaluation or treatment; persons with multiple sex partners in the past 6 months; sex partners and household contacts of HBsAg-positive persons; MSM; IDUs; health care and public safety personnel with potential exposure to blood; and persons with diabetes, HIV, renal failure on dialysis, and liver disease.[19,20]

Risk-Reduction Education and Counseling

Screening encounters are also excellent opportunities for risk-reduction education and counseling, which are evidence-based and recommended by the USPSTF.[21] Broaching the subject of sexuality and STIs can be challenging. However, there are several techniques to help clinicians do so while minimizing awkwardness and maximizing patient acceptability and responsiveness (**Box 5**).

EVIDENCE THAT CONDOMS AND COUNSELING WORK
Condoms

The male latex condom provides an almost impermeable barrier to most STI pathogens. Studies in HIV discordant couples suggest that consistent condom use will not eliminate

Box 4
Preventing HPV-related cervical cancer in women older than 26 years

1. HPV vaccination is not currently recommended by the CDC for women older than 26 years.

2. Clinical trials showed limited or no protection against HPV-related diseases in women older than 26 years.

3. To prevent cervical cancer for women older than 26 years, routine cervical cancer screening is recommended. See http://www.cdc.gov/std/hpv/stdfact-hpv-vaccine-young-women.htm

transmission, but will decrease it by up to 80%.[24,25] Condom use is the cornerstone of HIV prevention worldwide.[26] A study of 917 female sex workers in Peru found that consistent condom use decreased the risk of acquiring gonorrhea by 62% and *Chlamydia* by 26%.[27] A prospective study of condom use in 82 female college students who had not previously been sexually active demonstrated a significant reduction in acquisition of vaginal HPV infections, from 89 to 38 per 100 patient-years at risk.[28]

Female latex condoms are also theoretically effective for decreasing transmission of STIs; however, there are no controlled trials documenting the effectiveness of the female condom in reducing rates of STIs.[29]

Counseling and Patient Education

Low-intensity counseling (eg, brief counseling during an office visit along with provision of information on STI transmission) has not been associated with a decrease in new STIs. There is good evidence, however, that moderate-intensity or high-intensity behavioral counseling reduces the risk of infection. An example of high-intensity counseling would be attending multiple (up to 10) sessions of counseling.[30] Many of the studies were completed in STI clinics and not in primary care practices. There is limited evidence that behavioral interventions affect the HIV transmission rates among high-risk patients.[31]

Abstinence counseling in primary care settings has not been studied.[30] Although one smaller, school-based controlled trial showed modest decreases in reports of sexual initiation,[32] a large systematic review of abstinence counseling projects in the community and in health care settings showed no difference in self-reported incidence of STIs or pregnancy.[33]

CURRENT PRACTICE PATTERNS
Collaborating with Local Public Health

Public health departments often run publicly funded STI clinics. Although these clinics provide an important safety net for the medically underserved and uninsured, only about 5% of patients with STIs are treated in this setting. Most patients receive care for STIs in community-based practices.[34] A national survey of 7300 physicians in the United States showed that fewer than one-third routinely screened patients for STIs, and only slightly more than half of physicians were reporting cases of syphilis, HIV, and AIDS. Reporting of gonorrhea and *Chlamydia* was even lower.[35]

Primary care clinicians need to collaborate with local public health officials to enhance not only reporting but also partner notification and treatment. This collaboration is also crucial for the monitoring of community prevalence of STIs, thereby guiding screening strategies and aiding in allocation of resources for interventions.

Given the high incidence of gonorrhea and *Chlamydia* infections, and the limited financial and personnel resources of public health departments, partner-notification programs are often far from comprehensive. One study showed that only 17% of high-risk patients reported with gonorrhea and 12% of patients with *Chlamydia* were interviewed for partner-notification assistance.[36] However, 52% of patients with HIV and 89% of patients with syphilis received partner-notification services. The CDC strongly recommends that all new cases of HIV and early syphilis be referred to public health for active partner-notification services.

Expedited Partner Therapy

Ideally, high-risk partners would be evaluated by a clinician and screened for STIs; however, a study evaluating private-sector patients with STIs found that 65% had

Box 5
Talking about sexuality and STIs with patients

Raise the topic of STIs with patients in a neutral and nonjudgmental way:

1. General introduction for all patients:

   a. "STIs can affect anyone, often without any signs or symptoms."

   b. "Because STIs affect health and well-being, I ask all my patients about it."

2. For presumably low-risk teens:

   a. If the teen is a minor, start with a separate conversation with the parent[a]

      i. "I would like to know your thoughts about sexuality in teenagers and what kind of discussions—if any—you have had with your child."

      ii. "I respect your views and how you would like to raise your child."

      iii. "Teens have many questions and get a lot of misinformation from their peers and the media."

      iv. "I would suggest we ask your child about what s/he knows about sex, what s/he has heard, and what questions s/he may have."

      v. "I plan to talk about risks for sexually transmitted diseases and pregnancy and how to reduce those risks."

      vi. "Before the 3 of us talk, I would like to speak to s/he privately to ask what s/he wants to talk about and make sure s/he is comfortable with talking to us both."

      vii. "At the end, I can also direct you both to more information so you can continue this discussion at home."

   b. Then meet with and bring in the teen[a]

      i. "Could we talk a bit about sex and your health?"

      ii. "Is there anything that might make this discussion a little easier?"

      iii. "I want to make sure that you have accurate information, so you can make decisions that will keep you safe and healthy."

      iv. "Do you have any questions about things you've heard from your friends about sex or sexually transmitted diseases?"

      v. "I'm not going to make any assumptions about what you know or don't know."

      vi. "I don't want to contradict your parents, so let's bring them into the room now."

3. For high-risk or infected teens and adults:

   a. Ask about and recognize their knowledge about STIs and efforts to reduce risk

   b. Teach through stories that make participants feel at ease

   c. Avoid stereotypes of how sexual orientation, education, or cultural background may influence behavior

   d. Use the patient's own terms when possible

   e. Start conversation with "did you know..." to invite curiosity

   f. Build rapport with patients by using...[b]

      i. ...open-ended questions (eg, "Tell me about any new sex partners you've had since your last visit" or "What's your experience with using condoms been like?")

      ii. ...understandable language (eg, "Have you ever had a sore or scab on your penis?")

      iii. ...normalizing language (eg, "Some of my patients have difficulty using a condom with every sex act. How is it for you?")

Discuss a comprehensive list of topics, once the topic is raised and rapport is established (the 5 Ps):[c]

1. Partners:

    a. "Do you have sex with men, women, or both?"

    b. "In the past 2 months, how many partners have you had sex with?"

    c. "In the past 12 months, how many partners have you had sex with?"

    d. "Is it possible that any of your sex partners in the past 12 months had sex with someone else while they were still in a sexual relationship with you?"

2. Prevention of pregnancy (eg, "What are you doing to prevent pregnancy?")

3. Protection from STIs (eg, "What do you do to protect yourself from STIs and HIV?")

4. Practices

    a. "To understand your risks for STIs, I need to understand the kind of sex you have had recently."

    b. "Have you had vaginal sex, meaning 'penis in vagina sex'?" If yes, "Do you use condoms: never, sometimes, or always?"

    c. "Have you had anal sex, meaning 'penis in rectum/anus sex'?" If yes, "Do you use condoms: never, sometimes, or always?"

    d. "Have you had oral sex, meaning 'mouth on penis/vagina'?"

    e. For condom answers: If "never": "Why don't you use condoms?'

    f. If "sometimes": "In what situations (or with whom) do you not use condoms?"

5. Past history of STIs

    a. "Have you ever had an STI?"

    b. "Have any of your partners had an STI?"

    c. Additional questions to identify risk for HIV and viral hepatitis include:

        i. "Have you or any of your partners ever injected drugs?"

        ii. "Have any of your partners exchanged money or drugs for sex?"

        iii. "Is there anything else about your sexual practices that I need to know about?"

[a] *Adapted from* Pillai and colleagues.[22]
[b] *Adapted from* National Network of STD/HIV Prevention Training Center.[23]
[c] *Adapted from* Workowski KA, Berman S; Centers for Disease Control and Prevention (CDC).[3]

untreated partners. Ninety percent of those patients preferred to tell partners themselves of the need for treatment, and 76% agreed to deliver treatment to a partner.[37] To improve partner notification and treatment of gonorrhea and *Chlamydia*, the CDC recommends expedited partner therapy (EPT) as a second-line alternative.[38] Most commonly EPT involves clinicians dispensing or prescribing single-dose antibiotic regimens for the partners of their infected patients, and having the patients deliver the medications or prescriptions to their partners.

Because EPT involves clinicians treating people they have not directly evaluated, specific legal authority is required in most states. As of August 2013, EPT was legal in 35 states and potentially allowable in 9 states, but 6 states prohibited its use. For more information about the legal status of EPT by state, the reader is directed to http://www.cdc.gov/std/ept/legal/default.htm.

EPT is not routinely recommended in MSM because of the increased risk of undiagnosed HIV. Data for the use of EPT are less consistent for *Trichomonas* infection, but may also be used selectively if other options for direct partner evaluation are not possible. EPT is not recommended for syphilis treatment.

Confidentiality

STI reporting and related information is kept confidential and protected by state law in most circumstances. Patient involvement in partner notification is voluntary. Public health officials providing partner-notification services do not reveal information about the infected patient to partners, nor is information about public health contact with the partners provided to the patient. At the same time, clinicians must be aware of their state's laws regarding the "duty to warn" people known to be at risk for infection. Some laws require partner notification, whereas other states permit, but do not require, clinicians to warn those at risk. Clinicians can obtain information regarding local requirements by contacting the local or state health department.

Confidentiality is also a key issue in providing care for adolescent patients. All states allow minors to consent for STI testing and treatment. No state requires parental notification or requires that clinicians notify parents that an adolescent minor has received STI services, except in limited or unusual circumstances. Eleven states have placed a lower age limit on the ability to consent, usually age 12 or 14 years. Summaries of state-by-state policies have been compiled for easy reference by the Guttmacher Institute and are available at www.guttmacher.org/statecenter.

Private health insurance claims require written explanation of benefits (EOB). Clinicians should be aware of the possible breach in confidentiality for adolescents under their parents' private insurance if an EOB statement detailing testing is sent by the insurance company to the parents after a confidential visit. Clinicians can consider billing for symptoms (eg, vaginitis) instead of diagnosis (eg, trichomoniasis), and might review with parents that certain tests are routine for adolescents as a way to preemptively manage these confidentiality conflicts. In some states, adolescents may be eligible for family-planning individual insurance coverage, including STI testing, without consideration of their parents' incomes. In addition, some public health systems have dedicated STI clinics where teens can receive free or low-cost confidential services.

Suspected Child Abuse

If STI infection occurs in children after the neonatal period, this is highly suspicious of sexual abuse. However, as noted in the foregoing Confidentiality section, all states allow minors to consent for STI testing and treatment, and no state requires parental notification or requires that clinicians notify parents that an adolescent minor has received STI services, except in limited or unusual circumstances. Therefore, the clinician must exercise judgment in determining whether child abuse has occurred (eg, two 17-year-olds engaging in mutually uncoerced sex may or may not constitute child abuse).

Clinicians are required to report cases of suspected child abuse to their local or state child protective services agency in all 50 states. If possible, the evaluation of a child with a suspected STI should be conducted by a clinician with experience working with sexually abused or assaulted children, with the goal of minimizing pain and further psychological trauma in the examination process. Presumptive treatment of STI infection should be deferred in children until all testing is complete, as a clear diagnosis is important for social and legal follow-up. The CDC offers guidance in their 2010 Sexually Transmitted Diseases Treatment Guidelines as to the timing intervals for screening tests after suspected assault or abuse.[3]

IMPACT OF CHANGES WITHIN HEALTH CARE
Electronic Health Records

By improving record keeping, electronic health records (EHRs) have the potential to become a strong tool in the prevention of STIs. EHRs can track screening rates, provide reminders for screening of individuals, and include follow-up testing in best-practice order sets. For example, an electronic system was used to monitor quality indicators in 263 patients at 3 HIV/AIDS clinics.[39] The investigators found that the electronic monitoring was a powerful quality-improvement tool that led to improved care. Another study used an electronic checklist within an EHR to improve STI screening in a cohort of 882 HIV-infected patients.[40] Using the checklist led to twice the number of STI diagnoses. Other research showed that an EHR reminder led to increased HIV testing among an urban population.[41] Further research is needed to confirm the promising results of the use of EHR-based interventions to improve STI screening.

Mobile Phone Applications

Numerous mobile phone apps include information about STIs with which clinicians are able to communicate easily with patients; however, they are used infrequently.[42] Apps and text messages can provide both educational content and reminders about behaviors. Use of text messaging has been shown to change health behavior (mostly in diabetes, smoking, asthma, and weight loss).[43] Although not as rigorously evaluated when applied to STIs, text messaging has been used to inform patients of an STI diagnosis, find partners, and remind patients to practice safe sex.[44]

Patient-Centered Medical Home

The patient-centered medical home (PCMH) is a concept in primary care that focuses on team-based care and coordination of the care of populations. It has been applied to HIV/AIDS clinics as a comprehensive way to provide primary care to patients. In this setting, PCMH has been viewed as a key modality in providing quality care and improving patient satisfaction and retention.[45,46] By providing a medical home for patients with HIV, the PCMH enables people with HIV to obtain all of their health care in one place.

Primary care clinics can use the model of PCMH to improve STI screening in their patient populations by identifying high-risk populations. Improved documentation with EHRs can enable clinicians to better monitor these populations and ensure that screening recommendations are followed. The team-based care used in PCMH can be capitalized on to provide comprehensive education about STIs and screening recommendations. Patients who have improved continuity of care with a single clinician may be more open about their sexual risk behaviors, thereby being more open to STI screening. Improved follow-up and continuity can help in the monitoring of people with existing STIs, enabling clinicians to ensure that all treatment is completed and in provision of follow-up care. For people with chronic STIs (ie, hepatitis, HIV) the PCMH can be the place where patients receive all their necessary care, including from specialists. The primary care clinician can then be the point person in the overall treatment plan for these chronically ill patients.

Another tenet of the PCMH is making sure that care is accessible. Applied to STIs, this means a PCMH clinic should seek to accommodate all patients who are worried about STIs or STI symptoms. During these urgent visits, clinicians have the opportunity to provide STI education. Point-of-care testing for STIs is an emerging concept that enables the clinician to receive real-time STI results while the patient waits. At present, there are point-of-care tests available for HIV, hepatitis C, and syphilis. Having immediate access to test results has the potential to improve care by ensuring that all patients get their results and are treated promptly.

Accountable Care Organizations

Accountable care organizations (ACOs) are defined as groups of clinicians, hospitals, and other health care providers who work together to provide high-quality, coordinated care to a defined population. If an ACO meets quality standards, achieves savings, and meets or exceeds a Minimum Savings Rate, the ACO will share in savings based on the ACO quality score. The current focus of ACOs trends toward improving the management of chronic disease with Medicare populations. ACOs for HIV care would be a new model of accountability and comprehensive care management in a population with high medication costs and frequent hospitalizations. STI screening is not currently included in the 33 required quality measures that comprise ACO quality performance standards.[47]

Screening for *Chlamydia* has been an indicator in the Health Plan Employer Data and Information Set (HEDIS)[48] since 2000. The proportion of sexually active females between the ages of 15 and 25 years screened for chlamydial infection annually in commercial and Medicaid plans using this HEDIS measure has increased steadily over the past decade,[49] suggesting that the addition of STI screening as part of the ACO quality performance standards would have a beneficial effect on STI screening rates.

Affordable Care Act

Increasing the number of people with health insurance will facilitate STI screening by primary care clinicians, which will decrease the number of people who have undiagnosed disease. The Affordable Care Act (ACA) includes financial incentives for health systems to achieve population health goals, such as screening women age 25 years and younger annually for *Chlamydia*. The ACA requires Medicare and qualified commercial health plans to cover routine preventive services graded A and B by the USPSTF (see **Table 2**) at no cost to patients, including STI prevention and counseling. For a comprehensive list of preventive services that have a grade of A or B, the reader is referred to http://www.uspreventiveservicestaskforce.org/uspstf/uspsabrecs.htm.

SUMMARY

Primary care clinicians are in an ideal position to help decrease the incidence of STIs by screening effectively and implementing evidence-based prevention methods. Because many STIs may be asymptomatic, it is important for clinicians to implement these guidelines in practice to decrease the incidence of STIs. The clinician should be aware that certain populations have higher risk for STIs, and more rigorous screening is recommended.

By incorporating standardized, open-ended, and nonjudgmental questions about sexuality into routine patient encounters, clinicians can increase patients' comfort levels with this line of questioning and increase STI screening and detection. In addition, through communication and collaboration with local public health departments, clinicians can enhance their awareness about local STI prevalence to guide screening and improve community health through outreach to partners at risk.

REFERENCES

1. Centers for Disease Control and Prevention. STDs today. National Prevention Information Network. Available at: http://www.cdcnpin.org/scripts/std/std.asp. Accessed September 14, 2013.

2. European Centre for Disease Prevention and Control (ECDC). Sexually transmitted infections in Europe 1990-2010. ECDC. Available at: http://www.ecdc.europa.eu/en/publications/publications/201206-sexually-transmitted-infections-europe-2010.pdf. Accessed September 17, 2013.
3. Workowski KA, Berman S, Centers for Disease Control and Prevention (CDC). Sexually transmitted diseases treatment guidelines, 2010. MMWR Recomm Rep 2010;59(RR-12):1–110. Available at: http://www.cdc.gov/std/treatment/2010/specialpops.htm. Accessed September 17, 2013.
4. Petroll AE, Mosack KE. Physician awareness of sexual orientation and preventive health recommendations to men who have sex with men. Sex Transm Dis 2011;38(1):63–7.
5. Wiessing L, Likatavicius G, Klempová D, et al. Associations between availability and coverage of HIV-prevention measures and subsequent incidence of diagnosed HIV infection among injection drug users. Am J Public Health 2009; 99(6):1049–52.
6. Holtgrave DR, Crosby RA. Social capital, poverty, and income inequality as predictors of gonorrhoea, syphilis, chlamydia and AIDS case rates in the United States. Sex Transm Infect 2003;79(1):62–4.
7. Sharpe TT, Voûte C, Rose MA, et al. Social determinants of HIV/AIDS and sexually transmitted diseases among black women: implications for health equity. J Womens Health 2012;21(3):249–54.
8. Swain GR. Individualized approach to screening patients for STIs. Am Fam Physician 2011;83(4):350–2.
9. Community Collaboration on Healthcare Quality of the Medical Society of Milwaukee County. Sexually transmitted diseases in Milwaukee County and other high risk areas: screening, testing and treatment recommendations. City of Milwaukee Health Department. Available at: http://city.milwaukee.gov/ImageLibrary/Groups/healthAuthors/DCP/PDFs/STD_Screen_Tx_Guide_updated_20080121.pdf. Accessed September 19, 2013.
10. Meyers D, Wolff T, Gregory K, et al. USPSTF recommendations for STI screening. Am Fam Physician 2008;77:819–24. Available at: http://www.uspreventiveservicestaskforce.org/uspstf08/methods/stinfections.htm. Accessed September 19, 2013.
11. Land JA, Van Bergen JE, Morré SA, et al. Epidemiology of *Chlamydia trachomatis* infection in women and the cost-effectiveness of screening. Hum Reprod Update 2010;16(2):189–204.
12. Satcher D. Addressing sexual health: looking back, looking forward. Public Health Rep 2013;128(Suppl 1):111–4.
13. Branson BM, Handsfield HH, Lampe MA, et al. Revised recommendations for HIV testing of adults, adolescents, and pregnant women in health-care settings. MMWR Recomm Rep 2006;55(RR14):1–17. Available at: http://www.cdc.gov/mmwr/preview/mmwrhtml/rr5514a1.htm. Accessed September 23, 2013.
14. Association of Public Health Laboratories (APHL). Laboratory detection of trichomonas. Available at: http://www.aphl.org/AboutAPHL/publications/Documents/ID_2013August_Advances-in-Laboratory-Detection-of-Trichomonas-vaginalis.pdf. Accessed November 11, 2013.
15. Elwyn G, Frosch D, Thomson R, et al. Shared decision making: a model for clinical practice. J Gen Intern Med 2012;27(10):1361–7.
16. Charles C, Gafni A, Whelan T. Shared decision-making in the medical encounter: what does it mean? (or it takes at least two to tango). Soc Sci Med 1997;44:681–92.

17. Centers for Disease Control and Prevention (CDC). Recommendations on the use of quadrivalent human papillomavirus vaccine in males—Advisory Committee on Immunization Practices (ACIP), 2011. MMWR Morb Mortal Wkly Rep 2011;60(50):1705–8. Available at: http://www.cdc.gov/mmwr/preview/mmwrhtml/mm6050a3.htm. Accessed September 23, 2013.

18. Centers for Disease Control and Prevention (CDC). FDA licensure of bivalent human papillomavirus vaccine (HPV2, Cervarix) for use in females and updated HPV vaccination recommendations from the Advisory Committee on Immunization Practices (ACIP). MMWR Morb Mortal Wkly Rep 2010;59(20):626–9. Available at: http://www.cdc.gov/mmwr/preview/mmwrhtml/mm5920a4.htm. Accessed September 17, 2013.

19. Mast EE, Margolis HS, Fiore AE, et al, Advisory Committee on Immunization Practices (ACIP) Centers for Disease Control and Prevention (CDC). A comprehensive immunization strategy to eliminate transmission of hepatitis B virus infection in the United States: recommendations of the Advisory Committee on Immunization Practices (ACIP) part 1: immunization of infants, children, and adolescents. MMWR Recomm Rep 2005;54(RR-16):1–23. Available at: http://www.cdc.gov/mmwr/preview/mmwrhtml/rr5416a1.htm. Accessed November 26, 2013.

20. Mast EE, Weinbaum CM, Fiore AE, et al, Advisory Committee on Immunization Practices (ACIP) Centers for Disease Control and Prevention (CDC). A comprehensive immunization strategy to eliminate transmission of hepatitis B virus infection in the United States: recommendations of the Advisory Committee on Immunization Practices (ACIP) Part II: immunization of adults. MMWR Recomm Rep 2006;55(RR-16):1–33. Available at: http://www.cdc.gov/mmwr/preview/mmwrhtml/rr5516a1.htm. Accessed September 17, 2013.

21. U.S. Preventive Services Task Force. Behavioral counseling to prevent sexually transmitted infections: recommendation statement. Ann Intern Med 2008;149:491–6. Available at: http://www.uspreventiveservicestaskforce.org/uspstf08/sti/stiart2.htm. Accessed September 17, 2013.

22. Pillai AS, Sprockel PT, Barthmare SC. Tips for talking to teens about STDs. J Fam Pract 2009;58(2):76–81. Available at: http://www.jfponline.com/fileadmin/php/qhi/downloadPdf.php?fp=/jfp_archive/pdf/5802/5802JFP_Article3.pdf. Accessed September 17, 2013.

23. National Network of STD/HIV Prevention Training Centers (NNPTC). Resources: sexual history. NNPTC. Available at: http://nnptc.org/resourcetags/sexual-history/. Accessed September 14, 2013.

24. Davis KR, Weller SC. The effectiveness of condoms in reducing heterosexual transmission of HIV. Fam Plann Perspect 1999;31:272–9.

25. Weller SC, Davis-Beaty K. Condom effectiveness in reducing heterosexual HIV transmission. Cochrane Database Syst Rev 2002;(1):CD003255.

26. Holmes KK, Levine R, Weaver M. Effectiveness of condoms in preventing sexually transmitted infections. Bull World Health Organ 2004;82(6):454–61.

27. Sanchez J, Campos PE, Courtois B, et al. Prevention of sexually transmitted diseases (STDs) in female sex workers: prospective evaluation of condom promotion and strengthened STD services. Sex Transm Dis 2003;30:273–9.

28. Winer RL, Hughes JP, Feng Q, et al. Condom use and the risk of genital human papillomavirus infection in young women. N Engl J Med 2006;354(25):2645–54.

29. Gallo MF, Kilbourne-Brook M, Coffey PS. A review of the effectiveness and acceptability of the female condom for dual protection. Sex Health 2012;9:18–26.

30. Lin JS, Whitlock E, O'Connor E, et al. Behavioral counseling to prevent sexually transmitted infections: a systematic review for the U.S. Preventive Services Task Force. Ann Intern Med 2008;149:497–508.
31. Ota E, Wariki WM, Mori R, et al. Behavioral interventions to reduce the transmission of HIV infection among sex workers and their clients in high-income countries. Cochrane Database Syst Rev 2011;(12):CD006045.
32. Jemmott JB, Jemmott LS, Fong GT. Efficacy of a theory-based abstinence-only intervention over 24 months: a randomized controlled trial with young adolescents. Arch Pediatr Adolesc Med 2010;164(2):152–9. Available at: http://archpedi.jamanetwork.com/article.aspx?articleid=382798.
33. Underhill K, Montgomery P, Operario D. Abstinence-plus programs for HIV infection prevention in high-income countries. Cochrane Database Syst Rev 2008;(1):CD007006.
34. Brackbill R, Sternberg M, Fishbein M. Where do people go for treatment of sexually transmitted diseases? Fam Plann Perspect 1999;31:10–5.
35. St Lawrence JS, Montaño DE, Kasprzyk D, et al. STD screening, testing, case reporting, and clinical and partner notification practices: a national survey of US physicians. Am J Public Health 2002;92:1784–8.
36. Golden MR, Hogben M, Handsfield HH, et al. Partner notification for HIV and STD in the United States: low coverage for gonorrhea, chlamydial infection, and HIV. Sex Transm Dis 2003;30(6):490–6.
37. Golden MR, Whittington WL, Handsfield HH, et al. Partner management for gonococcal and chlamydial infection: expansion of public health services to the private sector and expedited sex partner treatment through a partnership with commercial pharmacies. Sex Transm Dis 2001;28(11):658–65.
38. Centers for Disease Control and Prevention (CDC). Expedited partner therapy. Atlanta (GA): CDC; 2013. Available at: http://www.cdc.gov/std/ept. Accessed September 22, 2013.
39. Virga PH, Jin B, Thomas J, et al. Electronic health information technology as a tool for improving quality of care and health outcomes for HIV/AIDS patients. Int J Med Inform 2012;81(10):e39–45.
40. Brooks G, McSorley J, Shaw A. Retrospective study of the effect of enhanced systematic sexually transmitted infection screening, facilitated by the use of electronic patient records, in an HIV-infected cohort. HIV Med 2013;14(6):347–53.
41. Avery AK, Del Toro M, Caron A. Increases in HIV screening in primary care clinics through an electronic reminder: an interrupted time series. BMJ Qual Saf 2014;23(3):250–6.
42. Muessig KE, Pike EC, Legrand S, et al. Mobile phone applications for the care and prevention of HIV and other sexually transmitted diseases: a review. J Med Internet Res 2013;15(1):e1.
43. Cole-Lewis H, Kershaw T. Text messaging as a tool for behavior change in disease prevention and management. Epidemiol Rev 2010;32:56–69.
44. Lom MS, Hocking JS, Hellard ME, et al. SMSSTI: a review of the uses of mobile phone text messaging in sexual health. Int J STD AIDS 2008;19:287–90.
45. Dang BN, Westbrook RA, Black WC, et al. Examining the link between patient satisfaction and adherence to HIV care: a structural equation model. PLoS One 2013;8(1):e54729.
46. Sitapati AM, Limmeos J, Bonet-Vazquez M, et al. Retention: building a patient-centered medical home in HIV primary care through PUFF (patients unable to follow-up found). J Health Care Poor Underserved 2012;23(Suppl 3):81–95.

47. Centers for Medicare & Medicaid Services (CMS). Accountable care organization 2013 program analysis: quality performance standards narrative measure specifications. CMS. Available at: http://www.cms.gov/Medicare/Medicare-Fee-for-Service-Payment/sharedsavingsprogram/Downloads/ACO-Narrative Measures-Specs.pdf. Accessed November 4, 2013.

48. National Committee for Quality Assurance (NCQA). What is HEDIS? NCQA. Available at: http://www.ncqa.org/HEDISQualityMeasurement/WhatisHEDIS. aspx. Accessed September 23, 2013.

49. Centers for Disease Control and Prevention (CDC). Chlamydia screening percentages reported by commercial and Medicaid plans by state and year. CDC. Available at: http://www.cdc.gov/std/chlamydia/female-enrollees-00-08. htm#figure1. Accessed September 23, 2013.

50. Centers for Disease Control and Prevention (CDC). CDC fact sheet: incidence, prevalence, and cost of sexually transmitted infections in the United States. CDC. Available at: http://www.cdc.gov/std/stats/STI-Estimates-Fact-Sheet-Feb-2013.pdf. Accessed November 23, 2013.

51. Centers for Disease Control and Prevention (CDC). HIV in the United States: at a glance. CDC. Available at: http://www.cdc.gov/hiv/statistics/basics/ataglance. html. Accessed November 23, 2013.

52. American Sexual Health Association (ASHA). Statistics on sexually transmitted infections. Available at: http://www.ashasexualhealth.org/std-sti/std-statistics. html. Accessed November 23, 2013.

53. U.S. Preventive Services Task Force (USPSTF). Recommendation statement. Screening for chlamydial infection (2007). USPSTF. Available at: http://www. uspreventiveservicestaskforce.org/uspstf/uspschlm.htm. Accessed September 20, 2013.

54. U.S. Preventive Services Task Force (USPSTF) Recommendation statement. Screening for gonorrhea (2005). USPSTF. Available at: http://www.uspreventiveser vicestaskforce.org/uspstf/uspsgono.htm. Accessed September 20, 2013.

55. U.S. Preventive Services Task Force (USPSTF) Recommendation statement. Screening for hepatitis B virus infection (2004). USPSTF. Available at: http:// www.uspreventiveservicestaskforce.org/uspstf/uspshepb.htm.   Accessed September 20, 2013.

56. U.S. Preventive Services Task Force (USPSTF) Recommendation statement. Screening for hepatitis B virus infection in pregnancy (2009). USPSTF. Available at: http://www.uspreventiveservicestaskforce.org/uspstf/uspshepbpg.htm. Accessed September 20, 2013.

57. U.S. Preventive Services Task Force (USPSTF) Recommendation statement. Screening for hepatitis C virus infection (2013). USPSTF. Available at: http://www. uspreventiveservicestaskforce.org/uspstf/uspshepc.htm. Accessed September 20, 2013.

58. U.S. Preventive Services Task Force (USPSTF) Recommendation statement. Screening for genital herpes (2005). USPSTF. Available at: http://www.uspreven tiveservicestaskforce.org/uspstf/uspsherp.htm. Accessed September 20, 2013.

59. U.S. Preventive Services Task Force (USPSTF) Recommendation statement. Screening for HIV (2013). USPSTF. Available at: http://www.uspreventiveservice staskforce.org/uspstf/uspshivi.htm. Accessed September 20, 2013.

60. U.S. Preventive Services Task Force (USPSTF) Recommendation statement. Screening for syphilis infection (2004). USPSTF. Available at: http://www. uspreventiveservicestaskforce.org/uspstf/uspssyph.htm. Accessed September 20, 2013.

61. U.S. Preventive Services Task Force (USPSTF) Recommendation statement. Screening for syphilis infection in pregnancy (2009). USPSTF. Available at: http://www.uspreventiveservicestaskforce.org/uspstf/uspssyphpg.htm. Accessed September 20, 2013.
62. U.S. Preventive Services Task Force (USPSTF) Recommendation statement. Screening for cervical cancer (2012). USPSTF. Available at: http://www.uspreventiveservicestaskforce.org/uspstf/uspscerv.htm. Accessed September 20, 2013.

Prevention of Unintended Pregnancy

A Focus on Long-Acting Reversible Contraception

Sarah Pickle, MD[a],*, Justine Wu, MD, MPH[a],
Edith Burbank-Schmitt, BA[b]

KEYWORDS

- Unintended pregnancy • Unplanned pregnancy • Contraception
- Long-acting reversible contraception • Family planning • Electronic health record

KEY POINTS

- Half of all pregnancies in the United States are unintended.
- Unintended pregnancies (UIPs) are more prevalent among minority and disadvantaged women and are associated with a higher risk for poor maternal and child health outcomes.
- With the recent passage of the Patient Protection and Affordable Care Act and its accompanying mandated contraceptive provision, there is an urgent need for more primary care providers to provide contraceptive services.
- Long-acting reversible contraceptives (LARC), specifically the intrauterine device and the subdermal progestin implant, are highly effective and safe for use in most women, yet remain underused in the United States.
- Providing LARC without patient cost sharing can decrease the rate of UIP and abortion.
- Clinicians should incorporate the use of Centers for Disease Control and Prevention Medical Eligibility Criteria for Contraceptive Use in their routine practice to provide evidence-based contraceptive services that are individually tailored to the user's characteristics or medical conditions.
- Clinicians should advise LARC as first-option contraceptive for most women, if they desire and can access these methods.

INTRODUCTION

Of the approximately 6 million pregnancies that occur annually in the United States, half are unintended.[1] Unintended pregnancy (UIP) is defined as a pregnancy that

Conflict of Interest: Dr J. Wu is a trainer for Nexplanon (Merck & Co, Inc, Whitehouse Station, NJ).
[a] Department of Family Medicine and Community Health, Rutgers Robert Wood Johnson Medical School, 1 Robert Wood Johnson Place, Medical Education Building Room 262, New Brunswick, NJ 08901, USA; [b] Rutgers Robert Wood Johnson Medical School, 1 Robert Wood Johnson Place, Medical Education Building Room 262, New Brunswick, NJ 08901, USA
* Corresponding author.
E-mail address: picklesr@rutgers.edu

0095-4543/14/$ – see front matter © 2014 Elsevier Inc. All rights reserved.

was mistimed (29% of all pregnancies) or unwanted (19% of all pregnancies).[2] Of those pregnancies that are unintended, half end in elective abortion.[1] Collectively, women who experience UIP are at increased risk of delaying prenatal care, experiencing maternal depression, and suffering physical violence during pregnancy.[3–7] Birth outcomes are less favorable as well, including low birth weight and increased risk of birth defects.[8] Children born as a result of UIP are more likely to live in poverty, experience adverse physical and psychological outcomes during childhood, and achieve lower educational attainment.[5,9,10] Although the overall US rate of UIP for all women has essentially been unchanged since 1994, teen pregnancy rate has declined, largely because of increased contraceptive use among adolescents, with a small contribution because of abstinence.[11] The rate of UIP is declining at a slower rate among minority women and lower-income women of all ages.[1,12] In 2006, the total cost of UIP in the United States was estimated to be $11.1 billion.[13]

The cornerstone to preventing UIP is widespread provision of contraception to women of childbearing age who do not currently desire pregnancy. Public funding for contraceptive services prevents 2.2 million unplanned pregnancies per year.[14] Family planning is among the core strategic areas in the Healthy People 2020 initiative, a 10-year agenda for improving the health and lives of Americans. Among the family planning goals for Healthy People 2020 are to increase the proportion of intended pregnancy from 51% (2002 data) to 56% and to reduce the number of women who become pregnant despite using a reversible form of contraception from 12.4% (2002 data) to 9.9%.[15] To achieve these outcomes, the Healthy People 2020 agenda calls for increased capacity in family planning services, particularly among publicly funded entities, to reach underserved and minority women at highest risk for UIP.[15]

Whether in the public or private sector, primary care providers (PCPs) have an important role to play in preventing UIP. In 2010, patients made 11.5 million visits to primary care offices for contraception and family planning counseling.[16] This number is expected to increase significantly with the implementation of the Affordable Care Act (ACA), which includes a provision that requires coverage for contraceptive counseling and services without patient cost sharing.[17]

This discussion is focused on reversible contraceptive methods, because women using reversible methods represent most women at risk for UIP. Although male partners can play an important role in prevention of UIP, this discussion is directed to contraceptive use in women. Currently available reversible contraceptive methods and emergency contraception (EC) are presented, accompanied by a discussion of their effectiveness and use patterns among US women. Although a detailed summary of all contraceptive methods is beyond the scope of this article, clinical tools to assist in patient-centered contraceptive selection are presented in the context of the patient-centered medical home (PCMH).

CURRENTLY AVAILABLE CONTRACEPTIVE METHODS IN THE UNITED STATES

Reversible forms of contraception can be divided into short-acting methods (user-dependent methods that must be used with each coital act, daily, weekly, monthly, or every 3 months) versus long-acting reversible devices (ie, user-independent methods that maintain efficacy without patient intervention) (**Table 1**). EC is postcoital contraception (**Table 2**), defined as any method that is used to prevent pregnancy after intercourse.[18,19] EC does not disrupt an implanted pregnancy[18] and is therefore not an abortifacient, as defined by the US Food and Drug Administration (FDA)[20] and the American Congress of Obstetricians and Gynecologists.[21] EC decreases the risk of pregnancy from 52% to 99%, depending on the method used for each coital

Table 1
Short-acting methods and long-acting reversible contraceptive methods

Long-Acting Reversible Contraceptive Methods	Short-Acting Methods
Copper T380A intrauterine device	Barrier methods (cervical cap, male/female condoms, diaphragm)
Levonogestrel intrauterine device	Oral contraceptive pills (combined estrogen and progestin, progestin only)
Subdermal progestin implant	Transdermal patch Vaginal ring Progestin injection

act.[18,19,22–33] There has been no proven population impact from EC use (no decrease in the rate of UIP), likely attributable to underuse of the method among women at the highest risk for UIP.[34–36]

CONTRACEPTIVE METHOD EFFECTIVENESS

The risk of pregnancy during 1 year of method use is summarized in **Table 3**.[40] The most effective methods (eg, implant, intrauterine device [IUD], sterilization) are associated with extremely low failure rates (<1%) with both perfect and typical use, because the methods are exceptionally effective and method success is not reliant on patient compliance.[41–43] For methods that require patient compliance, the rate of failure with typical use is significantly higher than that associated with perfect use.

Because the effectiveness of short-acting methods varies significantly depending on user adherence, clinicians should periodically assess compliance among all patients using these methods. To encourage complete disclosure and open discussion from patients' regarding typical use patterns, clinicians should normalize the fact that most users do not practice perfect compliance because of factors within and out of their control. **Table 4** provides suggested questions and talking points to promote patient-provider discussions about potential barriers to adherence and strategies to improve adherence within the context of the patient's situation.

Table 2
Forms of EC

Form	Comments
Copper intrauterine device	Most effect method of EC and only method that can be continued for routine contraception[24,37]
Ulipristal acetate	More effective than levonogestrel pills, prescription only[38]; decreased efficacy noted in women with a BMI ≥35 kg/m^2[39]
Levonogestrel pills	Several EC dedicated packages available over the counter, behind the counter, and prescription-only access, dependent on product and patient age; decreased efficacy noted in women with a BMI ≥26 kg/m^2[39]
Yuzpe method (using combined oral contraceptive pills)	Not as effective as levonogestrel pill products, and associated with higher rate of side effects (nausea, vomiting)[24]

Abbreviation: BMI, body mass index, calculated as weight in kilograms divided by the square of height in meters.

Table 3
Contraceptive effectiveness

	Proportion of Women Who Become Pregnant over 1 y of Use	
Method	Perfect Use	Typical Use
Implant	0.05	0.05
Vasectomy	0.10	0.15
Levonogestrel IUD	0.2	0.2
Copper IUD	0.6	0.6
Tubal sterilization	0.5	0.5
Injectable	0.2	6
Pill	0.3	9
Vaginal ring	0.4	9
Patch	0.3	9
Diaphragm	6	12
Sponge	9/20 (never given birth/given birth)	12/24 (never given birth/given birth)
Male condom	2	18
Female condom	5	21
Withdrawal	4	22
Fertility awareness methods	0.4–5	24
Spermicides	18	28
No method	85	85

Adapted from Trussell J. Contraceptive efficacy. In: Hatcher RA, Trussell J, Nelson AL, et al, editors. Contraceptive technology. 20th edition. New York: Ardent Media, Inc; 2011. p. 791.

CURRENT CONTRACEPTIVE PRACTICE PATTERNS AMONG REPRODUCTIVE AGE WOMEN (AGED 15–44 YEARS) IN THE UNITED STATES

As shown in **Table 5**, almost every woman who has ever had intercourse uses a form of contraception in her lifetime.[44] In 2010, 62% of reproductive age women used

Table 4
Suggested talking points for discussing contraceptive adherence

Question to Elicit Contraceptive Adherence	Suggested Talking Point
"It is very common to miss pills. At the end of the month, how many times have you typically missed a pill?"	Missed pills should be taken as soon as possible after the missed dose If 2 or more pills are missed, EC should be used if the patient has had unprotected sex, and the patient should use a backup method for the following 7 d If multiple pills are missed throughout the month due, consider switching to highly effective methods (ie, LARC) to increase compliance
"Sometimes partners can be resistant to condoms. For every 10 times you have sex, how many times does your partner use a condom?"	EC should be used after each episode of unprotected sex Consider LARC methods that do not require repeated patient or partner participation

Abbreviations: EC, emergency contraception; LARC, long-acting reversible contraceptives.

Table 5
Contraceptive method choice among US women, 2010

Method	Number of Users (in thousands)	Percentage of All Women, Age 15–44 y	Percentage of All Contraceptive Users
Pill (combined estrogen and progestin)	10,540	17.1	27.5
Tubal sterilization	10,200	16.5	26.6
Male condom	6280	10.2	16.3
Vasectomy	3860	6.2	10.0
IUD	2140	3.5	5.6
Withdrawal	1990	3.2	5.2
Injectable	1450	2.4	3.8
Vaginal ring	830	1.3	2.2
Fertility awareness methods	440	0.7	1.1
Patch	290	0.5	0.7
Implant	180	0.3	0.5
Other methods[a]	200	0.3	0.5
No method	23,260	37.8	—

[a] EC, female condoms, spermicides, diaphragm, and condoms.
Adapted from Jones J, Mosher W, Daniels K. Current contraceptive use in the United States, 2006–2010, and changes in patterns of use since 1995. National health statistics reports; no. 60. Hyattsville (MD): National Center for Health Statistics; 2012.

contraception.[45] The pill and permanent sterilization have remained the most popular methods among all users since 1982, with rates in 2010 at 27.5% and 26.5%, respectively.[46]

Although most women use some form of contraception in their lifetime, most unintended pregnancies can be attributed to women who use contraception inconsistently (inconsistent users) and those who use no contraception at all (nonusers), across all demographic groups. Most striking is that nonusers represent only 10% of all at-risk women,[47] yet account for 52% of the approximately 3 million unintended pregnancies annually.[48] This finding is not surprising considering that the annual risk of pregnancy associated with contraceptive nonuse is as high as 85%.[42] By adopting any method of contraception, even if one of the least effective methods (eg, withdrawal), the annual risk of pregnancy decreases significantly.[42] Hence, public health efforts would be most effective at reducing UIP if focused on increasing the uptake of any contraceptive method among nonusers (ideally, the most effective method possible), improving adherence among current users, ensuring continued contraceptive access to current users, and, when possible, switching to more effective methods among current users.

Recent trends in contraceptive practice among US women are worth noting and have direct implications for clinical practice. The percentage of women relying on condoms as their most effective method declined from 20% in 1995 to 16% in 2006 to 2010, with a concomitant increase in hormonal method use from 4.4% to 7.2%.[45] Use of long-acting reversible contraceptives (LARC) among women at risk for UIP increased steadily from 2.4% in 2002 to 8.5% in 2009.[49] The term LARC is almost synonymous with the IUD, because IUD use greatly overshadows implant use in the United States (8% vs <1%, respectively).[49] This increased use of LARC occurred across all subgroups, regardless of age, race and ethnicity, religion, income, education, and marital status.[49] Despite these trends, the rate of UIP in the United States is still higher than that of other industrialized nations.[50] Increasing LARC use among US women is a key strategy to narrowing the gap between the United States and other industrialized nations with respect to the rate of UIP.

CURRENT PRACTICE PATTERNS
The IUD: Underused in the United States

Special attention is focused on the IUD to highlight an underuse phenomenon that seems unique to the United States. Although IUDs are among the safest and most effective contraceptive methods, IUD use in the United States is only 8% among all women who use contraception, compared with 11% in the United Kingdom, 23% in France, and 41% in China.[49]

There are 3 IUDs currently approved by the FDA: (1) the copper T380A (ParaGard, Teva Women's Health, Sellersville, PA), approved for up to 10 years of use[51]; (2) the levonorgestrel intrauterine system (LNG-IUS) (Mirena, Bayer Health Care Pharmaceuticals Inc, Wayne, NJ), approved for up to 5 years of use[52]; and (3) a newer version of the LNG-IUS, which has a smaller frame and smaller total dose of LNG (Skyla, Bayer Health Care Pharmaceuticals Inc, Wayne, NJ), approved for up to 3 years of use.[53] Several large trials have shown that the copper T380A and the conventional LNG-IUS maintain efficacy beyond their FDA-approved periods and could be used safely by some women for extended use ($\geq$12 years of continuous use for the copper 380A,[54–56] and $\geq$7 years of continuous use for the LNG-IUS).[57–62] Despite the safety and efficacy of the IUD, cost, physician and patient misconceptions, and provider training in the insertion and removal of LARC methods challenge increased IUD use.

Barriers to IUD Use in the United States

Cost

Over time, LARC methods are highly cost-effective because of the associated long duration of action and almost 100% efficacy.[63] For each dollar spent on the IUD, $5 is saved.[64] The Mirena and ParaGard IUDs exceed the cost-effectiveness of oral contraceptive pills at approximately 1.25 and 1.5 years, respectively, and become the most cost-effective method compared with all hormonal methods and male condoms at 3 years. Male sterilization is the only contraceptive method that is slightly more cost-effective than the IUD at 5 years.[63]

LARC devices require significant out-of-pocket cost for those who are uninsured or underinsured.[63,65,66] Surveys of insurance companies show that coverage of IUD devices ranges from 40% to 98%, and insertion coverage ranges from 42% to 100%, with variations attributable to both the insurance plan and existing state mandates.[65,67] For women without health insurance that covers the cost of the IUD device and insertion, the out-of-pocket cost can reach $500 to $1000,[65,66] an amount prohibitive for many lower-income women and adolescents. Even among insured women, up-front costs can discourage adoption of LARC methods. A retrospective chart review in 2007 to 2008 of insured women requesting an IUD reported that women with an out-of-pocket cost of greater than $50 were 11 times less likely to choose an LARC method compared with insured women with an out-of-pocket cost of less than $50.[68] The high cost of LARC and the variability in insurance reimbursement for LARC services also deter providers from offering LARC services in their routine practice.[69]

Further evidence of the benefits of providing LARC at little to no cost is derived from the Contraceptive CHOICE Project in St Louis, MO. This large-scale prospective study offered a diverse group of nearly 10,000 adolescents and women at risk for UIP free access to any reversible contraceptive method of their choice.[70–72] After counseling, 75% of study participants chose a long-acting reversible method: 46% chose LNG-IUD, 12% copper IUD, and 17% subdermal implant.[70] Findings also reported a decrease in abortion rate, fewer repeat abortions, and a lower rate of adolescent births in the study cohort (6.3/1000) compared with national rates (34.3/1000).[70] This ecologic study provides compelling evidence that free access to the entire spectrum of contraceptive methods, accompanied by appropriate counseling, can substantially increase LARC use, decrease UIP, and reduce the number of abortions.

Clinician and patient misconceptions

Challenges to promoting IUD use in the United States are better understood in historical context. The IUD was popular initially among US women when introduced in the 1960s, until the Dalkon shield, an IUD on the market at the time, was linked to pelvic inflammatory disease and, more rarely, septic miscarriage and death.[73] Although currently available IUDs have resolved the design flaws and are safe,[74–76] negative memories of the Dalkon shield continue to linger among some patients and providers.[73]

Evidence suggests that many patients report low knowledge of and express misconceptions about IUD use, which limits acceptability of this method. For example, several studies over the past decade have shown that less than half of young women aged 14 to 25 years have ever heard of IUDs.[77–79] Other research suggests that although many (87%) women aged 18 to 29 years know that the IUD exists, most (56%–80%) have limited knowledge beyond its existence,[80] and both misconceptions and negative attitudes toward the method are prevalent.[79,80] However, patient education can help to create a more positive attitude toward the IUD,[71,79,81] emphasizing the need for clinicians to educate patients on LARC use, especially women at high risk for UIP.

Like patients, many health care providers also have misconceptions about IUD use, especially as it relates to adolescent and nulliparous women.[82] In a survey of more than 800 physicians, physician assistants, and nurse practitioners, almost half (46%) did not believe that nulliparous women or adolescents were appropriate candidates for the IUD,[69] despite a recommendation by the American College of Obstetricians and Gynecologists, Centers for Disease Control and Prevention (CDC), and Society of Family Planning that the IUD should be used as first-line contraception in adolescents and nulliparous patients.[83–85] Research has shown that clinicians who have misconceptions regarding the link between pelvic inflammatory disease and IUD use were less likely to provide IUDs.[78,86] Increased clinician knowledge of and positive attitudes about IUDs have been shown to correlate to increased comfort in recommending this method to patients.[87]

Provider training

A lack of clinician training in insertion and removal of LARC devices can limit patient access to these methods. Although most obstetrics and gynecology physicians report training in LARC insertion,[88] a national survey of family physicians reported that only a quarter of family physicians had inserted an IUD in the previous year.[89] Variables associated with increased provision of IUDs included residency training in IUD insertion, higher knowledge and comfort levels with IUDs, and increased belief in patient receptivity to IUDs.[89] Pediatricians have reported limited knowledge of and training in LARC counseling and insertion, which may lead to missed opportunity for discussing LARC use among adolescent patients.[90–92]

KEY CHARACTERISTICS OF PRACTICE ORGANIZATION THAT FACILITATE LARC UPTAKE

Clinician and patient attitudes and the availability of trained providers limit the uptake of LARC. Organizations that address all 3 of these barriers (cost, misconceptions, and training) have the highest likelihood of increasing LARC uptake among women who are at risk of UIP (**Boxes 1** and **2**).[70,92,97,98]

RECOMMENDATIONS FOR CONTRACEPTIVE COUNSELING

Most randomized controlled trials regarding interventions to improve patient adherence to hormonal and nonhormonal methods (in particular, oral contraceptive pills and injections) are of low to moderate quality and provide little evidence to support the benefit of contraceptive counseling.[99,100] Theory-based interventions to improve contraceptive compliance (eg, counseling sessions based on social cognitive theory or motivational interviewing) have shown more promising results but may be limited in application to general practice given the intensity and lengthier duration.[101] In contrast to studies reporting no effect of structured counseling on contraceptive uptake in specialized reproductive health settings,[102,103] other research suggests that counseling by primary care physicians can increase uptake of hormonal methods and LARC.[104] These collective findings suggest that the impact of counseling in primary care may be greater than that observed in specialized clinics.[105] Even with inconsistent evidence regarding the benefits of contraceptive counseling, multiple professional organizations recommend contraception counseling as a routine part of preventive care for women and men (**Table 6**).[106–111]

Given that no single method of counseling has proved effective over others, we present a framework for contraceptive counseling (GATHER [greet, ask, tell, help, explain, return][112]) as used in the CHOICE project, a large-scale study in the United States reporting an uptake of LARC by approximately 75% of participants.[70] The GATHER model emphasizes the provision of contraceptive information via a "client-centered process focused on the woman, her expressed needs, situation, problems, issues and concerns"; the model is based on a platform of trust and rapport developed between the provider (whether clinician, counselor, or other professional) and the patient at the onset of the session (**Table 7**).[81]

The CHOICE study reported no differences in LARC uptake between university-based sites using the GATHER model compared with community partner sites that provided usual counseling only, raising the question of whether structured counseling is necessary. One explanation for the high uptake of LARC in the usual counseling group may stem from the fact that all participants (whether they received GATHER or usual counseling) were provided with information on enrollment describing the high effectiveness of LARC. The GATHER model as implemented by the CHOICE project has practical applicability for primary care irrespective of its effect on LARC

Box 1
Purchasers, payers, and providers must be ready, willing, and able

The ACA requires most health plans to provide birth control (including LARC) without cost sharing to women; however, some employers and insurance providers seek exemptions based on religious or moral grounds, and legislation has been proposed to eliminate the mandate altogether.[93,94] Some offices serving economically disadvantaged women may find it cost prohibitive to stock LARC on site,[95,96] and many PCPs lack comfort in recommending LARC or placing IUDs.[89] Thus, increased use of LARC requires more than eliminating women's out-of-pocket costs. The purchasers, payers, and providers of health care must ensure adequate access to LARC for all women, all of the time.

Box 2
Key characteristics of practice organization that facilitate LARC use

Address clinician and patient misperceptions or sociocultural barriers to LARC uptake

Avoid unnecessary preprocedural protocols (eg, mandate Pap smear before IUD insertion)

Adopt and widely disseminate evidence-based eligibility criteria for appropriate IUD candidates (eg, explicitly acknowledge that nulliparous and adolescent women are candidates)

Ensure that devices are both readily available for insertion and at low to no cost to patients

Have access to providers trained in LARC insertion

Train support staff (nurses, medical assistants, office schedulers) to streamline processes

---

uptake. First, GATHER promotes and facilitates patient-centered care and shared decision making, principles widely valued in health care provision. Second, as shown by the CHOICE project, those without medical training can effectively use the GATHER model with only a modicum of training.[81] Although up-front investment of time and training of nonmedical staff is required, this model of counseling provision could prove cost-effective and pragmatic in busy primary care settings, by reducing the workload of licensed clinicians.

SCREENING FOR UIP

Although organizations have issued recommendations regarding contraceptive counseling, none has provided guidance about how clinicians should screen or risk stratify women for UIP. Kavanaugh and Schwarz[113] adapted a single-item and a multi-item measure of the London Measure of Unplanned Pregnancy for the purpose of prospectively assessing pregnancy intent among high-risk women requesting pregnancy tests. The single-item measure is outlined in **Table 8**; this question could be used during the clinical encounter to screen for UIP risk and guide subsequent contraceptive counseling.[113]

IMPACT OF CHANGES WITHIN HEALTH CARE
ACA

With the implementation of the ACA, an estimated 18.6 million women who previously lacked insurance will obtain coverage.[114] Most of these women will interface

---

Table 6
Key organizations' recommendations for counseling on UIP

Organization	Recommendation
American Association of Family Physicians[106]	Recommends counseling for men and women on prevention of UIP, including abstinence and the prescription of routine contraception and EC
American Academy of Pediatrics[107,108]	Recommends routine contraception and counseling, including EC, for all adolescents, regardless of sexual activity
American Congress of Obstetrics and Gynecology[109,110]	Recommends counseling on contraceptive options for prevention of unwanted pregnancy, including EC, for women aged 13–39 y
American Medical Association[111]	Recommends reducing UIP through family planning and education, and discussion of EC during routine contraceptive counseling

Table 7 Modified GATHER model for contraceptive counseling		
Step	**Provider's Action**	**Examples**
G = greet	Approach each patient in a respectful way to build trust and rapport	"Hello [patient's name]. Welcome to [facility name]. My name is ____ and I will be helping you explore birth control methods today."
A = ask	Ask the patient about her health and life circumstances, and elicit her contraceptive preferences using open-ended questions	"What methods did you have in mind today, if any at all?" "What is important to you when considering a birth control method?"
T = tell	Tell the patient about contraceptive methods and prevention of sexually transmitted infections, starting with LARC methods as first-line choices if appropriate. Address patient concerns about method side effects and safety up front. Gently correct any misperceptions about safety and side effects	"You said you did not want to be pregnant for at least a few years. I would like to start by first telling you about long-acting birth control methods..." "You mentioned you do not want any 'hormones'. Can you tell me more about your concerns?"
H = help	Help the patient navigate her contraceptive choices, if she expresses a desire to have provider input (eg, shared decision making)	"Because you said you wanted to avoid pregnancy for several years and really don't like the idea of hormones, I would suggest that you consider the copper T IUD..."
E = explain	Explain the patient's chosen method, including effectiveness, how to use, possible side effects and benefits	"You have chosen to use the copper T IUD, which is almost 100% effective at preventing pregnancy. Once it is placed in the uterus, you do not need to do anything to keep it working. Some women notice that their periods get heavier..."
R = return	All patients should be invited for a follow-up visit or phone call to assess the patient's satisfaction with her chosen method. The patient should not be forced to return to the office when not medically necessary	"We routinely offer a check-up visit to make sure you are happy with your method. However, you are welcome to come/call earlier if you have any concerns."

Adapted from Rinehart W, Rudy S, Drennan M. GATHER guide to counseling. Popul Rep J 1998;(48):1–31; and Madden T, Mullersman JL, Omvig KJ, et al. Structured contraceptive counseling provided by the Contraceptive CHOICE Project. Contraception 2013;88(2):243–9.

with a primary care clinician who can address contraceptive needs within the context of ongoing medical conditions, highlighting the critical role of the PCP in the prevention of UIP. The barriers of cost and access to highly effective contraception (eg, LARC) will decrease for many women, because the ACA requires most new and nongrandfathered private insurance plans to cover a full range of contraceptive services (including IUDs, contraceptive implants, oral contraception, injectables, the ring, diaphragms, cervical caps, nonsurgical permanent contraceptives, and sterilization) without cost sharing for women who participate in these plans.[114,115]

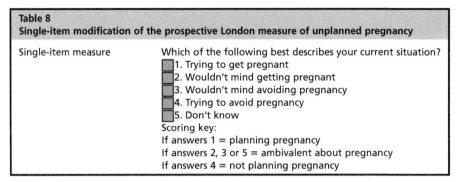

Table 8
Single-item modification of the prospective London measure of unplanned pregnancy

Single-item measure	Which of the following best describes your current situation?
	☐ 1. Trying to get pregnant
	☐ 2. Wouldn't mind getting pregnant
	☐ 3. Wouldn't mind avoiding pregnancy
	☐ 4. Trying to avoid pregnancy
	☐ 5. Don't know
	Scoring key:
	If answers 1 = planning pregnancy
	If answers 2, 3 or 5 = ambivalent about pregnancy
	If answers 4 = not planning pregnancy

Adapted from Kavanaugh ML, Schwarz EB. Prospective assessment of pregnancy intentions using a single- versus a multi-item measure. Perspect Sex Reprod Health 2009;41(4):238–43.

PCMH

The PCMH is a transformative health care delivery model that redefines the provision of health care in the United States. As primary care communities transition to the PCMH model, the focus of care is based on 5 key tenets: patient-centered, coordinated, accessible, comprehensive, and quality and safety.[116]

To address UIP prevention in primary care within a PCMH framework, each patient must be educated and activated to make informed decisions about contraception in a manner that recognizes her personal values, pregnancy intentions, and desired level of participation in her family planning decisions. Patient-centered care may involve a shared decision-making model, in which the patient's preference is incorporated with medical evidence to reach a mutually agreeable decision between patient and clinician.[117] However, patient-centered care may also take the form of clinician-directed decision making, in which the provider takes the predominant lead in making a clinical decision, or an informed choice model, in which the clinician provides only the necessary information for the patient to make an autonomous decision.[118] In a cross-sectional survey of a diverse, predominantly low-income group of women, autonomous decision making was more preferred (50%) than shared decision making (32%), followed by provider-led (18%) decision making as it relates to making contraceptive decisions.[119] Mixed evidence exists as to whether age, income, education, race, or ethnicity can reliably predict a patients' preferred decision-making style,[118–126] emphasizing the need for clinicians to explore each individual patient's desired level of participation in her contraceptive decisions.

To start a conversation about contraception decision making, clinicians can inquire about key elements of contraception that may be important to the patient, including ease of use, efficacy, cost, privacy, safety, effect on future fertility, and prevention of sexually transmitted infections. Patient-friendly tools to help guide this conversation are shown in **Box 3**.[127,128] The clinician can then provide information on the methods that may fit best with the patient's personal values, taking into account coexisting health conditions or other indications for hormonal contraception (eg, menorrhagia, polycystic ovarian syndrome), and initiate the contraception using a quick start method using the resources in **Box 3**.[129–133]

Electronic Health Record

The 2009 Health Information Technology for Economic and Clinical Health Act set forth payment incentives to encourage physician adoption of the electronic health

---

Box 3
Contraceptive education tools for patients and clinicians

For patients

Reproductive Health Access Project–Fact Sheets[a]

   http://www.reproductiveaccess.org/fact_sheets.htm

Reproductive Health Education in Family Medicine–Your Birth Control Choices[b]

   http://rhedi.org/contraception/contra_info.php

For clinicians

CDC Medical Eligibility Criteria for Initiating Contraception[c]

   http://www.cdc.gov/reproductivehealth/UnintendedPregnancy/USMEC.htm#a

CDC US Selected Practice Recommendations for Contraceptive Use[d]

   http://www.cdc.gov/mmwr/pdf/rr/rr62e0614.pdf

National Guideline Clearinghouse Quick Start[e]

   http://www.guideline.gov/content.aspx?id=24715#Section420

Reproductive Health Access Project Clinical Tools Contraception[f]

   http://www.reproductiveaccess.org/contraception/index.htm

Reproductive Health Education in Family Medicine–Quick Start Algorithm[g]

   http://rhedi.org/contraception/quick_start_algorithm.php

   [a] *Adapted from* Reproductive Health Access Project.[127]
   [b] *Adapted from* the Center for Reproductive Health Education in Family Medicine.[128]
   [c] *Adapted from* Centers for Disease Control and Prevention.[129]
   [d] *Adapted from* Center for Disease Control and Prevention.[130]
   [e] *Adapted from* Faculty of Sexual and Reproductive Healthcare.[131]
   [f] *Adapted from* Reproductive Health Access Project.[132]
   [g] *Adapted from* The Center for Reproductive Health Education in Family Medicine.[133]

---

record (EHR). There was a 50% increase in EHR use in outpatient offices from 2009 (48%) to 2012 (72%), indicating that EHR use is becoming the standard of care.[134] The use of EHRs in office-based settings offers the opportunity for patient-centered, safe, timely, efficient, effective, and equitable health care to be provided and measured in numerous domains.[135,136]

Although research investigating EHR-based interventions to promote family planning and contraception use is in its infancy, early findings have suggested promise. For example, 1 study found that a chart-based prompt including a list of contraceptive options, a contraceptive counseling checklist, and referral information for women with chronic medical conditions increased contraceptive counseling, although the prompt did not increase contraceptive prescriptions or referrals. Researchers suggest that the mixed findings may be attributable to the subspecialty practices receiving the prompt (neurology, rheumatology, and a diabetes clinic), where clinicians may have lacked comfort or familiarity with prescribing contraception.[137] Integration of a similar chart-based prompt into a primary care setting may prove more effective.

However, prompts alone may not be enough, because EHR alerts were not effective at promoting IUD use among adolescents who had recently given birth, despite some adolescents desire for a long-acting reversible form of contraception.[138] These findings are consistent with other research suggesting considerable variability in the effectiveness of automated alerts and clinical reminders in changing providers' behaviors.[139–141] EHR prompts that contain links to contraceptive resources may help improve their effectiveness, because the prompt would serve both as a reminder and as a potential toolbox.[142] Beyond prompts and alerts, EHRs can also be used to identify women who may face pregnancy-related risks. For example, using an electronic alert to identify reproductive-aged women who were prescribed potentially teratogenic medication, researchers found that contraceptive counseling was effective at motivating nearly a quarter of the identified women to consider switching from a less effective to a highly effective form of contraception.[143] However, EHR decision support may fall short of changing clinician behavior, as shown by research that found that almost half of women prescribed potential teratogens reported no contraceptive counseling, despite an EHR reminder to clinicians.[144] Research suggests that EHR technology could be harnessed to identify high-risk populations, thereby reducing unplanned high-risk pregnancies and, relatedly, health care costs, but it must be integrated at multiple levels to create meaningful behavioral change.

Given the nascent literature on EHR-based interventions in family planning, the verdict is still out in terms of the capacity of the technology to improve quality and outcomes and reduce costs. To improve generalizability, future studies should assess interventions across systems and among a diverse set of providers, focusing both on the structures and processes of care as well as on patient-centered outcomes.

Research investigating the use of EHRs to improve family planning, prevent unplanned pregnancies, and improve use of highly effective contraception such as LARC can learn from strategies that have proved successful in other areas of health care, such as the hard stop, in which the provider cannot continue until the alert is addressed.[145] Although these same strategies have not been studied in relation to contraception or prevention of UIP, and it is unclear if these same concepts can be generalized to family planning, a hard stop that directs the provider to address pregnancy intentions and contraceptive methods in reproductive-aged women may show promise.

As US medical practices move toward the PCMH model, high-functioning EHR systems that include embedded health reminders are key components to meeting the

Table 9
Suggested EHR-based interventions for family planning

EHR Decisions Support Function	Integrated Family Planning Function
Health resources for clinicians	Links to health resources for clinicians (see **Table 6**)
Protocols and clinical pathways	Decision tree for contraceptive method choice
Standing orders	Order sets for contraceptive choices including pills, patches, injectables, rings, LARC, and EC
Preventive service and wellness	Integration of contraceptive assessment tool,[147] and addition of last menstrual period and last unprotected sex into visit templates
Standard care guidelines and protocols	Hard stop prompt for pregnancy intention and contraceptive assessment at all visits for reproductive-aged women
Prescribing alerts	Alert flag when tetratogenic medication is prescribed in reproductive-aged women with link to contraceptive clinical decision tree
Laboratory test-related alerts	Alert flag for contraceptive assessment associated with screening for sexually transmitted infections

tenets of the PCMH.[146] The limited studies on EHR-based interventions on family planning and unintended pregnancies suggest that multiple innovations embedded in various layers of the EHR help facilitate measurable changes in behavior. Contraceptive management techniques may be best integrated into the EHR under the functionality of decision support, which includes health resources, protocols and clinical pathways, standing orders, and alert systems with reminders and warnings.[135,136] **Table 9** outlines several EHR-based interventions that may help align primary care practice with the PCMH model.

SUMMARY

Unintended pregnancies, which account for half of all pregnancies annually in the United States, are associated with higher rate risk of poor maternal and child health outcomes. Prevention of UIP includes the provision of highly effective contraception, including LARC. LARC, specifically the IUD and subdermal progestin implant, are highly effective and safe for use in most women, yet remain underused in the United States, largely because of patient and clinician misconceptions and high cost. Increased LARC uptake and decreased UIP can be achieved by providing LARC without patient cost sharing and by using clinical tools that provide PCPs with evidence-based information on patient eligibility for various contraceptive methods. Integrating these clinical tools into the EHR provides an opportunity for clinicians to further advance the tenets of the PCMH.

REFERENCES

1. Finer L, Zolna M. Unintended pregnancy in the United States: incidence and disparities. Contraception 2011;84(5):478–85.
2. Facts on unintended pregnancy in the United States. New York: Guttmacher Institute; 2013.
3. Altfeld S, Handler A, Burton D, et al. Wantedness of pregnancy and prenatal health behaviors. Women Health 1992;26(4):29–43.
4. Hellerstedt WL, Pirie PL, Lando HA, et al. Differences in preconceptional and prenatal behaviors in women with intended and unintended pregnancies. Am J Public Health 1998;88(4):663–6.
5. Joyce TJ, Kaestner R, Korenman S. The effect of pregnancy intention on child development. Demography 2000;37(1):83–94.
6. Gazmararian JA, Adams MM, Saltzman LE, et al. The relationship between pregnancy intendedness and physical violence in mothers of newborns. Obstet Gynecol 1995;85(6):1031–8.
7. Goodwin MM, Gazmararian JA, Johnson CH. Pregnancy intendedness and physical abuse around the time of pregnancy: findings from the Pregnancy Risk Assessment Monitoring System, 1996-1997. Matern Child Health J 2000; 4(2):85–92.
8. D'Angelo DV, Gilbert BC, Rochat RW, et al. Differences between mistimed and unwanted pregnancies among women who have live births. Perspect Sex Reprod Health 2004;36(5):192–7.
9. Marsiglio W, Mott FL. Does wanting to become pregnant with a first child affect the subsequent maternal behaviors and infant birth weight? J Marriage Fam 1988;50(4):1023–36.
10. Baydar N. Consequences for children of their birth planning status. Fam Plann Perspect 1995;27(6):228–34.

11. Santelli JS, Linberg LD, Singh S, et al. Explaining recent declines in adolescent pregnancy in the United States: the contribution of abstinence and improved contraceptive use. Am J Public Health 2007;97(1):150–6.
12. Jones RK, Kavanaugh ML. Changes in abortion rates between 2000 and 2008 and lifetime incidence of abortion. Obstet Gynecol 2011;117(6):1358–66.
13. Sonfield A, Kost K, Gold RB, et al. The public costs of births resulting from unintended pregnancies: national and state-level estimates. Perspect Sex Reprod Health 2011;43(2):94–102.
14. Guttmacher Institute. Contraceptive needs and services, 2010. New York: Guttmacher Institute; 2013.
15. Healthy People 2020. Family planning objectives. US Department of Health and Human Services. Washington, DC: Office of Disease Prevention and Health Promotion; 2011. Available at: http://healthypeople.gov/2020/topicsobjectives2020/objectiveslist.aspx?topicId=137%3E. Accessed October 20, 2013.
16. National Ambulatory Medical Care Survey: 2010 summary tables. Ambulatory and Hospital Care Statistics Branch. Atlanta (GA): Centers for Disease Control and Prevention; 2010.
17. Cuellar A, Simmons A, Finegold K. The Affordable Care Act and women. ASPE research brief. Washington, DC: Department of Health and Human Services; 2012.
18. Trussell J, Ellertson C. Efficacy of emergency contraception. Fertility Control Reviews 1995;4:8–11.
19. Trussell J, Raymond EG. Emergency contraception: a last chance to prevent unintended pregnancy. Princeton (NJ): Princeton University; 2013.
20. US Food and Drug Administration. Prescription drug products; certain combined oral contraceptives for use as postcoital emergency contraception. Fed Regist 1997;62(37):8609–12.
21. American College of Obstetricians and Gynecologists. Emergency contraception. Practice Bulletin no. 112. American College of Obstetricians and Gynecologists. Obstet Gynecol 2010;115:1100–9.
22. Randomised controlled trial of levonorgestrel versus the Yuzpe regimen of combined oral contraceptives for emergency contraception. Task Force on Postovulatory Methods of Fertility Regulation. Lancet 1998;352:428–33.
23. Arowojolu A, Okewole I, Adekunle A. Comparative evaluation of the effectiveness and safety of two regimens of levonorgestrel for emergency contraception in Nigerians. Contraception 2002;66:269–73.
24. Cheng L, Gülmezoglu A, Piaggio G, et al. Interventions for emergency contraception. Cochrane Database Syst Rev 2008;(2):CD001324.
25. Creinin M, Schlaff W, Archer D, et al. Progesterone receptor modulator for emergency contraception: a randomized controlled trial. Obstet Gynecol 2006;108:1089–97.
26. Glasier AF, Cameron ST, Fine PM, et al. Ulipristal acetate versus levonorgestrel for emergency contraception: a randomised non-inferiority trial and meta-analysis. Lancet 2010;375:555–62.
27. Hamoda H, Ashok PW, Stalder C, et al. A randomized trial of mifepristone (10 mg) and levonorgestrel for emergency contraception. Obstet Gynecol 2004;104:1307–13.
28. Ho PC, Kwan MS. A prospective randomized comparison of levonorgestrel with the Yuzpe regimen in post-coital contraception. Hum Reprod 1993;8:389–92.
29. Ngai SW, Fan S, Li S, et al. A randomized trial to compare 24 h versus 12 h double dose regimen of levonorgestrel for emergency contraception. Hum Reprod 2004;20:307–11.

30. Raymond E, Taylor D, Trussell J, et al. Minimum effectiveness of the levonorgestrel regimen of emergency contraception. Contraception 2004;69:79–81.

31. Trussell J, Rodríguez G, Ellertson C. Updated estimates of the effectiveness of the Yuzpe regimen of emergency contraception. Contraception 1999;59: 147–51.

32. von Hertzen H, Piaggio G, Ding J, et al. Low dose mifepristone and two regimens of levonorgestrel for emergency contraception: a WHO multicentre randomised trial. Lancet 2002;360:1803–10.

33. Wu S, Wang C, Wang Y, et al. A randomized, double-blind, multicenter study on comparing levonorgestrel and mifepristone for emergency contraception. J Reprod Med 1999;8(Supp 1):43–6.

34. Polis CB, Schaffer K, Blanchard K, et al. Advance provision of emergency contraception for pregnancy prevention [review]. Cochrane Database Syst Rev 2007;(2):CD005497.

35. Raine TR, Harper CC, Rocca CH, et al. Direct access to emergency contraception through pharmacies and effect on unintended pregnancy and STIs: a randomized controlled trial. JAMA 2005;293:54–62.

36. Raymond EG, Stewart F, Weaver M, et al. Impact of increased access to emergency contraceptive pills: a randomized controlled trial. Obstet Gynecol 2006; 108(5):1098–106.

37. Cleland K, Zhu K, Goldstuck N. The efficacy of intrauterine devices for emergency contraception: a systematic review of 35 years of experience. Hum Reprod 2012;27(7):1994–2000.

38. Brache V, Cochon L, Deniaud M, et al. Ulipristal acetate prevents ovulation more effectively than levonogestrel: analysis of pooled data from three randomized trials of emergency contraception regimen. Contraception 2013;88: 611–8.

39. Glasier A, Cameron ST, Blithe D, et al. Can we identify women at risk of pregnancy despite using emergency contraception? Data from randomized trials of ulipristal acetate and levonorgestrel. Contraception 2011;84(4):363–7.

40. Trussell J. Contraceptive efficacy. In: Hatcher RA, Trussell J, Nelson AL, et al, editors. Contraceptive technology. 20th edition. New York: Ardent Media; 2011. p. 791.

41. Trussell J. Estimates of contraceptive failure from the 1995 National Survey of Family Growth, letter to the editor. Contraception 2008;78(1):85.

42. Trussell J. Contraceptive failure in the United States. Contraception 2011;83(5): 397–404.

43. Kost K, Singh S, Vaughan B, et al. Estimates of contraceptive failure from the 2002 National Survey of Family Growth. Contraception 2008;77(1):10–21.

44. Daniels K, Mosher W, Jones J. Contraceptive methods women have ever used: United States, 1982–2010. Atlanta (GA): National Health Statistics Reports; 2013.

45. Jones J, Mosher W, Daniels K. Current contraceptive use in the United States, 2006–2010, and changes in patterns of use since 1995. National Health Statistics Reports; no. 60. Hyattsville (MD): National Center for Health Statistics; 2012.

46. Mosher WD, Jones J. Use of contraception in the United States: 1982–2008. National Center for Health Statistics. Vital Health Stat 23 2010;(29):1–44.

47. Wu J, Meldrum S, Dozier A, et al. Contraceptive nonuse among US women at risk for unplanned pregnancy. Contraception 2008;78(4):284–9.

48. Gold R, Sonfield A, Richards C, et al. Next steps for America's family planning program: leveraging the potential of Medicaid and title X in an evolving health care system. New York: Guttmacher Institute; 2009.

49. Finer LB, Jerman J, Kavanaugh ML. Changes in use of long-acting contraceptive methods in the United States, 2007–2009. Fertil Steril 2012;98(4): 893–7.
50. Singh S, Sedgh G, Hussain R. Unintended pregnancy: worldwide levels, trends, and outcomes. Stud Fam Plann 2010;41:241–50.
51. ParaGard [package insert]. Sellersville, PA: Teva Women's Health, Inc; 2011.
52. Mirena [package insert]. Wayne, NJ: Bayer Healthcare Pharmaceuticals; 2013.
53. Skyla [package insert]. Wayne, NJ: Bayer Healthcare Pharmaceuticals; 2013.
54. Bahamondes L, Faundes A, Sobreira-Lima B, et al. TCu 380A IUD: a reversible permanent contraceptive method in women over 35 years of age. Contraception 2005;72(5):337–41.
55. Sivin I. Utility and drawbacks of continuous use of a copper T IUD for 20 years. Contraception 2007;75(Suppl 6):S70–5.
56. United Nations Development Programme/United Nations Population Fund/ World Health Organization/World Bank Special Programme of Research, Development and Research Training in Human Reproduction. Long-term reversible contraception: twelve years of experience with the TCu380A and TCu220C. Contraception 1997;56:341–52.
57. Andersson K, Odlind V, Rybo G. Levonorgestrel-releasing and copper-releasing (Nova T) IUDs during five years of use: a randomized comparative trial. Contraception 1994;49(1):56–72.
58. Diaz J, Faundes A, Diaz M, et al. Evaluation of the clinical performance of a levonorgestrel-releasing IUD, up to seven years of use, in Campinas, Brazil. Contraception 1993;47(2):169–75.
59. Hidalgo MM, Hidalgo-Regina C, Bahamondes MV, et al. Serum levonorgestrel levels and endometrial thickness during extended use of the levonorgestrel-releasing intrauterine system. Contraception 2009;80(1):84–9.
60. Ronnerdag M, Odlind V. Health effects of long-term use of the intrauterine levonorgestrel-releasing system. A follow-up study over 12 years of continuous use. Acta Obstet Gynecol Scand 1999;78(8):716–21.
61. Sivin I, el Mahgoub S, McCarthy T, et al. Long-term contraception with the levonorgestrel 20 mcg/day (LNg 20) and the copper T 380Ag intrauterine devices: a five-year randomized study. Contraception 1990;42(4):361–78.
62. Sivin I, Stern J, Coutinho E, et al. Prolonged intrauterine contraception: a seven-year randomized study of the levonorgestrel 20 mcg/day (LNg 20) and the copper T380 Ag IUDS. Contraception 1991;44(5):473–80.
63. Trussell J, Lalla AM, Doan QV, et al. Cost effectiveness of contraceptives in the United States. Contraception 2009;79:5–14 [Erratum. Contraception 2009;80: 229–30; Update. Contraception 2010;82:391; Update and correction. Contraception 2012;85:218].
64. Frost J, Zolna M, Frohwirth L. Contraceptive needs and services, 2010. New York: Guttmacher Institute; 2013.
65. Quality of Healthcare Access for Women Survey. Executive summary, female reproductive health coverage. Available at: http://www.arhp.org/publications-and-resources/studies-and-surveys/healthcare-access-survey. Accessed October 27, 2013.
66. IUD. 2013. Available at: http://www.plannedparenthood.org/health-topics/birth-control/iud-4245.htm. Accessed October 27, 2013.
67. Sonfield A, Benson R, Gold JJ, et al. US insurance coverage of contraceptives and the impact of contraceptive coverage mandates, 2002. Perspect Sex Reprod Health 2002;36(2):72–9.

68. Gariepy AM, Simon EJ, Patel DA, et al. The impact of out-of-pocket expense on IUD utilization among women with private insurance. Contraception 2011;84(6): e39–42.

69. Harper CC, Blum M, de Bocanegra HT, et al. Challenges in translating evidence to practice: the provision of intrauterine contraception. Obstet Gynecol 2008; 111(6):1359–69.

70. Peipert JF, Madden T, Allsworth JE. Preventing unintended pregnancies by providing no-cost contraception. Obstet Gynecol 2012;120:1291–7.

71. Mestad R, Secura G, Allsworth J. Acceptance of long-acting reversible contraceptive methods by adolescent participants in the Contraceptive CHOICE Project. Contraception 2011;84(5):493–8.

72. Secura GM, Allsworth JE, Madden T. The contraceptive CHOICE project: reducing barriers to long-acting reversible contraception. Am J Obstet Gynecol 2010;203(2):115.e1–7.

73. Sonfield A. Popularity disparity: attitudes about the IUD in Europe and the United States. Guttmacher Institute Policy Review 2007;10(4).

74. Darney PD. Time to pardon the IUD? N Engl J Med 2001;345:608–10.

75. Grimes D. Intrauterine device and upper-genital-tract infection. Lancet 2000; 356:1013–9.

76. Shelton JD. Risk of clinical pelvic inflammatory disease attributable to an intrauterine device. Lancet 2001;357:443.

77. Fleming KL, Sokoloff A, Raine TR. Attitudes and beliefs about the intrauterine device among teenagers and young women. Contraception 2010;82(2): 178–82.

78. Stanwood NL, Garrett JM, Konrad TR. Obstetrician-gynecologists and the intrauterine device: a survey of attitudes and practice. Obstet Gynecol 2002;99: 275–80.

79. Whitaker AK, Johnson LM, Harwood B, et al. Adolescent and young adult women's knowledge of and attitudes toward the intrauterine device. Contraception 2008;78:211–7.

80. Kaye K, Suellentrop K, Sloup C. The fog zone: how misperceptions, magical thinking, and ambivalence put young adults at risk for unplanned pregnancy. Washington, DC: National Campaign to Prevent Teen and Unplanned Pregnancy; 2009.

81. Madden T, Mullersmann JL, Omvig KJ. Structured contraceptive counseling provided by the Contraceptive CHOICE Project. Contraception 2013;88(2): 243–9.

82. Diaz VA, Hughes N, Dickerson LM, et al. Clinician knowledge about use of intrauterine devices in adolescents in South Carolina AHEC. Fam Med 2011;43(6): 407–11.

83. US Medical Eligibility Criteria (US MEC) for contraceptive use, 2010. 2010. Available at: http://www.cdc.gov/reproductivehealth/unintendedpregnancy/ usmec.htm. Accessed November 2, 2013.

84. Adolescents and long-acting reversible contraception: implants and intrauterine devices. Committee Opinion. No. 539. American College of Obstetricians and Gynecologists. Obstet Gynecol 2012;120:963–8.

85. Lyus R, Lohr P, Prager S. Use of the Mirena LNG-IUS and Paragard CuT380A intrauterine devices in nulliparous women. Contraception 2010;81:367–71.

86. Madden T, Allsworth JE, Hladky KJ, et al. Intrauterine contraception in Saint Louis: a survey of obstetrician and gynecologists' knowledge and attitudes. Contraception 2010;81(2):112–6.

87. Postlethwaite D, Shaber R, Mancuso V, et al. Intrauterine contraception: evaluation of clinician practice patterns in Kaiser Permanente Northern California. Contraception 2007;75:177–84.

88. Tang J, Maurer R, Bartz D. Intrauterine device knowledge and practices: a national survey of obstetrics and gynecology residents. South Med J 2013;106(9): 500–5.

89. Rubin SE, Fletcher J, Stein T, et al. Determinants of intrauterine contraception provision among US family physicians: a national survey of knowledge, attitudes and practice. Contraception 2011;83(5):472–8.

90. Fox HB, McManus MA, Klein JD, et al. Adolescent medicine training in pediatric residency programs. Pediatrics 2010;125(1):165–72.

91. Hellerstedt WL, Smith AE, Shew ML, et al. Perceived knowledge and training needs in adolescent pregnancy prevention: results from a multidisciplinary survey. Arch Pediatr Adolesc Med 2000;154(7):679–84.

92. Rubin S, Davis K, McKee D. New York City physicians' view of providing long-acting reversible contraception to adolescents. Ann Fam Med 2013; 11:130–6.

93. Eisenberg D, McNicholas C, Peipert JF. Cost as a barrier to long-acting reversible contraceptive (LARC) use in adolescents. J Adolesc Health 2013;52(Suppl 4): S59–63.

94. Sonfield A, Pollack HA. The Affordable Care Act and reproductive health: potential gains and serious challenges. J Health Polit Policy Law 2013;38:373–91.

95. Beeson T, Wood S, Bruen B, et al. Accessibility of long-acting reversible contraceptives (LARCs) in Federally Qualified Health Centers (FQHCs). Contraception 2014;89(2):91–6.

96. Kavanaugh ML, Jerman J, Ethier K, et al. Meeting the contraceptive needs of teens and young adults: youth-friendly and long-acting reversible contraceptive services in US family planning facilities. J Adolesc Health 2013;52(3):284–92.

97. Hathaway M. Increasing long-acting reversible contraception uptake through the delivery of title X services at federally qualified health centers. Contraception 2013;88:301.

98. Teal SB, Romer SE. The BC4U service model: achieving astronomical LARC rates in adolescents. Association of Reproductive Health Care Professionals, Reproductive Health 2013. Denver, September 21, 2013.

99. Halpern V, Grimes DA, Lopez L, et al. Strategies to improve adherence and acceptability of hormonal methods for contraception. Cochrane Database Syst Rev 2006;(1):CD004317.

100. Arrowsmith ME, Aicken CR, Majeed A, et al. Interventions for increasing uptake of copper intrauterine devices: systematic review and meta-analysis. Contraception 2012;86(6):600–5.

101. Lopez LM, Tolley EE, Grimes DA, et al. Theory-based interventions for contraception. Cochrane Database Syst Rev 2013;(8):CD007249.

102. Simmons KB, Edelman AB, Li H, et al. Personalized contraceptive assistance and uptake of long-acting, reversible contraceptives by postpartum women: a randomized, controlled trial. Contraception 2013;88(1):45–51.

103. Langston AM, Rosario L, Westhoff CL. Structured contraceptive counseling–a randomized controlled trial. Patient Educ Couns 2010;81(3):362–7.

104. Lee JK, Parisi SM, Akers AY, et al. The impact of contraceptive counseling in primary care on contraceptive use. J Gen Intern Med 2011;26(7):731–6.

105. Landry DJ, Wei J, Frost JJ. Public and private providers' involvement in improving their patients' contraceptive use. Contraception 2008;78(1):42–51.

106. AAFP Statement of Policy on Contraceptive Advice. Updated 2007. Available at: http://www.aafp.org/online/en/home/policy/policies/c/contraceptiveadvice.html. Accessed October 27, 2013.

107. American Academy of Pediatrics Committee on Adolescence, Blythe MJ, Diaz A. Contraception and adolescents. Pediatrics 2007;120(5):1135–48.

108. Committee On Adolescence. Emergency Contraception. Pediatrics 2012;130: 1174–82.

109. Well-woman care: assessments and recommendations. 2013. Available at: http://www.acog.org/About_ACOG/ACOG_Departments/Annual_Womens_Health_ Care/Assessments_and_Recommendations. Accessed November 3, 2013.

110. Guidelines for adolescent health care. 2nd edition. Washington, DC: American College of Obstetricians and Gynecologists Committee on Adolescent Health Care; 2011.

111. AMA Women Physicians Congress. Policy compendium on issues relation to women physicians and women's health. Chicago: American Medical Association; 2013.

112. Rinehart W, Rudy S, Drennan M. GATHER guide to counseling. Popul Rep J 1998;(48):1–31.

113. Kavanaugh ML, Schwarz EB. Prospective assessment of pregnancy intentions using a single- versus a multi-item measure. Perspect Sex Reprod Health 2009;41(4):238–43.

114. Affordable Care Act and women. 2013. Available at: http://www.hhs.gov/healthcare/ facts/factsheets/2012/03/women03202012a.html. Accessed October 27, 2013.

115. Contraceptive cover in the new health care law: frequently asked questions. 2011. Available at: http://www.nwlc.org/sites/default/files/pdfs/contraceptive_ coverage_faq_11.9.11.pdf. Accessed October 27, 2013.

116. Patient-centered medical home resource center. Available at: http://pcmh.ahrq. gov/page/defining-pcmh. Accessed October 27, 2013.

117. Makoul G, Clayman ML. An integrative model of shared decision making in medical encounters. Patient Educ Couns 2006;60:301–12.

118. Murray E, Pollack L, White M, et al. Clinical decision-making: physicians' preferences and experiences. BMC Fam Pract 2007;8:10.

119. Dehlendorf C, Diedrich J, Drey E, et al. Preferences for decision-making about contraception and general health care among reproductive age women at an abortion clinic. Patient Educ Couns 2013;81(3):343–8.

120. Cassileth BR, Zupkis RV, Sutton-Smith K, et al. Information and participation preferences among cancer patients. Ann Intern Med 1980;92:832–6.

121. Deber RB, Kraetschmer N, Urowitz S, et al. Do people want to be autonomous patients? Preferred roles in treatment decision-making in several patient populations. Health Expect 2007;10:248–58.

122. Levinson W, Kao A, Kuby A, et al. Not all patients want to participate in decision making. A national study of public preferences. J Gen Intern Med 2005;20:531–5.

123. McKinstry B. Do patients wish to be involved in decision making in the consultation? A cross sectional survey with video vignettes. BMJ 2000;7(321): 867–71.

124. Schneider A, Korner T, Mehring M, et al. Impact of age, health locus of control and psychological co-morbidity on patients' preferences for shared decision making in general practice. Patient Educ Couns 2006;61:292–8.

125. Spies CD, Schulz CM, Weiss-Gerlach E, et al. Preferences for shared decision making in chronic pain patients compared with patients during a premedication visit. Acta Anaesthesiol Scand 2005;50:1019–26.

126. Wallberg B, Michelson H, Nystedt M, et al. Information needs and preferences for participation in treatment decisions among Swedish breast cancer patients. Acta Oncol 2000;39(4):467–76.

127. Reproductive Health Access Project. Facts sheets. Available at: http://www.reproductiveaccess.org/fact_sheets.htm. Accessed November 3, 2013.

128. The Center for Reproductive Health Education in Family Medicine (RHEDI). Clinical resources, patient education. Available at: http://rhedi.org/clinicians.php. Accessed November 3, 2013.

129. Centers for Disease Control and Prevention. US medical eligibility criteria for contraceptive use, 2010. MMWR Early Release 2010;59:52–63.

130. Division of Reproductive Health, National Center for Chronic Disease Prevention and Health Promotion, Centers for Disease Control and Prevention (CDC). US selected practice recommendations for contraceptive use, 2013: adapted from the World Health Organization selected practice recommendations for contraceptive use, 2nd edition. MMWR Recomm Rep 2013;62(RR05):1–46.

131. Clinical Effectiveness Unit. Quick starting contraception. London: Faculty of Sexual and Reproductive Healthcare (FSRH); 2010. Available at: http://www.guideline.gov/content.aspx?id=24715-Section420. Accessed November 3, 2013.

132. Reproductive Health Access Project. Contraception. Available at: http://www.reproductiveaccess.org/contraception/index.htm. Accessed November 3, 2013.

133. The Center for Reproductive Health Education in Family Medicine (RHEDI). Quick start algorithm. Available at: http://rhedi.org/contraception/quick_start_algorithm.php. Accessed November 3, 2013.

134. Hsiao CJ, Hing E. Use and characteristics of electronic health record systems among office-based physician practices: United States, 2001–2012. National Center for Health Statistics Brief. Hyattsville (MD): National Center for Health Statistics; 2012.

135. Institute of Medicine. Crossing the quality chasm: a new health system for the 21st century. Washington, DC: National Academy of Medicine; 2001.

136. Ferris TG, Johnson S, Jha A, et al. Health information technology in the United States: where we stand, 2008. A framework for measuring the effects of health information technology on health care quality. Princeton (NJ): Institute for Health Policy at Massachusetts General Hospital, School of Public Health and Health Services at George Washington University, and Robert Wood Johnson Foundation; 2008.

137. Benfield N, Berrios S, Harleman E, et al. Increasing contraception counseling in subspecialty medicine clinics with a chart-based prompt. Contraception 2012; 86:311.

138. Tocce K, Sheeder J, Python J, et al. Long acting reversible contraception in postpartum adolescents: early initiation of etonogestrel implant is superior to IUDs in the outpatient setting. J Pediatr Adolesc Gynecol 2012;25(1):59–63.

139. Bright TJ, Wong A, Dhurjati R, et al. Effect of clinical decision-support systems: a systematic review. Ann Intern Med 2012;157(1):29–43.

140. Holt TA, Thorogood M, Griffiths F. Changing clinical practice through patient specific reminders available at the time of the clinical encounter: systematic review and meta-analysis. J Gen Intern Med 2012;27(8):974–84.

141. Moxey A, Robertson J, Newby D. Computerized clinical decision support for prescribing: provision does not guarantee uptake. J Am Med Inform Assoc 2010;17(1):25–33.

142. Akers AY, Gold MA, Borrero S, et al. Providers' perspectives on challenges to contraceptive counseling in primary care. J Womens Health (Larchmt) 2010; 19(6):1163–70.

143. Mody S, Wu J, Ornelas M, et al. Utilizing the electronic medical records to refer women prescribed category D or X medications for contraceptive counseling. Contraception 2013;88:463.

144. Schwarz EB, Parisi SM, Handler SM, et al. Counseling about medication-induced birth defects with clinical decision support in primary care. J Womens Health (Larchmt) 2013;22(10):817–24.

145. Klatt T, Hopp E. Effect of a best-practice alert on the rate of influenza vaccination of pregnant women. Obstet Gynecol 2012;119(2):301–5.

146. Shortell S, Gillies R, Wu F. United States innovations in healthcare delivery. Public Health Review 2010;32(1):190–212.

147. Schwarz EB, Parisi SM, Williams SL, et al. Promoting safe prescribing in primary care with a contraceptive vital sign: a cluster-randomized controlled trial. Ann Fam Med 2012;10(6):516–22.

Intimate Partner Violence Victimization
Identification and Response in Primary Care

Vijay Singh, MD, MPH, MS[a,b,*], Ketti Petersen, MD[a,c],
Simone Rauscher Singh, PhD, MA[d]

KEYWORDS

- Intimate partner violence • Domestic violence • Victimization • Screening
- Assessment • Intervention • Documentation

KEY POINTS

- In the United States more than 1 out of 3 women experience intimate partner violence (IPV) victimization in their lifetime.
- Clinical conditions associated with IPV include mental health and substance use disorders, chronic pain, and traumatic injuries.
- Short screening instruments such as HITS (Hurt, Insult, Threaten, Scream) or the Abuse Assessment Screen can identify IPV victimization.
- Intervention includes referral to support services, treatment of associated health conditions, and mandatory reporting if required.
- Counseling that emphasizes danger assessment, safety behaviors, and information on community resources has been shown to reduce IPV victimization.
- Clinical guidelines recommend IPV screening for all or most women, and providing or referring victims to intervention.

DEFINITION OF INTIMATE PARTNER VIOLENCE

Intimate partner violence (IPV), domestic violence, and family violence have been used historically, and sometimes interchangeably, to refer to emotional, physical, and sexual violence within intimate partner relationships. IPV describes a pattern of coercive

Conflicts of Interest: None.

[a] Department of Family Medicine, University of Michigan, 1150 West Medical Center Drive, M7300 Med Sci I, Ann Arbor, MI 48109-5625, USA; [b] Department of Emergency Medicine, Institute for Healthcare Policy and Innovation, University of Michigan Injury Center, 2800 Plymouth Road, Suite B10-G080, Ann Arbor, MI 48109-2800, USA; [c] Department of Family Medicine, University of Michigan, 200 Arnet Street, Suite 200, Ypsilanti, MI 48109-1213, USA; [d] Department of Health Management and Policy, School of Public Health, University of Michigan, 1415 Washington Heights, M3533 SPH II, Ann Arbor, MI 48109-2029, USA

* Corresponding author. Departments of Family Medicine and Emergency Medicine, University of Michigan Injury Center, 2800 Plymouth Road, Suite B10-G080, Ann Arbor, MI 48109-2800.
E-mail address: vijaysin@umich.edu

behavior that establishes power and control in the context of a current or past intimate relationship, regardless of gender, sexual orientation, marital status, or living situation. IPV may include physical violence, sexual violence and assault, psychological and emotional violence, progressive isolation and stalking, deprivation, intimidation, and reproductive coercion.[1] IPV research and clinical guidelines have focused on violence against women, not men, and this review focuses on IPV against women. However, strategies for screening, assessment, intervention, and documentation described in this review can be adapted for male patients.

PREVALENCE, HEALTH SERVICE USE, AND COST OF IPV VICTIMIZATION IN THE UNITED STATES

Women have historically been and continue to be disproportionately affected by IPV. In the United States, 35.6% of women (42 million) within their lifetime will be victims of intimate partner rape, physical violence, or stalking, and 14.8% (17 million) will be injured as a result. By comparison, 28.5% of men, or about 32 million, within their lifetime will be victims of intimate partner rape, physical violence, or stalking.[2] Despite the high lifetime prevalence of IPV against men, most research remains focused on IPV against women. In part this may be due to gender differences in IPV impact and injury. The 2010 National Intimate Partner and Sexual Violence Survey defines "IPV-related Impact" as experiencing any of the following as a result of physical violence, stalking, or rape: being fearful or concerned for safety, having symptoms of posttraumatic stress disorder, being injured, needing health care, contacting a crisis help hotline, needing housing services, needing victim's advocate services, needing legal services, missing at least 1 day of work or school, or contracting a sexually transmitted infection or becoming pregnant if raped. Whereas 28.8% of women have a lifetime reported prevalence of experiencing the aforementioned IPV-related impact, only 9.9% of men do. In addition, whereas 14.8% of women during their lifetime experience an injury resulting from IPV, only 4% of men do.[2] There are similar gender differences in IPV-related homicide. Of victims killed by an intimate partner, women made up 70% whereas men constituted 30%.[3] In 2010 there were 1800 murders of women by men, with 94% killed by male acquaintances, and of those women killed, 65% (1017) were wives or intimate acquaintances.[4] Although gender differences in IPV-related homicide exist, women's risk of intimate partner homicide is greatest within the first year of leaving an abusive relationship.[5]

Women across the socioeconomic spectrum are at risk for IPV, regardless of race or ethnicity. Lifetime prevalence of physical violence, stalking, or rape among women is 35% among Caucasians, 37% among Hispanics, 44% among African Americans, 46% among Native American and Alaskan Natives, and 54% among those identified as multiracial.[2] Both lower and higher socioeconomic status has been associated with IPV. Of women in a large health plan, only 23% of those with an annual income greater than $75,000, compared with 54% of those with an annual income of less than $50,000, reported IPV victimization in the past year.[6] Of women in that same large health plan, 35% with a history of nonphysical IPV and 29% with a history of physical IPV reported an annual income greater than $75,000.[7]

IPV varies depending on the type of medical setting, and contributes to use of health services. Although no nationally representative data are available, a recent study across different health care sites in Boston, Massachusetts showed that IPV prevalence was highest among patients in an addiction recovery program (36%), followed by emergency departments (16.5%), obstetrics/gynecology clinics (12.7%), and primary care (8.6%).[8] IPV can be the precipitating reason for patients to present for medical care. Annually there are 320,000 outpatient and 480,000 emergency depart-ment visits directly attributable to IPV against women.[9] Of assault-related injuries seen at select emergency departments, 39% of women identified IPV as the cause.[10]

The health impacts of IPV extend beyond the period of a violent relationship. After documented exposures to controlling behaviors or physical or sexual violence, survi-vors have a 1.6- to 2.3-fold increase in health care use compared with those without IPV.[11] Compared with never-abused women, those with physical and nonphysical IPV made more use of mental health services for ongoing abuse, with lesser use for those with abuse in the past 5 years, and least use among those with abuse greater than 5 years in the past.[7] Compared with women without any history of IPV, health service utilization was still 20% higher 5 years after women's abuse ceased, and the effects on health care use could persist indefinitely.[12]

Health care costs are highest for IPV victims with current abuse. Women experi-encing past-year physical IPV have 42% higher annual health care costs than do never-abused women. Compared with women with no IPV history, women with phys-ical abuse in the past 5 years had 24% higher annual health care costs, and women with physical abuse greater than 5 years in the past had 19% higher annual health care costs.[7] These increased costs decrease over time since the last IPV exposure. Relative to women with no IPV history, total health care costs remained higher for 3 years following IPV exposure. Starting at 4 years after IPV ended, total health care costs were similar to those among women without IPV.[13] In the first year after an as-sault, the cost of health care for IPV survivors has been estimated to be between $2.3 billion and $7 billion.[14] A 2004 study estimated the social cost of IPV against women to be greater than $8.3 billion based on physical and mental health outcomes, premature death from violence, and lost productivity.[15] Based on a 44% prevalence of IPV, a 2007 longitudinal cohort study found that excess costs attributable to IPV measured in a health maintenance organization are $19.3 million per year for every 100,000 women enrollees aged 18 to 64 years.[12] The Centers for Disease Control and Preven-tion estimated the annual cost of IPV against women in the United States to be $5.8 billion in 2002, which translates into $10.4 billion in 2012.[14]

HEALTH CONDITIONS ASSOCIATED WITH IPV

Various clinical conditions and biopsychosocial factors are associated with IPV. These factors can serve as markers or red flags for IPV, and these conditions are routinely addressed by primary care providers. Primary care providers who are aware that IPV may underlie these conditions can improve identification of IPV and create oppor-tunities for intervention. As already noted, women experience higher rates of IPV and IPV-related impact in comparison with men. Among women, the period of greatest IPV risk is when younger than 26 years,[16] and 68% of women will first experience IPV be-tween the ages of 18 and 34 years.[2] Assessing family and social history can uncover factors associated with IPV. A family history of witnessing parental IPV increases the risk of experiencing physical or nonphysical IPV.[17] Social history elements that sug-gest IPV include lower income, low academic achievement, and unemployment.[18] Mental health conditions associated with IPV include depression, anxiety, posttrau-matic stress disorder, sleep disorders, substance abuse, and suicidality.[6,19,20] Women with a history of IPV, rape, or stalking by any perpetrator also have a higher prevalence of many common conditions including asthma, irritable bowel syndrome, unexplained chronic gastrointestinal symptoms, diabetes, frequent headaches, chronic pain, and overall poor physical and mental health.[2,21] In addition, women experiencing IPV or forced sexual intercourse have associations with numerous gynecologic conditions including sexually transmitted infections, vaginal bleeding, chronic pelvic pain, dyspareunia, sexual dysfunction, and multiple unintended pregnancies. IPV during pregnancy has been associated with infants of low birth weight.[22] Finally, head, neck, or facial injuries, especially ones that cannot be verified by an independent witness, are associated with IPV.[23]

IPV SCREENING

Comprehensive screening components are outlined in the National Consensus Guidelines (NCG) on Identifying and Responding to Domestic Violence Victimization in Health Care Settings,[24] and the World Health Organization (WHO) clinical and policy guidelines on responding to IPV and sexual violence against women.[20] Before beginning screening, primary care providers need to consider which female patients they will assess for IPV. The WHO guideline recommends targeted screening, meaning that clinicians ask about IPV only when associated clinical conditions are present. The United States Preventive Services Task Force (USPSTF) guideline recommends IPV screening for a broader group: all women aged 14 to 46 years.[25] The NCG recommends routine or universal screening, meaning that clinicians ask about IPV to an even broader group: all adolescents and adult patients, and include an assessment for both current and past IPV victimization. However, given time constraints in the primary care setting, and acknowledging differing views among guidelines, clinicians need a practical decision for whom to screen for IPV. This review recommends that primary care providers screen for current rather than past IPV among 2 groups: all women aged 14 to 46 years, and women older than 46 only when associated clinical conditions are present (first box of **Fig. 1**). Screening for current IPV can focus inquiry on those with a higher likelihood of leaving a relationship, which is the time of greatest risk for homicide.[5] Screening by primary care providers of all women aged 14 to 46 years follows USPSTF guidelines and incorporates part of the NCG guidelines. Screening women older than 46, only when assessing conditions caused or complicated by IPV, incorporates WHO guidelines and limits the burden of universal screening by overstretched primary care providers.

Within the primary care setting, screening begins with reviewing medical history for IPV-associated health conditions described earlier, and observing patient and partner behaviors. Such behaviors include vague or somatic complaints over repeated visits, injuries that are unexplained or inconsistent with history provided, or the presence of a partner who controls the patient's interview or will not leave patient alone with the primary care provider (**Box 1**).[24] When assessing for IPV, primary care providers should find a private place to discuss the topic with the patient. To ensure a more accurate response, clinicians should question the patient apart from partner, family, or friends. Primary care providers can develop a waiting-room sign stating that privacy of all patients will be respected and that patients will be seen alone for some portion of their visit. Having a sign like this helps primary care providers normalize the experience of seeing a patient alone without a friend or family member present.[26] A framing statement (**Table 1**) can introduce and further normalize patients being asked about IPV. An example statement is for primary care providers to say they routinely ask patients about abusive relationships, as some patients are too uncomfortable to bring it up themselves.[24]

Before directly questioning patients about IPV and related traumatic injuries, it is important to have knowledge of state-based mandatory reporting laws for IPV. Except for Alabama, New Mexico, and Wyoming, all states require primary care providers to report specified instances whereby a patient has an injury attributable to violence.

Screen if woman is either:

1. Of childbearing age 14–46

2. Over age 46 with clinical conditions associated with IPV:

   Mental health problems: depression, posttraumatic stress disorder, suicidal ideation

   Substance use: alcohol or illicit drugs

   Chronic unexplained pain, headaches

   Chronic unexplained gastrointestinal symptoms, irritable bowel syndrome

   Adverse reproductive symptoms: chronic pelvic pain, dyspareunia, sexual
      dysfunction

   Adverse reproductive outcomes: unintended pregnancies, low birth weight

   Traumatic injury

   See Box 1 for related list of patient and partner behaviors

Screen with HITS or AAS questions, after introductory statement (see Table 1)

Assess homicide risk and safety after the medical visit[37]:

   1. Has the physical violence increased over the past 6 months?

   2. Has your partner used a weapon or threatened you with a weapon?

   3. Do you believe your partner is capable of killing you?

   4. Have you been beaten while pregnant?

   5. Is your partner violently and constantly jealous of you?

Assess suicidal ideation

Assess for mental health or substance use disorders

Fig. 1. Screen, assess, intervene, and document (SAID) algorithm for primary care providers to identify and respond to intimate partner violence (IPV) victimization. AAS, Abuse Assessment Screen; HITS, Hurt, Insult, Threaten, Scream. (*Data from* Refs.[20,24,66–69])

Intervene with
1. Support: Be nonjudgmental and validating; Tell her "you are not alone and you do not deserve to be abused" (see Table 2)
2. Safety planning: Offer to call National Domestic Violence Hotline 1-800-799-SAFE or local IPV program for patient counseling, legal advice, or shelter (see Table 2)
3. Referrals: Provide referral to health system-based counseling for advocacy, support, and safety planning. If no trained service providers available on-site, describe national and community resources (see Box 2). Provide referral to home visitation programs.
4. Treatment as needed for suicidal ideation, mental health, or substance use disorders
5. Mandatory reporting to law enforcement if patient presents with an injury, according to state law
6. Follow-up care for IPV, safety reassessment, and associated clinical conditions

Document screening question responses or exactly what patient said using quotations
Document physical examination: behavior or injuries, using drawings or photographs
Document assessment of presence or absence of IPV
Document safety assessment, planning, and referrals
Document follow-up plans to address IPV and associated clinical conditions

Fig. 1. (continued)

A list of these reporting laws is available at http://www.futureswithoutviolence.org/userfiles/file/HealthCare/Compendium%20Final.pdf.[27] If a report is mandated, law enforcement will generally require the following information: (1) name of IPV victim; (2) residence, if known, of IPV victim; (3) cause, character, and extent of injury; and (4) identification of perpetrator, if known. Primary care providers are not violating the privacy rule of the Health Insurance Portability and Accountability Act (HIPAA) when releasing patient information as part of mandatory reporting to authorities.[28] Benefits of mandatory reporting include potential prosecution of the perpetrator, improved responsiveness of primary care provider, and lifting the burden of reporting from the IPV victim.[20,29] Barriers to mandatory reporting include provider time and

> **Box 1**
> **Patient and partner behaviors that may indicate intimate partner violence (IPV)**
>
> - Failure to keep medical appointments or comply with medical recommendations
> - An unusually high number of visits to health care providers
> - Vague or somatic complaints over repeated visits
> - Injuries that are unexplained, inconsistent with history provided, or during pregnancy
> - Secrecy or obvious discomfort when asked about relationships or IPV
> - The presence of a partner who comes into examination room, controls interview, or will not leave patient alone with primary care provider
>
> *Data from* Family Violence Prevention Fund. National Consensus Guidelines on identifying and responding to domestic violence victimization in health care settings. San Francisco (CA): Family Violence Prevention Fund; 2004.

resource requirements, women's discouragement from reporting IPV, confidentiality and autonomy being compromised, and risk of retaliation or injury by the perpetrator.[20,29,30] These barriers lead some IPV victims to not support mandatory reporting, and, given safety risks for potentially increased violence, these women may suggest that they should decide when to report.[31] Accounting for these risks, the WHO guidelines do not support mandatory reporting of IPV because it can impinge on women's autonomy and decision making.

Despite the legal obligation to report injuries resulting from violence, primary care providers can share decision making with patients. Clinicians can inform patients about the limits of confidentiality if a violence-related injury has occurred (see **Table 1**). An example confidentiality statement is for a primary care provider to say "Before we get started, I want you to know that everything you share with me is confidential, unless (fill in state law here) or you have been injured by a weapon. I would have to report that situation, ok?"[26]

When asked about IPV, patients often need time to give their answers, as disclosing a personal history of IPV can be emotionally difficult. Even when an initial inquiry does not yield an IPV disclosure, using a caring, empathetic tone may open the door for discussing the topic at some later time. Despite evidence supporting the use of IPV screening tools in the primary care setting, patients may have many reasons for not disclosing violence. For example, victims of IPV may subscribe to religious or cultural beliefs that focus on keeping their family together, have feelings of embarrassment or shame, fear retaliation by their partner, lack trust in others, depend economically on their abusive partner, be unaware of alternatives, or lack an adequate support system.[32] In addition, primary care providers should consider not screening for IPV if they are unable to obtain an appropriate interpreter or secure a private space in which to conduct an inquiry.

There are many different IPV screening tools, and no one tool is best.[33] For a comprehensive list of screening tools, primary care providers can refer to *IPV and Sexual Violence Victimization Assessment Instruments for Use in Healthcare Settings*, published by the Centers for Disease Control and Prevention, and available online at http://www.cdc.gov/ncipc/pub-res/images/ipvandsvscreening.pdf.[34] Among many screening tools to choose from, this review focuses on 2 with characteristics needed by primary care providers. These characteristics include having few questions and therefore saving time, previous testing in primary care and outpatient settings, and high sensitivity and specificity.

Table 1
Screening questions for primary care providers to identify intimate partner violence (IPV) victimization among patients

Example statements for introducing the topic of IPV into the clinical encounter	
Introductory or framing statements	1. Violence is a problem for many patients. Because it affects health and well-being, I ask all my patients about it.[24]
	2. We've started talking to all of our patients about safe and healthy relationships because it can have such a large impact on your health.[1]
Confidentiality statement	Before we get started, I want you to know that everything here is confidential, meaning that I won't talk to anyone else about what is said unless you tell me that...(insert your state mandatory reporting law, listed at http://www.futureswithoutviolence.org/userfiles/file/HealthCare/Compendium%20Final.pdf).[1,27]
HITS screening tool[34]	
Questions	How often does your partner... 1. Hurt you physically 2. Insult you or talk down to you 3. Threaten you with harm 4. Scream or curse at you?
Scoring	5-point scale: never (1 point), rarely (2 points), sometimes (3 points), fairly often (4 points), frequently (5 points). Scores >10 points are positive for IPV
Sensitivity (%)	86–96
Specificity (%)	86–99
Abuse Assessment Screen[34]	
Questions	1. Have you ever been emotionally or physically abused by your partner or someone important to you? 2. Within the last year, have you been hit, slapped, kicked, or otherwise physically hurt by someone? 3. Since you've been pregnant, have you been hit, slapped, kicked, or otherwise physically hurt by someone? 4. Within the last year, has anyone forced you to have sexual activities? 5. Are you afraid of your partner or anyone you listed above?
Scoring	Yes to any question is positive for IPV
Sensitivity (%)	93–94
Specificity (%)	55–99

Adapted from Rabin RF, Jennings JM, Campbell JC, et al. Intimate partner violence screening tools: a systematic review. Am J Prev Med 2009;36(5):439–45.e4; with permission. HITS reprinted with permission from Kevin Sherin, MD, MPH (Kevin_Sherin@doh.state.fl.us). Copyright 2003.

HITS

A 4-question screening tool called HITS (Hurt, Insult, Threaten, Scream)[35] is not only an acronym for the subject matter it addresses but also a mnemonic for physical violence, making it easy to remember for busy primary care providers (see **Table 1**). The 4 HITS questions are "how often does your partner: hurt you physically, insult or talk down to you, threaten you with harm, or scream or curse at you?" Questions are answered on a 5-point scale from never (1 point) to frequently (5 points). A score of more than 10 is positive and has a 91% positive predictive value. For studies including women, the HITS sensitivity is 86% to 96% and specificity is 86% to 99%.[33,34] These sensitivity and specificity levels are nearly the highest of all available

IPV screening tools. Primary care providers should note that HITS does not include assessment for sexual abuse. A question on forced sex can be gleaned from the Abuse Assessment Screen, described next.

The Abuse Assessment Screen

The Abuse Assessment Screen (AAS)[36] includes 5 questions covering emotional, physical, and sexual abuse, and can be used with pregnant patients (see **Table 1**). Given this review's and USPSTF guideline inclusion of screening women of child-bearing age, the AAS provides an IPV screening tool that assesses forced sexual activity as well as violence during pregnancy. The 5 AAS questions are: (1) have you ever been emotionally or physically abused by your partner or someone important to you, (2) within the last year, have you been hit, slapped, kicked, or otherwise physically hurt by someone, (3) since you've been pregnant, have you been hit, slapped, kicked, or otherwise physically hurt by someone, (4) within the last year, has anyone forced you to have sexual activities, and (5) are you afraid of your partner or anyone you listed above? Yes to any question is positive for IPV. The AAS has sensitivity of 93% to 94% with specificity of 55% to 99%.[33,34] Of note, the AAS includes a body map on which primary care providers can document the location of any patient injuries (Appendix 1). This body map assists in injury documentation in the medical record.

Screening, Assessment, Intervention, and Documentation

An algorithm for identification and response to IPV includes Screening, Assessment, Intervention, and Documentation (SAID) (see **Fig. 1**). The first step is screening (see earlier discussion). The second step, assessment, occurs if a patient has a positive screen or self-discloses IPV. Primary care providers must assess for safety after the medical visit, given the risk of homicide when a woman leaves an abusive relationship. Safety assessment should include 5 questions. (1) Has the physical violence increased over the past 6 months? (2) Has your partner used a weapon or threatened you with a weapon? (3) Do you believe your partner is capable of killing you? (4) Have you been beaten while pregnant? (5) Is your partner violently and constantly jealous of you?[37] Yes to 3 or more questions denotes high risk of harm or injury, with sensitivity of 83% and specificity of 56%. The assessment concludes with determining the presence of suicidal ideation, mental health disorders, or substance use disorders.

As highlighted in **Fig. 1** and **Table 2**, the intervention phase of the algorithm starts with nonjudgmental, validating, and supportive statements, such as "you are not alone, and help is available".[24] The intervention step also includes developing a safety plan, particularly for those whose safety assessment reveals a greater risk of injury. Safety planning includes strategies during a violent incident, when preparing to leave a violent relationship, in a patient's home, and through legal means (Appendix 2). Appendix 2 can be given as a handout for patients who disclose current IPV and whose safety assessment shows greater risk of injury. The intervention phase also includes making referrals to on-site or other easily accessible resources (**Box 2**). Primary care providers can refer women to IPV advocates from their health system, local shelters, or the National Domestic Violence Hotline 1-800-799-SAFE. An additional referral can be to home visitation programs. Such a nurse-based program for pregnant, low-income, first-time mothers is the Nurse-Family Partnership (NFP), with locations listed by state at http://www.nursefamilypartnership.org/locations. The SAID intervention phase concludes with treatment of associated health conditions, mandatory reporting if required, and developing follow-up plans.

The documentation phase includes a detailed recording of the patient encounter including responses to screening questions, results from the physical examination,

Table 2 Supportive statements and safety planning for primary care providers to use with patients experiencing intimate partner violence (IPV)		
Supportive statements[24]	1.	This is not your fault.
	2.	No one deserves to be treated this way.
	3.	I'm sorry you've been hurt.
	4.	Do you want to talk about it?
	5.	I am concerned about your and your family's safety.
	6.	Help is available to you.
Safety planning[24]	1.	Pack a bag in advance
	2.	Have personal documents ready
	3.	Hide extra sets of house and car keys
	4.	Establish a code with family or friends
	5.	Plan where to go
Other support by primary care providers[20]	1.	Ask about history of IPV, listening carefully, but do not pressure patient to talk
	2.	Provide practical care and support that responds to patient concerns, but does not intrude
	3.	Remember that risk of homicide is highest within year of patient leaving IPV perpetrator; The patient alone is in the best position to determine what to do, and may prefer to stay with perpetrator
	4.	If unable to provide first-line support or safety planning, ensure that someone else within health care setting or by phone (see **Box 2**) is immediately available to do so

safety assessment, safety planning, referrals, and follow-up plans. Primary care providers can document screening responses and injury locations in the patient's medical record by incorporating Appendix 1 in paper or electronic format. Documentation is important, as IPV victims may use medical records to substantiate reports of abuse, obtain personal protective orders, or gain access to health and human service resources. The medical record can serve as unbiased evidence and factual information, particularly if documented shortly after IPV occurs.[38] However, patients who have previously given their spouse or partner access to their medical record should be aware that this IPV information is at risk of being released unless access is revoked. Primary care providers can use HIPAA to refuse disclosure of health information to family members or patient representatives, if clinicians suspect that the family member or representative has been the perpetrator of IPV or other forms of abuse or neglect.[24]

IPV SCREENING OUTCOMES AND GUIDELINES

There is good support for the ability of screening tools to detect abuse.[25,39] All of the IPV screening instruments include questions for patients, which are administered in various ways: self-administered, on paper or by computer, or via interviews by primary care providers. Maximum sensitivity should be the goal for IPV screening tools, so as to avoid missing affected patients.[33] Both HITS and AAS show high diagnostic accuracy, with sensitivity of 86% or higher.[34] IPV screening tools used by primary care providers should be brief, comprehensive, and tested in diverse populations. Both HITS and AAS have 5 or fewer questions, and each has been tested against more comprehensive measures, including provider interview. The HITS screening tool has been tested with Hispanic and African American women, and includes a Spanish version.

Box 2
Intimate partner violence (IPV) resources for patients and primary care providers

National Domestic Violence Hotline: 800-799-SAFE (7233) and http://www.ndvh.org/

- Provides crisis intervention, information, safety planning, and referral for IPV victims, perpetrators, friends, and families
- Staffed 24 hours a day in English, Spanish, and more than 170 different languages through interpreter services
- IPV resources listed by state are at http://www.thehotline.org/help/resources/

National Coalition Against Domestic Violence: http://www.ncadv.org/

- An advocacy organization working to eliminate IPV and empower victims
- Patients can create a safety plan at http://www.ncadv.org/protectyourself/MyPersonalSafety Plan.php

American Bar Association:

- Offers safety planning and general legal information for primary care providers to use with patients: http://apps.americanbar.org/tips/publicservice/safetipseng.html

Futures Without Violence: http://www.futureswithoutviolence.org/

- Works to prevent violence within the home, and in the community
- Primary care providers can order posters, brochures, safety planning cards, and buttons from health material index at http://www.futureswithoutviolence.org/section/our_work/health/_ health_material

Office on Violence Against Women: http://www.ovw.usdoj.gov/

- US Department of Justice organization that facilitates programs to end IPV
- IPV resources listed by state are at http://www.ovw.usdoj.gov/statedomestic.htm

Adapted from Cronholm PF, Fogarty CT, Ambuel B, et al. Intimate partner violence. Am Fam Physician 2011;83(10):1165–72.

The AAS screening tool has been tested in women with a range of ethnicities, including international settings.[33]

The evidence base is growing for positive patient outcomes from screening. Of 6743 women in a large randomized controlled trial (RCT) evaluating IPV screening versus no screening, no harms were demonstrated.[40] IPV identification questions and a resource list alone do not improve general health outcomes.[41] However, in an RCT of 1044 African American patients who were pregnant or postpartum, the intervention group had IPV counseling that emphasized danger assessment, safety behaviors, and information on community resources. Women in the intervention group had fewer recurrent episodes of IPV during pregnancy and postpartum (adjusted odds ratio, 0.48; 95% confidence interval, 0.29–0.80).[42] In another RCT 360 abused women were randomly assigned to receive either a referral card with a safety plan and resources for IPV services, or a 20-minute nurse case management protocol that included a brochure with a 15-item safety plan, supportive care, anticipatory guidance, and guided referrals. At 2 years both study groups reported fewer threats of abuse, assaults, danger risks for homicide, and increased safety behaviors when compared with their baseline assessment.[43] Home visitation programs have also been shown to improve IPV victimization. An RCT of 643 mothers who gave birth to an infant determined to be at high risk for child maltreatment received a 3-year home visitation program by paraprofessionals from community agencies. The intervention group, which received referrals to IPV shelters, had lower rates of IPV victimization and lower rates of physical assault victimization.[44] The NFP home visitation program for pregnant first-time mothers was shown in an RCT to reduce past 6-month IPV from 13% under control conditions to 6% in the intervention group.[45] The NFP has recently incorporated an IPV curriculum similar to the SAID algorithm.[46] This nurse-based IPV intervention is currently being tested in a 15-site RCT.[47]

The NCG, WHO, and USPSTF guidelines, though differing, recommend SAID as integrated in this review. The NCG advocates for IPV screening at most patient encounters, including new patient encounters or chief complaints, and comprehensive health visits.[24] The WHO and USPSTF guidelines do not describe how frequently primary care providers should screen patients.[20,25] Guidelines from medical organizations present various methods to identify IPV victims, as shown in **Table 3**. The American College of Obstetrics and Gynecology (ACOG) states that health care providers should routinely screen all women at periodic intervals, including at the first prenatal visit, at least once per trimester, and at the postpartum checkup.[1] The American Academy of Family Physicians (AAFP) directly follows USPSTF guidelines, and therefore recommends routine screening of all women of childbearing age.[48] The American Medical Association (AMA) encourages routine screening[49] while the American Academy of Pediatrics (AAP) advises targeted or routine IPV screening.[50] The ACOG, AAFP, AMA, and AAP each recommend assessment, intervention, and documentation as outlined in the SAID algorithm. Without definitive evidence or guidance on how frequently to screen patients, primary care providers can screen annually all women aged 14 to 46 years. Women aged 46 and older may be screened on an annual basis, although screening may be less frequent depending on the presence or absence of associated clinical conditions.

Table 3
Medical organization[a] guidelines for primary care providers to identify intimate partner violence (IPV) victimization[b]

Medical Organization	American College of Obstetrics and Gynecology[1]	American Academy of Family Physicians[48]	American Medical Association[49]	American Academy of Pediatrics[50]
Population	All women	All women age 14–46	All patients	All or some caregivers
Routine or targeted screening	Routine	Routine	Routine	Routine or targeted
Screening tool(s)	AAS and others	HITS and others	c	HITS and others
Frequency of screening	First prenatal visit, at least once per trimester, and at postpartum checkup	c	c	c

Abbreviations: AAS, Abuse Assessment Screen IPV screening instrument; HITS, Hurt, Insult, Threaten, Scream IPV screening instrument.
    [a] Note that National Consensus Guidelines,[24] World Health Organization,[20] and US Preventive Services Task Force[25] guidelines are not listed here, as they are not a specific medical organization. Please refer to text for these guidelines.
    [b] Each medical organization recommends same response to identifying IPV victimization. This response is to address assessment, intervention, and documentation as outlined in SAID (Screening, Assessment, Intervention, and Documentation) algorithm (see **Fig. 1**).
    [c] Not described in guidelines.

CURRENT PRACTICE PATTERNS AND OPTIMIZING PRACTICE ORGANIZATION

Research from the past 2 decades suggests that screening for IPV within primary care settings remains low, ranging from 3% to 10% for routine inquiry in patients without injury[51–55] to as much as 79% when patients present with injuries. More recent data show that fewer than 25% of female patients report that health care professionals ask about IPV.[56,57] These low rates of IPV screening reflect barriers to delivery. IPV screening barriers include primary care providers' lack of comfort with the subject, fear of offending the patient, powerlessness or loss of control, and insufficient time or training.[58,59] Lack of comfort with IPV screening may stem from 12% to 15% of physicians reporting witnessing IPV in their childhood, or experiencing IPV as an adult. Patient barriers to screening include fear of retaliation from an abusive partner, lack of disclosure, fear of police involvement, and cultural differences.[52,59]

There are several key characteristics of practice organization that can improve IPV screening rates. First, primary care offices should develop policies to address IPV victimization among patients, and these office guidelines should include information on mandatory reporting and confidentiality.[60] Second, primary care offices should display educational posters, brochures, and safety planning and resource cards in common areas and private patient locations such as bathrooms.[1] Third, practices should develop and have available IPV referral lists with resources for patients (see **Box 2**). Fourth, clinical staff with patient contact should receive IPV training, often available from local IPV programs.[1,60] Finally, primary care offices can download an IPV quality assessment tool at http://www.futureswithoutviolence.org/section/our_work/health/_family_violence_quality_assessment_tool. This tool for primary care offices addresses IPV screening, assessment, intervention, documentation, and practice organization.[61]

IMPACT OF CHANGES WITHIN HEALTH CARE
The Affordable Care Act

Since August 2012, the Affordable Care Act has required insurance coverage to include IPV screening and counseling at no additional cost to women.[62] Since the beginning of 2013, the Affordable Care Act has mandated that Medicare, Medicaid, and new group and individual insurance plans cover USPSTF-recommended preventive services, which includes IPV screening and counseling for women 14 to 46 years of age.[63] This expanded coverage will likely increase women aged 14 to 46 seeking health services, thereby creating time and workload challenges for primary care providers. Rather than screening all women, primary care providers can inquire routinely for women aged 14 to 46, but screen women aged 46 and older only if the patient has clinical conditions associated with IPV. IPV screening intervals, though not well defined, could be taken as annually for women aged 14 to 46, and for those aged 46 and older only if related clinical conditions develop. Primary care offices can consider saving time by administering the HITS or AAS screening tools before the patient visit, such as while the woman is waiting in private for the provider to meet with her in the examination room. If primary care practices do not have IPV-trained service providers on-site for counseling interventions, they may be able to partner with local IPV programs for access to such resources.

The Patient-Centered Medical Home and Electronic Health Records

The attributes of the patient-centered medical home (PCMH) of improving the quality and safety of health care and making care more patient-centered, comprehensive, and coordinated[64] do not yet have measured effects on IPV identification and response. However, PCMH will likely build long-term provider-patient relationships, and through this women may be more willing to disclose IPV when screened. For example, PCMH concepts of patient-centered and coordinated care can inform how patients are referred to IPV advocates locally or nationally. First, primary care providers should meet with local IPV program professionals, as well as call the National Domestic Violence Hotline, to understand the services they provide. This care coordination can give clinicians a specific name or person to contact when referring patients. Office-based familiarity with community services can increase the likelihood that a patient follows through with a referral, especially when primary care providers offer a patient use of a clinic phone to call an IPV hotline or advocate. Next, when speaking to a woman who discloses IPV, primary care providers can say "I want you to know that there are national hotline numbers with folks who are available 24/7 if you want to talk. They can connect you to local services if you need more urgent help. Also, I know (insert name of local advocate) who I can put you on the phone with right now if you would like to talk to her."[26]

PCMH concepts of patient-centered and coordinated care can also ease the burden of mandatory reporting when a patient does not want it. First, primary care providers should recognize that a report made against a patient's wishes may lead to feelings of helplessness and frustration. Clinicians should inform patients about the process of reporting to help them understand what to expect, and involve them in making the report. These actions can minimize the untoward effects of reporting and give a patient more of a sense of control throughout the process. For example, a primary care provider can say "I do have to make a report, but you are welcome to listen as I call in the report, so you know what is being said and there are no surprises. I can also put in the report any concerns you have about what will happen if your partner finds out about the report." The primary care provider can offer to connect the patient to an IPV advocate on the phone so as to create a safety plan around potential retaliation by her partner after the report is made.[26]

Electronic health records (EHRs) will be central in operationalizing key features of PCMH. Primary care practices could build efficiency by creating EHR-based IPV screening prompts given annually for female patients aged 14 to 46 years.[20] The use of an EHR may improve the accuracy and thoroughness of documentation in instances of suspected or reported abuse. Historically, admission of medical records in court has been limited by legibility and lack of substantial documentation, including timing of abuse, photographs, or body maps of injuries.[38] Documentation in an EHR can eliminate the concern regarding both legibility and accurate timing of the medical evaluation. Many EHRs include integrated "body maps," or outlines of the human body or face, which can be used to draw and document injuries.[38] The AAS screening tool with body map of injury (see Appendix 1) can be used as a template. More recently, EHRs are developing ways to integrate digital images, including using smart-phone or hand-held device applications to directly connect clinical images into the patient record. In addition, primary care providers can use their EHR to generate IPV resource lists for patients.

Both PCMH and EHR can be used to develop and record IPV quality or performance indicators. The quality assessment tool for primary care offices described earlier can be used to define quality measures. In addition, the Joint Commission on Accreditation of Healthcare Organizations (Joint Commission) requires hospitals to identify, refer, and report, as mandated by state law, patients experiencing IPV.[65] The Joint Commission requirements largely follow the SAID algorithm, which can be used as an additional basis for quality or performance indicators in primary care offices.

SUMMARY

IPV encompasses emotional, physical, and sexual violence. In the United States more than 1 out of 3 women experiences IPV victimization in their lifetime, at an annual cost of more than $10 billion. Clinical conditions associated with IPV include mental health and substance use disorders, chronic pain, adverse reproductive outcomes, and traumatic injuries. Short screening instruments such as HITS or the AAS can identify IPV victimization. Nonjudgmental statements that validate an IPV victim's experience should be followed by safety assessment and planning. Intervention includes referral to support services, treatment of associated health conditions, mandatory reporting if required, and documentation. Counseling that emphasizes danger assessment, safety behaviors, and information on community resources has been shown to reduce IPV victimization. Clinical guidelines recommend IPV screening for all or most women, and providing or referring victims to intervention. Low rates of primary care provider IPV screening reflect barriers that may be addressed by practice organization. Changes brought about by the Affordable Care Act will increase coverage for IPV victimization screening and counseling. Although this review limits its focus to IPV against women, many of the strategies for SAID described herein can be adapted for male patients.

ACKNOWLEDGMENTS

The authors thank Cameron Shultz, PhD, MSW and Mack Ruffin IV, MD, MPH for reviewing this article.

REFERENCES

1. ACOG Committee Opinion No. 518: intimate partner violence. Obstet Gynecol 2012;119(2 Pt 1):412–7.
2. Black MC, Basile KC, Breiding MJ, et al. National Intimate Partner and Sexual Violence Survey (NISVS): 2010 summary report. Atlanta (GA): National Center for Injury Prevention and Control, Division of Violence Prevention and Control. Center for Disease Control and Prevention; 2011.
3. Catalano SS, Erica S, Snyder H, et al. Female victims of violence. Washington, DC: U.S. Department of Justice Publications and Materials; 2009. Paper 7.
4. Violence Policy Center. When men murder women: an analysis of 2010 Homicide Data: females murdered by males in single victim/single offender incidents. Washington, DC: 2012. Available at: http://www.vpc.org/studies/wmmw2012. pdf. Accessed March 14, 2014.
5. Campbell JC, Webster D, Koziol-McLain J, et al. Risk factors for femicide in abusive relationships: results from a multisite case control study. Am J Public Health 2003;93(7):1089–97.
6. Bonomi AE, Anderson ML, Reid RJ, et al. Medical and psychosocial diagnoses in women with a history of intimate partner violence. Arch Intern Med 2009; 169(18):1692–7.
7. Bonomi AE, Anderson ML, Rivara FP, et al. Health care utilization and costs associated with physical and nonphysical-only intimate partner violence. Health Serv Res 2009;44(3):1052–67.
8. McCloskey LA, Lichter E, Ganz ML, et al. Intimate partner violence and patient screening across medical specialties. Acad Emerg Med 2005;12(8):712–22.
9. Tjaden P, Thoennes N. Extent, nature and consequences of intimate partner violence: findings from the National Violence Against Women Survey.

Washington, DC: National Institute of Justice and the Centers for Disease Control and Prevention; 2000.

10. Biroscak BJ, Smith PK, Roznowski H, et al. Intimate partner violence against women: findings from one state's ED surveillance system. J Emerg Nurs 2006; 32(1):12–6.

11. Ulrich YC, Cain KC, Sugg NK, et al. Medical care utilization patterns in women with diagnosed domestic violence. Am J Prev Med 2003;24(1):9–15.

12. Rivara FP, Anderson ML, Fishman P, et al. Healthcare utilization and costs for women with a history of intimate partner violence. Am J Prev Med 2007;32(2): 89–96.

13. Fishman PA, Bonomi AE, Anderson ML, et al. Costs changes following cessation of IPV. J Gen Intern Med 2010;25(9):920–5.

14. Liebschutz JM, Rothman EF. Intimate-partner violence—what physicians can do. N Engl J Med 2012;367(22):2071–3.

15. Max W, Rice DP, Finkelstein E, et al. The economic toll of intimate partner violence against women in the United States. Violence Vict 2004;19(3): 259–72.

16. Walton-Moss BJ, Manganello J, Frye V, et al. Risk factors for intimate partner violence and associated injury among urban women. J Community Health 2005;30(5):377–89.

17. Ernst AA, Nick T, Weiss S, et al. Domestic violence in an inner-city ED. Ann Emerg Med 1997;30(2):190–7.

18. Krug EG, Dahlberg LL, Mercy JA, et al. World report on violence and health. Geneva (Switzerland): World Health Organization; 2002.

19. Grisso JA, Schwarz DF, Hirschinger N, et al. Violent injuries among women in an urban area. N Engl J Med 1999;341(25):1899–905.

20. World Health Organization. Responding to intimate partner violence and sexual violence against women: WHO clinical and policy guidelines. Geneva (Switzerland): World Health Organization; 2013.

21. Black MC. Intimate partner violence and adverse health consequences: implications for clinicians. Am J Lifestyle Med 2011;5(5):428–39.

22. Campbell JC. Health consequences of intimate partner violence. Lancet 2002; 359(9314):1331–6.

23. Wu V, Huff H, Bhandari M. Pattern of physical injury associated with intimate partner violence in women presenting to the emergency department: a systematic review and meta-analysis. Trauma Violence Abuse 2010;11(2):71–82.

24. Family Violence Prevention Fund. National Consensus Guidelines on identifying and responding to domestic violence victimization in health care settings. San Francisco (CA): Family Violence Prevention Fund; 2004.

25. Moyer VA. Screening for intimate partner violence and abuse of elderly and vulnerable adults: a U.S. Preventive Services Task Force Recommendation Statement. Ann Intern Med 2013;158(6):478–86.

26. Chamberlain LL, Levenson R. Addressing intimate partner violence, reproductive and sexual coercion: a guide for obstetric, gynecologic and reproductive health care settings. San Francisco (CA): Futures Without Violence; 2012.

27. Durborow N, Lizdas KC, O'Flaherty A, et al. Compendium of state statutes and policies on domestic violence and health care. San Francisco (CA): Family Violence Prevention Fund; 2010. p. 73.

28. Office of Civil Rights. HIPAA Privacy, Disclosures for Public Health Activities. 45 CFR 164.512(b). 2003. Available at: http://www.hhs.gov/ocr/privacy/hipaa/understanding/coveredentities/publichealth.html. Accessed November 23, 2013.

29. Feldhaus KM, Houry D, Utz A, et al. Physicians' knowledge of and attitudes toward a domestic violence mandatory reporting law. Ann Emerg Med 2003;41(1): 159.
30. Smith JS, Rainey SL, Smith KR, et al. Barriers to the mandatory reporting of domestic violence encountered by nursing professionals. J Trauma Nurs 2008;1: 9–11.
31. Sullivan CM, Hagen LA. Survivors' opinions about mandatory reporting of domestic violence and sexual assault by medical professionals. Affilia 2005; 20(3):346–61.
32. Ganley AL. Improving the health care response to domestic violence: a trainer's manual for health care providers. San Francisco (CA): Family Violence Prevention Fund; 1998.
33. Rabin RF, Jennings JM, Campbell JC, et al. Intimate partner violence screening tools: a systematic review. Am J Prev Med 2009;36(5):439–45.e4.
34. Basile KC, Hertz MF, Back SE. Intimate partner violence and sexual violence victimization assessment instruments for use in healthcare settings: version 1. Atlanta (GA): Centers for Disease Control and Prevention, National Center for Injury Prevention and Control; 2007.
35. Sherin KM, Sinacore JM, Li X, et al. HITS: a short domestic violence screening tool for use in a family practice setting. Fam Med 1998;30(7):508–12.
36. Parker B, McFarlane J, Soeken K, et al. Physical and emotional abuse in pregnancy: a comparison of adult and teenage women. Nurs Res 1993;42(3):173–8.
37. Snider C, Webster D, O'Sullivan CS, et al. Intimate partner violence: development of a brief risk assessment for the emergency department. Acad Emerg Med 2009;16(11):1208–16.
38. Isaac NE, Enos VP. Documenting domestic violence: how heath care providers can help victims. Washington, DC: National Institute of Justice; 2001. Research in Brief.
39. Wathen CN, MacMillan HL. Interventions for violence against women: scientific review. JAMA 2003;289(5):589–600.
40. MacMillan HL, Wathen CN, Jamieson E, et al. Screening for intimate partner violence in health care settings: a randomized trial. JAMA 2009;302(5):493–501.
41. Klevens J, Kee R, Trick W, et al. Effect of screening for partner violence on women's quality of life a randomized controlled trial. JAMA 2012;308(7):681–9.
42. Kiely M, El-Mohandes A, El-Khorazaty M, et al. An integrated intervention to reduce intimate partner violence in pregnancy: a randomized controlled trial. Obstet Gynecol 2010;115(2 Pt 1):273–83.
43. McFarlane JM, Groff JY, O'Brien JA, et al. Secondary prevention of intimate partner violence: a randomized, controlled trial. Nurs Res 2006;55:52–61.
44. Bair-Merritt MH, Jennings JM, Chen R, et al. Reducing maternal intimate partner violence after the birth of a child: a randomized, controlled trial of the Hawaii Healthy Start Home Visitation Program. Arch Pediatr Adolesc Med 2010;164: 16–23.
45. Olds DL, Robinson J, Pettitt L, et al. Effects of home visits by paraprofessionals and by nurses: age 4 follow-up results of a randomized trial. Pediatrics 2004; 114:1560–8.
46. Jack SM, Ford-Gilboe M, Wathen CN, et al. Development of a nurse home visitation intervention for intimate partner violence. BMC Health Serv Res 2012;12:50.
47. Olds D, Donelan-McCall N, O'Brien R, et al. Improving the nurse-family partnership in community practice. Pediatrics 2013;132(Suppl 2):S110–7.

48. American Academy of Family Physicians, AAFP clinical recommendations. Intimate partner violence and abuse of elderly and vulnerable adults. 2013. Available at: http://www.aafp.org/patient-care/clinical-recommendations/all/domestic-violence.html?cmpid=_van_280. Accessed November 23, 2013.

49. American Medical Association, H-515.965 Family and intimate partner violence. 2009. Available at: http://www.ama-assn.org/ama1/pub/upload/mm/PolicyFinder/policyfiles/HnE/H-515.965.HTM. Accessed November 23, 2013.

50. Thackeray JD, Hibbard R, Dowd MD. Intimate partner violence: the role of the pediatrician. Pediatrics 2010;125(5):1094–100.

51. Taliaferro E, Salber P. The physician's guide to domestic violence: how to ask the right questions and recognize abuse. Another way to save a life. Volcano (CA): Volcano Press; 1995.

52. Rodriguez MA, Bauer HM, McLoughlin E, et al. Screening and intervention for intimate partner abuse: practices and attitudes of primary care physicians. JAMA 1999;282(5):468–74.

53. Sitterding HA, Adera T, Shields-Fobbs E. Spouse/partner violence education as a predictor of screening practices among physicians. J Contin Educ Health Prof 2003;23(1):54–63.

54. Elliott L, Nerney M, Jones T, et al. Barriers to screening for domestic violence. J Gen Intern Med 2002;17(2):112–6.

55. Chamberlain L, Perham-Hester KA. The impact of perceived barriers on primary care physicians' screening practices for female partner abuse. Women Health 2002;35(2–3):55–69.

56. Kramer A, Lorenzon D, Mueller G. Prevalence of intimate partner violence and health implications for women using emergency departments and primary care clinics. Womens Health Issues 2004;14(1):19–29.

57. Klap R, Tang L, Wells K, et al. Screening for domestic violence among adult women in the United States. J Gen Intern Med 2007;22(5):579–84.

58. Sugg NK, Inui T. Primary care physicians' response to domestic violence. Opening Pandora's box. JAMA 1992;267(23):3157–60.

59. Sprague S, Madden K, Simunovic N, et al. Barriers to screening for intimate partner violence. Women Health 2012;52:587–605.

60. O'Campo P, Kirst M, Tsamis C, et al. Implementing successful intimate partner violence screening programs in health care settings: evidence generated from a realist-informed systematic review. Soc Sci Med 2011;72(6):855–66.

61. Zink T, Fisher BS. Family violence quality assessment tool for primary care offices. Qual Manag Health Care 2007;16(3):265–79.

62. James L, Schaeffer S. Futures without violence. Interpersonal and domestic violence screening and counseling: understanding new federal rules and providing resources for health providers. 2012. http://www.futureswithoutviolence.org/userfiles/file/HealthCare/FWV-screening_memo_Final.pdf. Accessed November 24, 2013.

63. Health Affairs. Health policy brief: preventive services without cost sharing. Bethesda (MD): Health Affairs; 2010. Available at: http://healthaffairs.org/healthpolicybriefs/brief_pdfs/healthpolicybrief_37.pdf. Accessed November 24, 2013.

64. American Academy of Family Physicians, American Academy of Pediatrics, American College of Physicians, American Osteopathic Association. Joint principles of the patient-centered medical home. 2007. Available at: http://www.aafp.org/dam/AAFP/documents/practice_management/pcmh/initiatives/PCMHJoint.pdf. Accessed November 24, 2013.

65. Futures without violence, comply with the joint commission standard PC.01.02.09 on Victims of Abuse. 2009. Available at: http://www.futureswithoutviolence.org/section/our_work/health/_health_material/_jcaho. Accessed November 24, 2013.
66. Singh V. Academic men's health: case studies in clinical practice intimate partner violence perpetration. J Men Health 2009;6(4):383–92.
67. Kimberg LS. Addressing intimate partner violence with male patients: a review and introduction of pilot guidelines. J Gen Intern Med 2008;23(12):2071–8.
68. Maryland Department of Health and Mental Hygiene. Intimate partner violence. a guide for health care providers. 2013. Available at: http://phpa.dhmh.maryland.gov/mch/Documents/IPV%20Guide%20for%20providers.January.pdf. Accessed November 24, 2013.
69. Cronholm PF, Fogarty CT, Ambuel B, et al. Intimate partner violence. Am Fam Physician 2011;83(10):1165–72.

APPENDIX 1: ABUSE ASSESSMENT SCREEN QUESTIONS AND BODY MAP

1) Have you ever been emotionally or physically abused by your partner or someone important to you?

    Yes ☐   No ☐

    If yes by whom? _____

    Total number of times _____

2) Within the last year, have you been hit, slapped, kicked or otherwise physically hurt by someone?

    Yes ☐   No ☐

    If yes by whom? _____

    Total number of times _____

3) Since you've been pregnant, have you been hit, slapped, kicked, or otherwise physically hurt by someone?

    Yes ☐   No ☐

    If yes by whom? _____

    Total number of times _____

4. Within the last year, has anyone forced you to have sexual activities?

    Yes ☐   No ☐

    If yes by whom? _____

    Total number of times _____

5. Are you afraid of your partner or anyone you listed above?

    Yes ☐   No ☐

MARK THE AREA OF INJURY ON A BODY MAP AND SCORE EACH INCIDENT ACCORDING TO THE FOLLOWING SCALE.

If any of the descriptions for the higher number apply, use the higher number.

1 = Threats of abuse including use of a weapon

2 = Slapping, pushing; no injuries and/or lasting pain

3 = Punching, kicking, bruises, cuts, and/or continuing pain

4 = Beating up, severe contusions, burns, broken bones

5 = Head injury, internal injury, permanent injury

6 = Use of weapon; wound from weapon

From Family Violence Prevention Fund. National Consensus Guidelines on identifying and responding to domestic violence victimization in health care settings. San Francisco (CA): Family Violence Prevention Fund; 2004.

APPENDIX 2: SAFETY PLANNING HANDOUT FOR PATIENTS WHO DISCLOSE IPV

Step 1:

Safety during a violent incident. I can use some or all of the following strategies:

A. If I have/decide to leave my home, I will go _____

B. I can tell _____ (neighbors) about the violence and request they call the police if they hear suspicious noises coming from my house.

C. I can teach my children how to use the telephone to contact the police.

D. I will use _____ as my code word so someone can call for help.

E. I can keep my purse/car keys ready at (place)_____, in order to leave quickly.

F. I will use my judgment and intuition. If the situation is very serious, I can give my partner what he/she wants to calm him/her down. I have to protect myself until I/we are out of danger.

Step 2:

Safety when preparing to leave. I can use some or all of the following safety strategies:

A. I will keep copies important documents, keys, clothes and money at _____

B. I will open a savings account by _____ , to increase my independence.

C. Other things I can do to increase my independence include: _____.

D. I can keep change for my phone calls on me at all times. I understand that if I use my telephone credit card, the telephone bill will show my partner those numbers that I called after I left.

E. I will check with _____ and my advocate to see who would be able to let me stay with them or lend me some money.

F. If I plan to leave, I won't tell my abuser in advance face-to-face, but I will call or leave a note from a safe place.

Step 3:

Safety in my own residence. Safety measures I can use include:

A. I can change the locks on my doors and windows as soon as possible.

B. I can replace wooden doors with steel/metal doors.

C. I can install additional locks, window bars, poles to wedge against doors, and electronic systems etc.

D. I can install motion lights outside.

E. I will teach my children how to make a collect call to _____ if my partner takes the children.

F. I will tell people who take care of my children that my partner is not permitted to pick up my children.

G. I can inform _____ (neighbor) that my partner no longer resides with me and they should call the police if he is observed near my residence.

Step 4.

Safety with a protection order. The following are steps that help the enforcement of my protection order.

A. Always carry a certified copy with me and keep a photocopy.

B. I will give my protection order to police departments in the community where I work and live.

C. I can get my protection order to specify and describe all guns my partner may own and authorize a search for removal.

From Family Violence Prevention Fund. National Consensus Guidelines on identifying and responding to domestic violence victimization in health care settings. San Francisco (CA): Family Violence Prevention Fund; 2004.

An Update on Breast Cancer Screening and Prevention

Maria Syl D. de la Cruz, MD[a],*, Mona Sarfaty, MD, MPH[a],
Richard C. Wender, MD[a,b]

KEYWORDS

- Breast cancer risk assessment • Breast cancer screening • Breast cancer prevention
- Mammography • Breast MRI • Guidelines

KEY POINTS

- Risk assessment is a key component for determining an individual's options for breast cancer screening and prevention.
- A primary care clinician needs to be able to identify risk factors that place a woman at higher-than-average risk for breast cancer, and if needed, place the appropriate referral for genetic counseling and risk-reduction assessment.
- Mammography is universally recommended for women ages 50 to 74, with the frequency of screening (annually or biennially) to be determined by individual patient preferences and a balance of net harms and benefits.
- Although guidelines generally recommend offering screening for women ages 40 to 49, some place additional emphasis on a shared decision-making model between patient and providers.
- Preventive measures, such as physical activity, tobacco cessation, limiting alcohol use, and maintaining a healthy weight, should be encouraged for all women to reduce breast cancer risk, and chemoprevention with selective estrogen receptor modulators is an important consideration for women at high risk from breast cancer.

INTRODUCTION

Breast cancer, the most common noncutaneous cancer among women in the United States, kills more women every year than nearly all other cancers, falling second only to lung cancer.[1,2] Surveillance estimates suggest more than 230,000 women will be diagnosed with breast cancer in 2014, and the disease will claim an estimated 40,000 lives.[3]

Conflict of Interest: None.
[a] Department of Family and Community Medicine, Thomas Jefferson University, 833 Chestnut Street, Suite 301, Philadelphia, PA 19107, USA; [b] American Cancer Society, 250 Williams Street, Atlanta, GA 30303, USA
* Corresponding author.
E-mail address: MariaSyl.delaCruz@jefferson.edu

Prim Care Clin Office Pract 41 (2014) 283–306
http://dx.doi.org/10.1016/j.pop.2014.02.006
0095-4543/14/$ – see front matter © 2014 Elsevier Inc. All rights reserved.
primarycare.theclinics.com

In the 1980s and 1990s, the incidence of diagnosed breast cancer rose because of an increase in mammography screening. The incidence then decreased sharply from 2002 to 2003, largely attributable to a reduction in the use of hormone replacement therapy following findings from the Women's Health Initiative.[4] Since 2003, the incidence of diagnosed breast cancer has remained relatively stable.[1]

Mortality rates from breast cancer have declined steadily since 1990. Among women younger than 50, death rates have decreased on average by 3.2% per year; the rate of decline has been slightly lower in women older than 50, at approximately 2.0% per year.[5] Continued improvements in cancer detection and treatment are the primary reasons for this drop[6]; however, not all segments of the population have benefited equally. Mortality rates, for example, have declined more slowly among blacks than whites, despite blacks' lower incidence rate. Age-adjusted mortality based on 2006 to 2010 surveillance data show the breast cancer incidence rate was 121.4 cases per 100,000 black women versus 127.4 cases per 100,000 white women; mortality, however, was 30.8 deaths per 100,000 black women versus 22.1 deaths per 100,000 white women.[5] The 5-year (2003–2009) relative survival rate is also lower for black women versus white women, at 78.7% versus 90.4%, respectively.[5] This disparity has been attributed to multiple factors, including more aggressive tumors, social conditions, access to high-quality health care, differences in detection (including screening behaviors), health system factors, and treatment differences.[7–12]

RISK ASSESSMENT FOR BREAST CANCER

Risk factor assessment is critically important for breast cancer screening. Women should be divided into high-risk or average-risk categories to guide screening options and risk-reduction strategies. Although screening programs traditionally use age as the primary risk factor, the individual's collective risk factors determine the net benefits and harms of additional screening, such as genetic testing, or interventions to reduce risk, such as chemoprevention.

Risk Factors

Age
The most important risk factor for breast cancer is age. Approximately 10% of women are diagnosed between ages 35 and 44, 22% are diagnosed between ages 45 and 54, and 25% are diagnosed between ages 55 and 64. Median age for diagnosis is 61 years, and the median age at death is 68 years.[5]

Family history and heritable gene mutations
Family history of breast or ovarian cancers on either the maternal or paternal side are also important risk factors, particularly in women diagnosed at younger than 45 years.[13] Women who have one first-degree female relative with breast cancer have a 1.8 times higher risk of developing breast cancer compared with women with no family history. Having 2 first-degree relatives with breast or ovarian cancer increases breast cancer risk by almost threefold; for women with 3 or more relatives, risk jumps by almost fourfold.[14] An estimated 10% of breast cancers can be attributed to an inherited gene mutation. BRCA1 and BRCA2 gene mutations are involved in hereditary breast and ovarian cancers, which occur with higher frequency in certain ethnic groups, such as the Ashkenazi Jewish population. Other more rare mutations include TP53 and PTEN, which are associated with Li-Fraumeni syndrome and Cowden syndrome, both of which lead to an increased risk for breast cancer. The mutation in the CDH1 gene involved with hereditary diffuse gastric cancer also predisposes women to an increased risk for lobular breast cancer.[13]

Clinical factors
Clinical factors that increase the risk of breast cancer include a history of proliferative lesions with atypia, history of chest irradiation, and breast density. Atypical ductal hyperplasia and atypical lobular hyperplasia increase risk by about 4 to 5 times compared with the average woman.[15] Risk is approximately doubled to 8 to 10 times for women with lobular carcinoma in situ (LCIS).[16] Women who received high-dose chest radiation at a younger age (≤30 years), such as for Hodgkin lymphoma, have higher incidence rates, starting about 8 years after radiation treatment.[17] High breast tissue density, a measure of the amount of glandular tissue relative to fatty tissue in the breast, has been shown to be a strong risk factor for the development of breast cancer.[18] Women with high breast tissue density have a 4 to 6 times increased risk of breast cancer compared with women with less-dense breast tissue.[19–21] High-density breast tissue also makes the detection of breast cancer by mammography more difficult.[20]

Reproductive factors
Factors that involve prolonged hormonal exposure may increase the risk for developing breast cancer, including early menarche, low parity, older age at first live birth, late menopause, and hormone replacement therapy (estrogen plus progestins). Conversely, factors that may be associated with decreased hormonal exposure, such as premature menopause (before age 40), may decrease the risk for developing breast cancer.[22] Other factors that may confer a protective effect include a younger age at first full-term pregnancy (<30 years), a higher number of pregnancies,[23] and breastfeeding, particularly for more than 1 year.[24] A summary of the important risk factors for breast cancer is listed in **Table 1**.

Risk Factor Tools

The National Cancer Institute developed a tool based on the Gail model to estimate a woman's 5-year risk and lifetime risk of invasive breast cancer.[25] This instrument, the Breast Cancer Risk Assessment Tool, includes reproductive risk factors (age of menarche, parity, age at first birth, breastfeeding, age at menopause), first-degree relatives with breast cancer, previous breast biopsies with or without atypical hyperplasia, and race. It is accessible online for free at http://cancer.gov/bcrisktool/default.aspx. However, the model cannot be applied to women who are younger than 35 years or who have LCIS, ductal carcinoma in situ, or invasive cancer. It is also not appropriate for women with a strong family history of breast cancer, as it does not include maternal second-degree or third-degree relatives with breast cancer, paternal family history, male breast cancer, or ovarian cancer.[26] For women with a strong family history of breast or ovarian cancer, other statistical models should be used (BRCAPRO, http://bcb.dfci.harvard.edu/bayesmendel/brcapro.php, or BOADICEA, http://ccge.medschl.cam.ac.uk/boadicea/).[27] For more information about the various instruments, go to the following National Cancer Institute Web page: http://www.cancer.gov/cancertopics/pdq/genetics/breast-and-ovarian/HealthProfessional/page1. If the lifetime risk for an individual woman is 20% or higher, then increased surveillance with different imaging studies and risk-reduction options should be reviewed with a health care professional.[13]

The primary care clinician
The primary care clinician's role involves identifying women who have a greater-than-average lifetime risk of developing breast cancer and designing a screening and risk-reduction strategy in concert with the patient. The identification of women who meet criteria to consider genetic testing and their referral to a genetic counselor constitutes

Table 1 Risk factors for breast cancer	
Relative Risk	**Factor**
>4.0	• Age (65+ vs <65 y, although risk increases across all ages until age 80) • Biopsy-confirmed atypical hyperplasia • Certain inherited genetic mutations for breast cancer (*BRCA1* and/or *BRCA2*) • Lobular carcinoma in situ • Mammographically dense breasts • Personal history of early onset (<40 y) breast cancer • Two or more first-degree relatives with breast cancer diagnosed at an early age
2.1–4.0	• Personal history of breast cancer (40+ y) • High endogenous estrogen or testosterone levels (postmenopausal) • High-dose radiation to chest • One first-degree relative with breast cancer
1.1–2.0	• Alcohol consumption • Ashkenazi (Eastern European) Jewish heritage • Diethylstilbestrol (DES) exposure • Early menarche (<12 y) • Height (tall) • High socioeconomic status • Late age at first full-term pregnancy (>30 y) • Late menopause (>55 y) • Never breastfed a child • No full-term pregnancies • Obesity (postmenopausal)/adult weight gain • Personal history of endometrium, ovary, or colon cancer • Recent and long-term use of menopausal hormone therapy containing estrogen and progestin • Recent oral contraceptive use

Adapted from American Cancer Society. Breast Cancer Facts & Figures 2013–2014. Atlanta (GA): American Cancer Society, Inc. 2013. p. 12.

a clear primary care responsibility. The referral criteria for genetic testing for hereditary breast and ovarian cancer syndrome and further genetic risk assessment is reviewed in **Box 1** and **Table 2**. Additional online resources on how to order genetic testing and how to find a genetic counselor are available in **Box 2**.

BREAST CANCER PREVENTION

A summary of recommendations for the primary prevention of breast cancer is outlined in **Box 3**.

Obesity, Physical Activity, Dietary Content

Obesity is a risk factor for postmenopausal breast cancer, as a higher amount of fat tissue increases estrogen levels and subsequent risk. Weight gain specifically has been associated with an increased risk for breast cancer.[28] In a prospective cohort of more than 80,000 women, those who gained 55 pounds or more after age 18 years had an almost 50% higher risk of breast cancer. After menopause, women who gained 22 pounds or more had an 18% higher risk.[29] Data on weight loss in relation to breast cancer risk is less clear. The Nurses' Health Study showed women with a sustained weight loss of 22 pounds or more since menopause and who had never used postmenopausal hormone replacement therapy had a lower breast cancer risk than women

---

Box 1
National Comprehensive Cancer Network criteria for referral for genetic testing for hereditary breast and/or ovarian cancer syndrome

- Individual from family with known *BRCA1/BRCA2* mutation
- Personal history of breast cancer plus 1 or more of the following:
  - Diagnosed at age ≤45 years
  - Presence of 2 primary breast cancers when first breast cancer diagnosis occurred at age ≤50 years
  - Diagnosed age ≤50 years with ≥1 close relative[a] with breast cancer at any age or with limited family history
  - Diagnosed age ≤60 years with a triple negative breast cancer
  - Diagnosed any age with ≥1 close relative[a] with breast cancer age ≤50 years
  - Diagnosed any age with ≥2 close relatives[a] with breast cancer at any age
  - Diagnosed any age with ≥1 close relative[a] with epithelial ovarian cancer[b]
  - Diagnosed any age with ≥2 close relatives[a] with pancreatic cancer or prostate cancer[c] at any age
  - Close male relative[a] with breast cancer
  - For individual of Ashkenazi Jewish heritage, no additional family history may be required
- Personal history of epithelial ovarian cancer[b]
- Personal history of male breast cancer
- Personal history of pancreatic cancer or prostate cancer[c] at any age with ≥2 close relatives[a] with breast and/or ovarian[b] and/or pancreatic or prostate cancer[c] at any age
- Family history only[d]
  - First-degree or second-degree relative meeting any of above criteria
  - Third-degree relative with breast cancer and/or ovarian cancer[a] with ≥2 close relatives[a] with breast cancer (at least one age ≤50 years) and/or ovarian cancer[b]

[a] First-, second-, or third-degree relative.
[b] Includes fallopian tube and primary peritoneal cancers.
[c] Gleason score ≥7.
[d] Significant limitations of interpreting test results for an unaffected individual should be discussed. Testing of unaffected individuals should be considered only when an appropriate affected family member is unavailable for testing. Clinical judgment should be used to determine if the patient has reasonable likelihood of a mutation, considering the unaffected patient's current age and the age of female unaffected relatives who link the patient with the affected relatives.

Adapted with permission from the NCCN Clinical Practice Guidelines in Oncology (NCCN Guidelines®) for Genetic/Familial Risk Assessment: Breast and Ovarian V.4.2013. © 2013 National Comprehensive Cancer Network, Inc. All rights reserved. The NCCN Guidelines® and illustrations herein may not be reproduced in any form for any purpose without the express written permission of the NCCN. To view the most recent and complete version of the NCCN Guidelines, go online to NCCN.org. NATIONAL COMPREHENSIVE CANCER NETWORK®, NCCN®, NCCN GUIDELINES®, and all other NCCN Content are trademarks owned by the National Comprehensive Cancer Network, Inc.

---

who simply maintained their weight.[29] However, another prospective cohort study in postmenopausal women found no association between a median weight loss of 11 pounds and a reduction in breast cancer, although this weight loss was not sustained in all women during the 5-year follow-up.[30] Studies in women who have undergone

Table 2
National Comprehensive Cancer Network criteria for referral for genetic risk assessment

An Affected Individual with 1 or More of the Following	An Unaffected Individual with a Family History of 1 or More of the Following
• A known mutation in a breast cancer susceptibility gene within the family	• A known mutation in a breast cancer susceptibility gene within the family
• Early age-at-onset breast cancer	• ≥2 breast primaries in single individual
• Triple negative (ER-/PR-/HER2-) breast cancer	• ≥2 individuals with breast primaries on same side of family
• Two breast cancer primaries in a single individual	• ≥1 ovarian cancer[a] primary from the same side of family
• Breast cancer at any age, and ○ ≥1 close relative[b] with breast cancer age ≤50 y, or ○ ≥1 close relative[b] with epithelial ovarian cancer[a] at any age ○ ≥2 close relatives[b] with breast cancer and/or pancreatic cancer at any age ○ From a population at increased risk	• First- or second-degree relative with breast cancer age ≤45 y
• ≥1 family member on same side of family with a combination of breast cancer and ≥1 of the following: pancreatic cancer, prostate cancer,[c] sarcoma, adrenocortical carcinoma, brain tumors, endometrial cancer, leukemia/lymphoma, thyroid cancer, dermatologic manifestations and/or macrocephaly, hamartomatous polyps of gastrointestinal tract, diffuse gastric cancer	• ≥1 family member on same side of family with a combination of breast cancer and ≥1 of the following: pancreatic cancer, prostate cancer,[c] sarcoma, adrenocortical carcinoma, brain tumors, endometrial cancer, leukemia/lymphoma, thyroid cancer, Cowden syndrome, hamartomatous polyps of gastrointestinal tract, diffuse gastric cancer
• Ovarian cancer[a]	• Male breast cancer
• Male breast cancer	

[a] Includes fallopian tube and primary peritoneal cancers.
[b] First-, second-, or third-degree relative.
[c] Gleason score ≥7.

Adapted with permission from the NCCN Clinical Practice Guidelines in Oncology (NCCN Guidelines®) for Genetic/Familial Risk Assessment: Breast and Ovarian V.4.2013. © 2013 National Comprehensive Cancer Network, Inc. All rights reserved. The NCCN Guidelines® and illustrations herein may not be reproduced in any form for any purpose without the express written permission of the NCCN. To view the most recent and complete version of the NCCN Guidelines, go online to NCCN.org. NATIONAL COMPREHENSIVE CANCER NETWORK®, NCCN®, NCCN GUIDELINES®, and all other NCCN Content are trademarks owned by the National Comprehensive Cancer Network, Inc.

bariatric surgery suggest that surgical weight loss may be associated with a decreased risk of breast cancer.[31,32] Using simulation modeling data, approximately 5.5% of breast cancer cases expected to occur in 2025 will be attributable to obesity. By 2025, the investigators estimated there would be approximately 3300 to 5700 fewer breast cancer deaths in women age 25 years or older if obesity was eradicated.[33]

There is growing evidence of a decreased risk of breast cancer with increased physical activity, particularly for postmenopausal women and women with hormone receptor–negative tumors.[34,35] The European Prospective Investigation into Cancer and Nutrition, a large prospective cohort study including more than 250,000 women, found an inverse association between breast cancer risk and moderate to high levels of total physical activity compared with those lowest in physical activity. For women

---

Box 2
Resources for genetic testing and genetic counseling

American Cancer Society—Genetic Testing: What You Need to Know

- http://www.cancer.org/cancer/cancercauses/geneticsandcancer/genetictesting/genetic-testing-what-you-need-to-know-toc

National Society for Genetic Counselors—The "Consumer Information" link on the Web site has information on genetic counseling, questions to ask before genetic testing, a guide to collecting family history, information on genetic testing and genetic counselors, and a directory of genetic counselors

- www.nsgc.org

American Board for Genetic Counseling—Additional information on how to find a genetic counselor

- http://www.abgc.net/ABGC/AmericanBoardofGeneticCounselors.asp

National Cancer Institute—List of services related to cancer genetics (cancer risk assessment, genetic counseling, genetic susceptibility testing)

- www.cancer.gov/cancertopics/genetics/directory

---

diagnosed after age 50 years, the largest risk reduction was associated with the highest amount of physical activity; for women diagnosed before age 50 years, the largest risk reduction was associated with moderate total physical activity. Both estrogen receptor–positive and progesterone receptor–positive cancers were inversely associated with moderate and high physical activity, suggesting that increased activity may lower concentrations of hormones and their related effect on estrogen-sensitive tumors. Other mechanisms through which physical activity may mitigate risk include reduced chronic inflammation, increased antioxidant enzymes, and an improved immune system.[36]

The data linking dietary factors to breast cancer risk remains inconclusive and inconsistent. Three large reviews including prospective studies did not show a strong association between dietary factors (fruit and vegetables, total fat intake, fat

---

Box 3
Summary of recommendations for primary prevention for breast cancer

Factors that are associated with an *increased risk* of breast cancer:

- Obesity (weight gain important, weight loss less clear)
- Tobacco (current and previous use)
- Alcohol use (3–14 drinks/week)

Factors that are associated with a *decreased risk* of breast cancer:

- Physical activity (moderate to high levels)
- Chemoprevention with SERMS (recommended for women age 35 or older at high risk for breast cancer and at low risk for medication adverse events, such as thromboembolic disease)

Factors that are associated with an *unknown relation to risk* of breast cancer:

- Dietary content (fruits; vegetables; total fat; vitamins A, C, E; beta-carotene; antioxidants; carbohydrates; dairy soy)

From Refs.[27–62]

biomarkers, vitamins [A, C, E, and beta-carotene], antioxidants, carbohydrates, dairy, soy) and risk for breast cancer.[37–39] A recent prospective study specifically looked at the role of total dietary fiber and its main food sources (vegetables, fruit, cereals, and legumes) with relation to breast cancer risk. After a median follow-up of 11.5 years, the investigators found that a high dietary intake of total fiber and a high intake of fiber from vegetables were both associated with a decreased breast cancer risk, but not fiber from fruit, cereals, or legumes. The association between fiber and breast cancer risk was not modified by body mass index, waist-hip ratio, or alcohol consumption. The role of dietary fiber still remains unclear in breast cancer risk, and further studies are needed to elucidate the relationship between dietary content and breast cancer prevention.[40]

Tobacco

Studies have shown a strong association between current and previous tobacco use and risk of breast cancer. In a prospective cohort study of almost 80,000 women, current smokers had a 16% higher risk of breast cancer and former smokers had a 9% increased risk over nonsmokers. This increased breast cancer risk remained up to 20 years after smoking cessation. For nonsmokers, a very high exposure to passive smoking (defined as ≥10 years' exposure in childhood, ≥20 years' exposure as an adult at home, and ≥10 years' exposure as an adult at work) resulted in a 32% increased risk of breast cancer compared with those never exposed to secondhand smoke.[41] Another study including nearly 3000 women found a significant increased risk of all-cause mortality in women who smoked either 15 to 24 cigarettes or 25+ cigarettes per day, with the highest risk for women who smoked the highest quantity. Overall, women who smoked for 20+ pack-years had a 54% increase in breast cancer mortality and an 81% increase in all-cause mortality.[42]

Alcohol

Alcohol use has been found to be associated with an increased risk of breast cancer in a number of studies.[43–45] Women who consumed 3 to 14 drinks per week had a 12% increased risk of breast cancer for every drink (10 g of alcohol) consumed per day[46]; this dose-dependent risk is independent of the specific type of alcoholic beverage.[43,45,46] The mechanism linking alcohol consumption to increased breast cancer risk may be alcohol's capacity to raise circulating concentrations of sex hormones.[46–48] Evidence does not support an association between alcohol intake and increased breast cancer risk among women who were past users or are current users of hormone replacement therapy when compared with those never using the therapy.[46,49–51]

Chemoprevention for Patients at High Risk: Selective Estrogen Receptor Modulators

Randomized trials have shown that chemoprevention with drugs like tamoxifen and raloxifene reduces breast cancer risk. In 1998, the first randomized trial with more than 13,000 women demonstrated that tamoxifen could reduce the risk of breast cancer in high-risk women with estrogen receptor–positive tumors.[52] Breast cancer risk was decreased by 42% in the tamoxifen group after an average of 7 years of follow-up compared with the control group. This protective effect continued for up to 10 years after completion of the 5-year treatment. Although tamoxifen was associated with a lower risk of breast cancer, the net benefit was reduced as a result of an increase in the risks of endometrial cancer, stroke, venous thromboembolism, cataracts, and vasomotor symptoms. However, tamoxifen also demonstrated the potential benefit of fracture reduction, particularly in postmenopausal women.[53,54] Despite this decrease in breast cancer risk, no trials with tamoxifen have shown an effect on all-cause mortality or breast cancer–specific mortality.[55–58]

Raloxifene, a drug originally studied for osteoporosis prevention, was also observed to decrease the risk of breast cancer.[59] In the Study of Tamoxifen and Raloxifene trial, raloxifene was nearly as effective as tamoxifen in preventing invasive breast cancer and had a lower risk of side effects. As observed with tamoxifen, this risk reduction effect applies only to the development of estrogen receptor–positive breast cancer. No difference was found in the number of deaths between tamoxifen and raloxifene.[60] Other trials also have failed to show a mortality benefit for raloxifene, but, notably, they lacked sufficient power to detect significant differences in mortality over their course of follow-up.[61,62]

An updated meta-analysis of more than 80,000 women found that 4 selective estrogen receptor modulators (SERMS) (tamoxifen, raloxifene, arzoxifene, and lasofoxifene) reduced breast cancer by 38% compared with the control group. An increased rate of endometrial cancer was mostly limited to the tamoxifen trials. Risk for venous thromboembolism was similar between tamoxifen and raloxifene, with a slightly increased rate with arzoxifene and lasofoxifene. All SERMS had similar risk reduction for fractures, and no effect of SERMs was found for myocardial infarction, stroke, or transient ischemic attacks.[54]

Because of the risk of adverse effects, SERMS are recommended only for women at high risk for breast cancer. The National Comprehensive Cancer Network Clinical Practice Guidelines In Oncology (NCCN Guidelines) for Breast Cancer Risk Reduction recommend tamoxifen as an option in women 35 years or older, with a life expectancy of 10 years or longer, who have had LCIS, or have a 1.7% or higher 5-year risk for breast cancer by the modified Gail model.[63] Tamoxifen is the more favorable choice of a risk-reduction agent compared with raloxifene for most postmenopausal women, based on results that showed less continued benefit of raloxifene compared with tamoxifen after cessation.[60,63]

BREAST CANCER SCREENING FOR WOMEN AT AVERAGE RISK

A summary of recommendations for breast cancer screening in average-risk women is listed in **Table 3**.

Mammography

Ages 40 to 49 years

Multiple studies have evaluated the benefits and harms of screening in women ages 40 years and older, but few have specifically evaluated the age group of women aged 40 to 49. The Age Trial looked specifically at women between the ages of 39 and 41 years, who were randomized to participate in annual mammography until age 48. The reduction in breast cancer mortality in the test group was not statistically significant after 10.7 years of follow-up; however, adjusting for noncompliance in women actually screened showed an estimated 24% reduction in mortality risk. Moreover, a meta-analysis of 8 trials (including the Age Trial) showed a 16% reduced risk in breast cancer mortality.[64] Some of this benefit is likely attributable to the inclusion of women up to age 49 years at entry in all studies except the Age Trial.[50] In a reanalysis of the Gothenburg trial looking at women aged 39 to 49 years, screening mammography was found to reduce risk by 31% for breast cancer mortality after 13 years of follow-up.[65] After combining data from 7 randomized trials, only 3 of which used adequate randomization, an updated Cochrane review found a 19% risk reduction in breast cancer mortality after 7 years and a 20% reduction after 13 years; however,

Table 3
Summary of screening recommendations for women at average risk from breast cancer

Screening Modality	US Preventive Services Task Force	Canadian Task Force on the Periodic Health Examination	American Cancer Society	National Comprehensive Cancer Network[a]	American Academy of Family Physicians	American College of Obstetricians and Gynecologists	American College of Radiology
Breast self-examination	Do not recommend	Do not recommend	Breast self-awareness encouraged	Breast self-awareness encouraged	Do not recommend	Breast self-awareness encouraged	—
Clinical breast examination	Insufficient evidence	Every 1–2 y starting at age 40	Every 3 y from ages 20 to 39, then annually	Every 1–3 y from ages 20 to 39, then annually	Insufficient evidence	Every 1–3 y from ages 20 to 39, then annually	—
Mammography	Every 2 y for women ages 50 to 74	Annually for women ages 50 to 74	Annually beginning at age 40	Annually beginning at age 40	Every 2 y for women ages 50 to 74	Annually beginning at age 40	Annually beginning at age 40

[a] Referenced with permission from the NCCN Clinical Practice Guidelines in Oncology (NCCN Guidelines®) for Breast Cancer Screening and Diagnosis V.2.2013. © National Comprehensive Cancer Network, Inc 2013. All rights reserved. To view the most recent and complete version of the guideline, go online to www.nccn.org. Accessed November 19, 2013. NATIONAL COMPREHENSIVE CANCER NETWORK®, NCCN®, NCCN GUIDELINES®, and all other NCCN Content are trademarks owned by the National Comprehensive Cancer Network, Inc.

Data from Tria Tirona M. Breast cancer screening update. Am Fam Physician 2013;87(4):277.

when the 3 trials with adequate randomization were examined alone, no statistically significant effect was detected.[66]

Conducting its own systematic review, the US Preventative Services Task Force (USPSTF) reported that mammography reduces breast cancer mortality by 15% for women aged 40 to 49 years, with overdiagnosis estimates varying between 1% and 10%[67]; these findings are similar to those reported by the Canadian Task Force on Preventive Health Care (CTFPHC).[68] Both the USPSTF and CTFPHC report an increased rate of false positives in women aged 40 to 49 years; hence, they both recommend that women ages 40 to 49 make an informed and shared decision on whether or not to participate in mammography screening. Neither group endorses routine screening of all women aged 40 to 49 years in the absence of shared decision making.[67,68] Other groups, notably, the American College of Obstetricians and Gynecologists (ACOG), the American Cancer Society (ACS), and the NCCN, continue to recommend routine screening in women 40 to 49. These groups cite evidence that the mortality risk reduction associated with screening younger women is comparable to the benefit observed in screening older women.[69–71] They also judged that the balance of benefits and harms favored a strategy of routine screening for all younger women. In addition, a large case-control study published after release of the USPSTF and CTFPHC guidelines suggests a lack of screening in women aged 40 to 49 years is associated with a higher death rate from breast cancer. Among 609 confirmed breast cancer deaths, 71% occurred in women who were not screened regularly, whereas 29% occurred in women who had been screened with mammography. In this study, the death rate from breast cancer was actually higher in women younger than 50 years compared with women 50 years or older.[72]

Ages 50 to 69 years
Screening mammography in women aged 50 to 69 years has been proven in multiple randomized trials to reduce breast cancer mortality from 15% to 20%.[65–68,73–79] Based on the higher incidence of breast cancer in this age group and the evidence of reduction on breast cancer mortality, cancer screening guidelines continue to recommend screening mammography. However, there is still debate over the frequency at which screenings should occur. The USPSTF commissioned screening models by 6 independent groups within the Cancer Intervention and Surveillance Modeling Network to identify the most efficient screening strategy. The investigators found that the method of starting screening at age 50 years and continuing biennially to age 69 years strikes the right balance between decreasing breast cancer mortality against potential harms.[80] However, some guideline groups continue to recommend offering annual screening, whereas others emphasize that the decision about screening frequency should be shared with the patient, based on their personal values.

Ages 70 years and older
Results from the Swedish Two-County trial of women aged 70 to 74 years showed no reduction in mortality with breast cancer screening.[77] However, the CTFPHC notes that the absolute benefits of mammography in women aged 70 to 74 years are likely comparable to those for women aged 50 to 69 years because of the higher absolute risk in older women. The CTFPHC therefore recommends routine mammography every 2 to 3 years in women aged 70 to 74 years as a weak recommendation based on low-quality evidence.[68] Similarly, the USPSTF continues to recommend biennial screening until age 74 for women who are in good health.[67] Overall, the decision to continue screening beyond the age of 75 years should take into account individual patient circumstances and preferences.

Breast Ultrasound

Breast ultrasound has been studied particularly for screening women with high breast density due to the lower sensitivity of mammography in these patients. One study found that 42% of all women with nonpalpable invasive breast cancer had their cancers detected only with screening ultrasound, and 37% of all cancers in women with dense breasts were detected only with screening ultrasound.[81] In another study of women with dense breast tissue who received either mammography plus ultrasound or mammography alone, supplemental ultrasound detected an additional 4.2 cancers per 1000 women.[82] Although these studies show promising results for the use of ultrasound in women with high breast density, at this time there is no recommendation for performing ultrasound as part of routine breast cancer screening.

Breast Self-Examination

A few large trials have analyzed the effect of instructing women in breast self-examination (BSE) on reducing breast cancer mortality. The UK Trialists study, a nonrandomized study with 16 years of follow-up, showed no significant difference in breast cancer mortality between the BSE and control groups.[83] A Cochrane review included randomized trials comparing BSE with control groups in both Russia[84] and Shanghai,[85] with each study showing no significant differences in breast cancer mortality after 13 and 11 years, respectively.[86] Furthermore, these trials show women performing BSE had an increased number of breast biopsies (53%) and they were not more likely to be diagnosed with breast cancer compared with women who were not taught BSE after 5 years of follow-up.[87] Another study showed that women 40 and older who performed more frequent or longer BSE were more likely to have a diagnostic mammography or ultrasound.[88] Overall, these findings do not support regular BSE as an effective screening method for decreasing breast cancer mortality.

Although no screening organization now recommends routine instruction of women in BSE, several organizations making recommendations do promote the concept of breast self-awareness. The ACS, the NCCN, and ACOG all promote teaching patients about breast self-awareness, the concept that a woman should be familiar with her own breasts and bring any changes to the attention of her health provider. Women should still be encouraged to report new breast changes, but they are not advised to perform a specific self-examination technique.[69–71]

Clinical Breast Examination

The efficacy of the clinical breast examination (CBE) has been investigated in a few large trials. In community settings assessing CBE as part of the National Early Detection Program, CBE detected 5.1% of breast cancers that were not detected by mammography and therefore could have been missed with mammography alone. The procedure for conducting a CBE was not reported, but the estimated sensitivity (ability of the test to correctly identify those patients with the disease[89]) for CBE was 58.8% and specificity (ability of the test to correctly identify those patients without the disease[89]) was 93.4%,[90] similar to previous estimates. In a Canadian study of 300,000 women aged 50 to 69, CBE increased the rate of detection of small invasive cancers over mammography alone by a small amount, between 2% and 6%. Trained nurses or physicians performed the CBE, which included visual inspection followed by a systematic 10-minute examination.[91] None of these trials showed a significant difference in breast cancer mortality between screening with combined mammography and CBE compared with mammography alone.[92]

The USPSTF found a lack of evidence to recommend for or against breast cancer screening with CBE apart from mammography.[93] The utility of CBE as a detection method, however, has relied on its performance characteristics. The variation of CBE techniques performed by clinicians makes it challenging to assess the efficacy of the clinical examination in routine practice, which may not meet the standards of the Canadian trial. Most professional guideline groups advocate incorporating CBE as long as it is performed correctly. Per the ACS recommendations, after visual inspection and palpation of lymph nodes, the examiner should use the pads of the middle 3 fingers using circular motions, to cover the area down the midaxillary line, across the inframammary ridge at the fifth/sixth rib, up the lateral edge of the sternum, across the clavicle, and back to the midaxilla. A vertical strip pattern is preferred over the concentric circle pattern, and the examination should palpate at increasing levels of pressure (superficial, intermediate, and deep).[94]

BREAST CANCER SCREENING FOR WOMEN AT HIGH RISK

The recommendations for screening and risk reduction for women at high risk from breast cancer are summarized in **Table 4**.

Magnetic Resonance Imaging

In April 2007, the ACS released guidelines on the use of annual breast magnetic resonance imaging (MRI) in addition to mammography for breast cancer screening in women at high risk. This includes women who have an approximate lifetime risk of 20% or higher; namely, those who are *BRCA* mutation carriers, first-degree relatives of known *BRCA* mutation carriers who have not undergone genetic testing, women who received chest irradiation between 10 and 30 years ago, Li-Fraumeni syndrome and first-degree relatives, and Cowden and Bannayan-Riley-Ruvalcaba syndromes and their first-degree relatives. Insufficient evidence for screening with MRI exists for LCIS, atypical ductal hyperplasia, heterogeneously dense breasts, women with a personal history of breast cancer, or women with a lifetime risk of less than 20%.[95]

Although not exclusive to *BRCA* 1 and 2 carriers, MRI combined with mammography has a higher sensitivity compared with mammography alone (70%–97% and 23%–41%, respectively)[96]; however, specificity is lower with the combined method (75%–97%) versus mammography alone (93%–99%) because of the high number of false positives with MRI.[96] Although studies show that breast MRI screening of *BRCA1* and *BRCA2* mutation carriers detects breast cancer earlier and more frequently than mammography, none has demonstrated an improvement in mortality or survival, largely related to the difficulty in conducting adequately large clinical trials.[96–103]

NCCN recommendations, for women who are *BRCA1/BRCA2* mutation carriers, include breast awareness starting at age 18, a CBE every 6 to 12 months, annual mammogram and MRI starting at age 25, a discussion of risk-reducing mastectomy and risk-reducing salpingo-oophorectomy, and consideration of chemoprevention.[13] For a more detailed discussion, see NCCN Guidelines Genetic/Familial Risk Assessment for Breast Cancer.[13]

CURRENT PRACTICE PATTERNS

The release of the 2009 USPSTF recommendations instigated public debate among advocacy and specialty organizations regarding the changes to individualized consultation and decision making for screening mammography for the 40 to 49 age group. Initial studies have assessed changes to practice patterns since the new recommendation. The National Health Interview Survey asked 27,829 women aged 40 and older to

Table 4
Screening and risk-reduction recommendations for women at high risk from breast cancer

Risk Factor	Clinical Breast Examination	Breast Self-Awareness	Mammography	MRI	Risk-Reduction Options
BRCA mutation carrier	Every 6 mo	Yes	Annually starting at age 25	Annually starting at age 25	Mastectomy bilateral salpingo-oophorectomy Tamoxifen/raloxifene
20% or greater lifetime risk	Every 6–12 mo	Yes	Annually starting 5–10 y before youngest breast cancer diagnosis in family	Offer	Tamoxifen/raloxifene
5-y risk 1.7% or greater based on modified Gail model	Every 6–12 mo	Yes	Annually beginning at age 40	Offer	Tamoxifen/raloxifene
History of thoracic ionizing radiation	Every 6–12 mo	Yes	Annually beginning at age 25 or 8–10 y after radiation exposure	Offer	
Biopsy with LCIS or atypical hyperplasia	Every 6–12 mo	Yes	Annually beginning at time of diagnosis	Offer	Tamoxifen/raloxifene Mastectomy for LCIS (controversial)

Abbreviations: LCIS, lobular carcinoma in situ; MRI, magnetic resonance imaging.
Adapted from Griffin JL, Pearlman MD. Breast cancer screening in women at average risk and high risk. Obstet Gynecol 2010;116(6):1417; with permission.

self-report mammography screening in the past year. Although there was a slight increase in the age-adjusted rates of self-reported mammography from 2008 to 2011, 2011 rates were not significantly different compared with 2008 for women in any age group.[104] Similarly, the Medical Expenditure Panel Surveys analyzed the biennial mammography rate for almost 30,000 women in 3 different age groups (40–49, 50–74, and 75 and older), and found no statistically significant difference in mammography rates between 2010 and earlier years (pooled rate 2006–2009) for any age group.[105]

Various studies also have evaluated screening preferences and differences based on specialty. In a web-based survey[106] of 11,922 primary care physicians, more than 95% recommended screening mammography to women aged 50 to 69 years, regardless of specialty. However, for women 40 to 49 years old, 94% of obstetrician gynecologists always recommended mammography compared with 81% of internal medicine physicians and 84% of family medicine physicians. Similarly, for women ages 70 and older, 86% of obstetrician gynecologists always recommended screening mammography compared with 67% for internal medicine and 59% for family medicine physicians.

Another survey[107] led by the National Cancer Institute asked 1212 primary care physicians about their breast cancer screening practices. The ACS guidelines were cited as the most influential (56%), followed by ACOG (47%), USPSTF (42%), American Academy of Family Physicians (32%), and American College of Physicians (25%) guidelines. More than two-thirds of all physicians recommended mammography to women aged 40 to 49 annually compared with more than 90% of all physicians who recommended annual mammography to women 50 years and older. Also, both family medicine and internal medicine physicians were more likely to no longer recommend screening at a certain age (30.2% and 37.8%, respectively) than obstetrician gynecologists (14.0%). Despite the varying recommendations, ultimately it is the responsibility of the provider to discuss the net harms and benefits of breast cancer screening with each patient to determine individual screening preferences.

BARRIERS TO DELIVERY

Despite having access to health care, many women are not being screened.[108] National Medicare data demonstrate that only 64% of eligible woman (65 and older) have had a mammogram within the previous 2 years. Screening rates in Medicare-eligible women who have family incomes less than 100% of the federal poverty rate are even lower (51%).[109] Furthermore, use of screening mammography varies by race and ethnicity. Hispanic, Asian, and foreign-born women who have lived in the United States for less than 10 years have lower rates of screening compared with other women.[108]

Several factors influence a woman's decision to obtain screening services. According to one systematic review, barriers that affect a woman's decision to obtain screening include concerns about mammography safety, pain associated with the procedure, language and cultural differences, provider biases, lack of social support, and lack of knowledge.[110] A report by the Institute of Medicine in 2003 revealed a major influencing factor was a woman's knowledge about the risk of breast cancer and the benefits of screening.[111] In a study of 20 focus groups with women from multiple racial and ethnic backgrounds,[112] the major reasons for not getting a repeat mammogram included concerns about test efficacy, time needed to schedule appointments, competing family demands, and concern about radiation exposure. Regardless of age, some women did not think they were at high risk for breast cancer because of a negative family history. The most commonly cited barriers to breast cancer screening in a 2006 survey of primary care physicians[113] included a lack of patient follow-through on mammography, lack of insurance coverage for screening, and lack of time to discuss screening. These barriers could be better addressed if providers were aware of the aforementioned patient concerns and the lack of education on screening.

Another challenge to breast cancer screening is ensuring appropriate follow-up of abnormal results. Minority women and those with poorer socioeconomic status are less likely to have timely follow-up after abnormal screening results and are more often diagnosed with late-stage disease. In a study of women with late-stage breast cancer at the time of diagnosis, 52% were not screened according to guidelines and 8% did not receive timely follow-up of their abnormal mammograms.[114] However, a wide variability in quality of care exists for cancer screening diagnosis and follow-up of abnormal tests, even among patients with insurance.[115]

Racial disparities in breast cancer include the discrepancy in mortality rates between blacks compared with whites. Cook County (Illinois, USA) investigators who analyzed 25,900 cases of breast cancer found that black women were more likely to be diagnosed at later stages than white women at any age after evaluating by stage, geocode, race/ethnicity, and socioeconomic status. Hispanic women were also likely to have a later diagnosis than white women up until approximately age 68. Poverty also was a predictor of being diagnosed with breast cancer at a later stage.[116] In another study, black women had a statistically significant lower 5-year survival rate (55.9%) compared with white women (68.8%). After matching for presentation characteristics, white patients were more likely to receive treatment compared with black patients, mean time from diagnosis to treatment was longer for black patients, and black patients were less likely to receive treatment with chemotherapy and more likely to receive breast-conserving surgery without other treatment compared with white patients. These presentation characteristics accounted for most of the difference in the absolute survival rates between black and white women. Compared with white patients, black patients had a poorer state of health at time of diagnosis with a higher number of comorbidities, more advanced disease, and worse prognostic features (eg, estrogen receptor status).[117]

IMPACT OF CHANGES WITHIN HEALTH CARE
Affordable Care Act

A review including 195 research studies with 4.8 million US women found that a lack of health insurance was a major predictor of women not obtaining mammography.[110] As the Affordable Care Act is fully implemented, the expansion of Medicaid along with subsidized state insurance exchanges and elimination of cost sharing is expected to improve access to breast cancer screening for many women. The US Census Bureau's 2009 American Community Survey of adults aged 18 to 64 estimated that approximately 2.8 million low-income women aged 40 to 64 will gain health insurance as a result of the Affordable Care Act.[118] This translates into an additional 500,000 women who will receive breast cancer screening in the first year of the act, and an estimated additional 1 million more over the subsequent 2 years.[116]

Patient-Centered Medical Home and the Electronic Health Record

The creation of a patient-centered medical home (PCMH) focused on preventive health and care coordination will help deliver cost-effective, efficient primary care. To accomplish this goal, PCMH approaches to care need to effectively identify women who are eligible to be screened, particularly targeting underscreened groups, such as racial and ethnic minorities. Health assessment tools, detailing a complete family history, the clinical team, and electronic health record (EHR) systems, can help to identify people who should be screened. The EHR can flag patients who are at high risk based on personal and family risk factors entered into the system by the clinical team. Outreach efforts can be conducted through electronic reminders, mail, or telephone to assist with scheduling and addressing screening concerns.[119] The collection of data on screening practices and breast cancer trends within the medical home can guide the delivery of preventive services, especially regarding current mammography use and geographic disparities. For example, women who live in rural areas of the United States have a significantly lower rate of breast cancer screening compared with women living in urban areas.[120] Because there is limited time in an office visit, the use of multicultural and multilingual decision aids (video, online, and print education tools) can help address the barriers of health literacy and lack of knowledge about the benefits and risks of screening. Patient navigators, defined as those assigned to helping patients overcome barriers to care, can assist with patient education, language and cultural issues, scheduling appointments, transportation, or other logistical problems. The use of the EHR also can contribute to more effective cancer-screening outreach efforts, such as identifying screening-eligible women and triggering follow-up of abnormal screening results.[119,121] In a study investigating EHR use and quality measures, investigators found that breast cancer screening improved by nearly 4.5% in sites using EHRs.[122]

SUMMARY

Risk stratification in breast cancer prevention and screening is a key component to reduce breast cancer mortality. Preventive measures, such as physical activity, tobacco cessation, limiting alcohol use, and maintaining a healthy weight, should continue to be emphasized as part of a healthy lifestyle and to minimize breast cancer risk. Chemoprevention with selective estrogen receptor modulators is also an important consideration for women who are at high risk for developing breast cancer. Identifying women who have a greater-than-average lifetime risk of breast cancer and referring them for genetic testing or counseling is a significant responsibility of the primary care provider. Given the variable guideline recommendations, a shared decision-making model will increasingly become an essential tool for primary care providers in counseling patients on cancer-screening options. Primary care providers will need to incorporate patients' personal and family risk factors, individual preferences, and recommended guidelines to provide their patients with appropriate screening and risk-reduction recommendations. Although implementation of the Affordable Care Act provides an opportunity to increase screening rates, public health efforts should continue to develop a comprehensive and collaborative model to reduce health disparities in breast cancer screening, prevention, and treatment.

ACKNOWLEDGMENTS

The authors thank Amy Burzinski for her assistance with the preparation of this article.

REFERENCES

1. Centers for Disease Control and Prevention. Cancer prevention and control: cancer in women. Available at: http://www.cdc.gov/cancer/dcpc/data/women.htm. Accessed November 18, 2013.

2. United States cancer statistics: 1999–2010 incidence and mortality web-based report. Atlanta (GA): U.S. Department of Health and Human Services, Centers for Disease Control and Prevention and National Cancer Institute; 2013.

3. Cancer facts and figures 2014. Atlanta (GA): American Cancer Society; 2014.

4. Ravdin PM, Cronin KA, Howlader N, et al. The decrease in breast-cancer incidence in 2003 in the United States. N Engl J Med 2007;356(16):1670–4.

5. Howlader N, Noone AM, Krapcho M, et al. SEER cancer statistics review, 1975-2010. Bethesda (MD): National Cancer Institute; 2013.

6. Berry DA, Cronin KA, Plevritis SK, et al. Effect of screening and adjuvant therapy on mortality from breast cancer. N Engl J Med 2005;353(17):1784–92.

7. DeSantis C, Siegel R, Bandi P, et al. Breast cancer statistics, 2011. CA Cancer J Clin 2011;61(6):409–18.

8. Virnig BA, Baxter NN, Habermann EB, et al. A matter of race: early- versus late-stage cancer diagnosis. Health Aff (Millwood) 2009;28(1):160–8.

9. Smith GL, Shih YC, Xu Y, et al. Racial disparities in the use of radiotherapy after breast-conserving surgery: a national Medicare study. Cancer 2010;116(3):734–41.

10. Ademuyiwa FO, Edge SB, Erwin DO, et al. Breast cancer racial disparities: unanswered questions. Cancer Res 2011;71(3):640–4.

11. Sheppard VB, Isaacs C, Luta G, et al. Narrowing racial gaps in breast cancer chemotherapy initiation: the role of the patient-provider relationship. Breast Cancer Res Treat 2013;139(1):207–16.

12. Wheeler SB, Reeder-Hayes KE, Carey LA. Disparities in breast cancer treatment and outcomes: biological, social, and health system determinants and opportunities for research. Oncologist 2013;18(9):986–93.

13. NCCN Clinical Practice Guidelines in Oncology (NCCN Guidelines®) for Genetic/Familial Risk Assessment: Breast and Ovarian V.4.2013. © National Comprehensive Cancer Network, Inc 2013. Available at: www.nccn.org. Accessed November 18, 2013.

14. Collaborative Group on Hormonal Factors in Breast Cancer. Familial breast cancer: collaborative reanalysis of individual data from 52 epidemiological studies including 58,209 women with breast cancer and 101,986 women without the disease. Lancet 2001;358(9291):1389–99.

15. Collins LC, Baer HJ, Tamimi RM, et al. Magnitude and laterality of breast cancer risk according to histologic type of atypical hyperplasia: results from the nurses' health study. Cancer 2007;109(2):180–7.

16. Page DL, Kidd TE Jr, Dupont WD, et al. Lobular neoplasia of the breast: higher risk for subsequent invasive cancer predicted by more extensive disease. Hum Pathol 1991;22(12):1232–9.

17. Breast cancer facts and figures 2013-2014. Atlanta (GA): American Cancer Society, Inc; 2013.

18. McCormack VA, dos Santos Silva I. Breast density and parenchymal patterns as markers of breast cancer risk: a meta-analysis. Cancer Epidemiol Biomarkers Prev 2006;15(6):1159–69.

19. Cummings SR, Tice JA, Bauer S, et al. Prevention of breast cancer in postmenopausal women: approaches to estimating and reducing risk. J Natl Cancer Inst 2009;101(6):384–98.

20. Boyd NF, Guo H, Martin LJ, et al. Mammographic density and the risk and detection of breast cancer. N Engl J Med 2007;356(3):227–36.

21. Harvey JA, Bovbjerg VE. Quantitative assessment of mammographic breast density: relationship with breast cancer risk. Radiology 2004;230(1):29–41.

22. Pearlman MD, Griffin JL. Benign breast disease. Obstet Gynecol 2010;116(3): 747–58.
23. Kelsey JL, Gammon MD, John EM. Reproductive factors and breast cancer. Epidemiol Rev 1993;15(1):36–47.
24. Collaborative Group on Hormonal Factors in Breast Cancer. Breast cancer and breastfeeding: collaborative reanalysis of individual data from 47 epidemiological studies in 30 countries, including 50,302 women with breast cancer and 96,973 women without the disease. Lancet 2002;360(9328): 187–95.
25. Breast cancer risk assessment tool. Available at: http://www.cancer.gov/bcrisktool/about-tool.aspx#gail. Accessed November 18, 2013.
26. Griffin JL, Pearlman MD. Breast cancer screening in women at average risk and high risk. Obstet Gynecol 2010;116(6):1410–21.
27. Claus EB, Risch N, Thompson WD. The calculation of breast cancer risk for women with a first degree family history of ovarian cancer. Breast Cancer Res Treat 1993;28(2):115–20.
28. Food, nutrition, physical activity, and the prevention of cancer: a global perspective. Washington, DC: AICR; 2007. Report No: World Cancer Research Fund/American Institute for Cancer Research.
29. Eliassen AH, Colditz GA, Rosner B, et al. Adult weight change and risk of postmenopausal breast cancer. JAMA 2006;296(2):193–201.
30. Teras LR, Goodman M, Patel AV, et al. Weight loss and postmenopausal breast cancer in a prospective cohort of overweight and obese US women. Cancer Causes Control 2011;22(4):573–9.
31. Christou NV, Lieberman M, Sampalis F, et al. Bariatric surgery reduces cancer risk in morbidly obese patients. Surg Obes Relat Dis 2008;4(6):691–5.
32. McCawley GM, Ferriss JS, Geffel D, et al. Cancer in obese women: potential protective impact of bariatric surgery. J Am Coll Surg 2009;208(6):1093–8.
33. Mandelblatt J, van Ravesteyn N, Schechter C, et al. Which strategies reduce breast cancer mortality most: a collaborative modeling of optimal screening, treatment, and obesity prevention. Cancer 2013;119(14):2541–8, 34.
34. Peters TM, Schatzkin A, Gierach GL, et al. Physical activity and postmenopausal breast cancer risk in the NIH-AARP diet and health study. Cancer Epidemiol Biomarkers Prev 2009;18(1):289–96.
35. Friedenreich CM, Cust AE. Physical activity and breast cancer risk: impact of timing, type and dose of activity and population subgroup effects. Br J Sports Med 2008;42(8):636–47.
36. Steindorf K, Ritte R, Eomois PP, et al. Physical activity and risk of breast cancer overall and by hormone receptor status: the European prospective investigation into cancer and nutrition. Int J Cancer 2013;132(7):1667–78.
37. Smith-Warner SA, Spiegelman D, Yaun SS, et al. Intake of fruits and vegetables and risk of breast cancer: a pooled analysis of cohort studies. JAMA 2001; 285(6):769–76.
38. Michels KB, Mohllajee AP, Roset-Bahmanyar E, et al. Diet and breast cancer: a review of the prospective observational studies. Cancer 2007;109(Suppl 12): 2712–49.
39. van Gils CH, Peeters PH, Bueno-de-Mesquita HB, et al. Consumption of vegetables and fruits and risk of breast cancer. JAMA 2005;293(2):183–93.
40. Ferrari P, Rinaldi S, Jenab M, et al. Dietary fiber intake and risk of hormonal receptor-defined breast cancer in the European prospective investigation into cancer and nutrition study. Am J Clin Nutr 2013;97(2):344–53.

41. Luo J, Margolis KL, Wactawski-Wende J, et al. Association of active and passive smoking with risk of breast cancer among postmenopausal women: a prospective cohort study. BMJ 2011;342:d1016.

42. Saquib N, Stefanick ML, Natarajan L, et al. Mortality risk in former smokers with breast cancer: pack-years vs. smoking status. Int J Cancer 2013;133(10): 2493–7.

43. Key J, Hodgson S, Omar RZ, et al. Meta-analysis of studies of alcohol and breast cancer with consideration of the methodological issues. Cancer Causes Control 2006;17(6):759–70.

44. Baan R, Straif K, Grosse Y, et al. Carcinogenicity of alcoholic beverages. Lancet Oncol 2007;8(4):292–3.

45. Smith-Warner SA, Spiegelman D, Yaun SS, et al. Alcohol and breast cancer in women: a pooled analysis of cohort studies. JAMA 1998;279(7):535–40.

46. Allen NE, Beral V, Casabonne D, et al. Moderate alcohol intake and cancer incidence in women. J Natl Cancer Inst 2009;101(5):296–305.

47. Dorgan JF, Baer DJ, Albert PS, et al. Serum hormones and the alcohol–breast cancer association in postmenopausal women. J Natl Cancer Inst 2001;93(9): 710–5.

48. Rinaldi S, Peeters PH, Bezemer ID, et al. Relationship of alcohol intake and sex steroid concentrations in blood in pre- and post-menopausal women: the European prospective investigation into cancer and nutrition. Cancer Causes Control 2006;17(8):1033–43.

49. Hamajima N, Hirose K, Tajima K, et al. Alcohol, tobacco and breast cancer—collaborative reanalysis of individual data from 53 epidemiological studies, including 58 515 women with breast cancer and 95 067 women without the disease. Br J Cancer 2002;87(11):1234–45.

50. Tjonneland A, Christensen J, Olsen A, et al. Alcohol intake and breast cancer risk: the European prospective investigation into cancer and nutrition (EPIC). Cancer Causes Control 2007;18(4):361–73.

51. Terry MB, Zhang FF, Kabat G, et al. Lifetime alcohol intake and breast cancer risk. Ann Epidemiol 2006;16(3):230–40.

52. Fisher B, Costantino JP, Wickerham DL, et al. Tamoxifen for prevention of breast cancer: report of the National Surgical Adjuvant Breast and Bowel Project P-1 study. J Natl Cancer Inst 1998;90(18):1371–88.

53. Fisher B, Costantino JP, Wickerham DL, et al. Tamoxifen for the prevention of breast cancer: current status of the National Surgical Adjuvant Breast and Bowel Project P-1 study. J Natl Cancer Inst 2005;97(22):1652–62.

54. Cuzick J, Sestak I, Bonanni B, et al. Selective oestrogen receptor modulators in prevention of breast cancer: an updated meta-analysis of individual participant data. Lancet 2013;381(9880):1827–34.

55. Cuzick J, Forbes JF, Sestak I, et al. Long-term results of tamoxifen prophylaxis for breast cancer—96-month follow-up of the randomized IBIS-I trial. J Natl Cancer Inst 2007;99(4):272–82.

56. Veronesi U, Maisonneuve P, Rotmensz N, et al. Tamoxifen for the prevention of breast cancer: late results of the Italian randomized tamoxifen prevention trial among women with hysterectomy. J Natl Cancer Inst 2007;99(9):727–37.

57. Powles TJ, Ashley S, Tidy A, et al. Twenty-year follow-up of the Royal Marsden randomized, double-blinded tamoxifen breast cancer prevention trial. J Natl Cancer Inst 2007;99(4):283–90.

58. Cuzick J, Powles T, Veronesi U, et al. Overview of the main outcomes in breast-cancer prevention trials. Lancet 2003;361(9354):296–300.

59. Cummings SR, Eckert S, Krueger KA, et al. The effect of raloxifene on risk of breast cancer in postmenopausal women: results from the MORE randomized trial. JAMA 1999;281(23):2189–97.
60. Vogel VG, Costantino JP, Wickerham DL, et al. Update of the National Surgical Adjuvant Breast and Bowel Project study of tamoxifen and raloxifene (STAR) P-2 trial: preventing breast cancer. Cancer Prev Res (Phila) 2010;3(6):696–706.
61. Martino S, Cauley JA, Barrett-Connor E, et al. Continuing outcomes relevant to evista: breast cancer incidence in postmenopausal osteoporotic women in a randomized trial of raloxifene. J Natl Cancer Inst 2004;96(23):1751–61.
62. Barrett-Connor E, Mosca L, Collins P, et al. Effects of raloxifene on cardiovascular events and breast cancer in postmenopausal women. N Engl J Med 2006; 355(2):125–37.
63. NCCN Clinical Practice Guidelines in Oncology (NCCN Guidelines®) for Breast Cancer Risk Reduction V.1.2013. © National Comprehensive Cancer Network, Inc 2013. Available at: www.nccn.org. Accessed November 18, 2013.
64. Moss SM, Cuckle H, Evans A, et al. Effect of mammographic screening from age 40 years on breast cancer mortality at 10 years' follow-up: a randomised controlled trial. Lancet 2006;368(9552):2053–60.
65. Bjurstam N, Bjorneld L, Warwick J, et al. The Gothenburg breast screening trial. Cancer 2003;97(10):2387–96.
66. Gotzsche PC, Jorgensen KJ. Screening for breast cancer with mammography. Cochrane Database Syst Rev 2013;(6):CD001877.
67. Nelson HD, Tyne K, Naik A, et al. Screening for breast cancer: an update for the U.S. Preventive Services Task Force. Ann Intern Med 2009;151(10):727–37, W237–42.
68. Tonelli M, Connor Gorber S, Joffres M, et al, Canadian Task Force on Preventive Health Care. Recommendations on screening for breast cancer in average-risk women aged 40-74 years. CMAJ 2011;183(17):1991–2001.
69. American College of Obstetricians-Gynecologists. Practice bulletin no. 122: breast cancer screening. Obstet Gynecol 2011;118(2 Pt 1):372–82.
70. Smith RA, Brooks D, Cokkinides V, et al. Cancer screening in the United States, 2013. CA Cancer J Clin 2013;63(2):87–105.
71. NCCN Clinical Practice Guidelines in Oncology (NCCN Guidelines®) for Breast Cancer Screening and Diagnosis V.2.2013. © National Comprehensive Cancer Network, Inc 2013. Available at: www.nccn.org. Accessed November 19, 2013.
72. Webb ML, Cady B, Michaelson JS, et al. A failure analysis of invasive breast cancer: most deaths from disease occur in women not regularly screened. Cancer 2013. [Epub ahead of print].
73. Independent UK Panel on Breast Cancer Screening. The benefits and harms of breast cancer screening: an independent review. Lancet 2012;380(9855): 1778–86.
74. Andersson I, Aspegren K, Janzon L, et al. Mammographic screening and mortality from breast cancer: the Malmo mammographic screening trial. BMJ 1988; 297(6654):943–8.
75. Frisell J, Lidbrink E, Hellstrom L, et al. Followup after 11 years—update of mortality results in the Stockholm mammographic screening trial. Breast Cancer Res Treat 1997;45(3):263–70.
76. Miller AB, To T, Baines CJ, et al. Canadian National Breast Screening Study-2: 13-year results of a randomized trial in women aged 50-59 years. J Natl Cancer Inst 2000;92(18):1490–9.

77. Nystrom L, Andersson I, Bjurstam N, et al. Long-term effects of mammography screening: updated review of the Swedish randomised trials. Lancet 2002; 359(9310):909–19.
78. Shapiro S. Periodic screening for breast cancer: the HIP (Health Insurance Plan) randomized controlled trial. J Natl Cancer Inst Monogr 1997;22:27–30.
79. Tabar L, Vitak B, Chen HH, et al. The Swedish two-county trial twenty years later: updated mortality results and new insights from long-term follow-up. Radiol Clin North Am 2000;38(4):625–51.
80. Mandelblatt JS, Cronin KA, Bailey S, et al. Effects of mammography screening under different screening schedules: model estimates of potential benefits and harms. Ann Intern Med 2009;151(10):738–47.
81. Kolb TM, Lichy J, Newhouse JH. Comparison of the performance of screening mammography, physical examination, and breast US and evaluation of factors that influence them: an analysis of 27,825 patient evaluations. Radiology 2002;225(1):165–75.
82. Berg WA, Blume JD, Cormack JB, et al. Combined screening with ultrasound and mammography vs mammography alone in women at elevated risk of breast cancer. JAMA 2008;299(18):2151–63.
83. 16-year mortality from breast cancer in the UK trial of early detection of breast cancer. Lancet 1999;353(9168):1909–14.
84. Semiglazov VF, Manikhas AG, Moiseenko VM, et al. Results of a prospective randomized investigation [Russia (St. Petersburg)/WHO] to evaluate the significance of self-examination for the early detection of breast cancer. Vopr Onkol 2003;49(4):434–41.
85. Thomas DB, Gao DL, Ray RM, et al. Randomized trial of breast self-examination in Shanghai: final results. J Natl Cancer Inst 2002;94(19):1445–57.
86. Kosters JP, Gotzsche PC. Regular self-examination or clinical examination for early detection of breast cancer. Cochrane Database Syst Rev 2003;(2):CD003373.
87. Hackshaw AK, Paul EA. Breast self-examination and death from breast cancer: a meta-analysis. Br J Cancer 2003;88(7):1047–53.
88. Tu SP, Reisch LM, Taplin SH, et al. Breast self-examination: self-reported frequency, quality, and associated outcomes. J Cancer Educ 2006;21(3):175–81.
89. Lalkhen AG, McCluskey A. Clinical tests: sensitivity and specificity. Cont Educ Anaesth Crit Care Pain 2008;8(6):221–3.
90. Bobo JK, Lee NC, Thames SF. Findings from 752 081 clinical breast examinations reported to a national screening program from 1995 through 1998. J Natl Cancer Inst 2000;92(12):971–6.
91. Bancej C, Decker K, Chiarelli A, et al. Contribution of clinical breast examination to mammography screening in the early detection of breast cancer. J Med Screen 2003;10(1):16–21.
92. Kerlikowske K, Grady D, Rubin SM, et al. Efficacy of screening mammography: a meta-analysis. JAMA 1995;273(2):149–54.
93. Humphrey LL, Helfand M, Chan BK, et al. Breast cancer screening: a summary of the evidence for the U.S. Preventive Services Task Force. Ann Intern Med 2002;137(5 Part 1):347–60.
94. Saslow D, Hannan J, Osuch J, et al. Clinical breast examination: practical recommendations for optimizing performance and reporting. CA Cancer J Clin 2004;54(6):327–44.
95. Saslow D, Boetes C, Burke W, et al. American Cancer Society guidelines for breast screening with MRI as an adjunct to mammography. CA Cancer J Clin 2007;57(2):75–89.

96. Warner E, Messersmith H, Causer P, et al. Systematic review: using magnetic resonance imaging to screen women at high risk for breast cancer. Ann Intern Med 2008;148(9):671–9.

97. Kriege M, Brekelmans CT, Boetes C, et al. Efficacy of MRI and mammography for breast-cancer screening in women with a familial or genetic predisposition. N Engl J Med 2004;351(5):427–37.

98. Kuhl CK, Schrading S, Leutner CC, et al. Mammography, breast ultrasound, and magnetic resonance imaging for surveillance of women at high familial risk for breast cancer. J Clin Oncol 2005;23(33):8469–76.

99. Leach MO, Boggis CR, Dixon AK, et al. Screening with magnetic resonance imaging and mammography of a UK population at high familial risk of breast cancer: a prospective multicentre cohort study (MARIBS). Lancet 2005;365(9473): 1769–78.

100. Kriege M, Brekelmans CT, Boetes C, et al. Differences between first and subsequent rounds of the MRISC breast cancer screening program for women with a familial or genetic predisposition. Cancer 2006;106(11):2318–26.

101. Warner E, Plewes DB, Hill KA, et al. Surveillance of BRCA1 and BRCA2 mutation carriers with magnetic resonance imaging, ultrasound, mammography, and clinical breast examination. JAMA 2004;292(11):1317–25.

102. Sardanelli F, Podo F, Santoro F, et al. Multicenter surveillance of women at high genetic breast cancer risk using mammography, ultrasonography, and contrast-enhanced magnetic resonance imaging (the High Breast Cancer Risk Italian 1 study): final results. Invest Radiol 2011;46(2):94–105.

103. Le-Petross HT, Whitman GJ, Atchley DP, et al. Effectiveness of alternating mammography and magnetic resonance imaging for screening women with deleterious BRCA mutations at high risk of breast cancer. Cancer 2011;117(17): 3900–7.

104. Pace LE, He Y, Keating NL. Trends in mammography screening rates after publication of the 2009 US preventive services task force recommendations. Cancer 2013;119(14):2518–23.

105. Howard DH, Adams EK. Mammography rates after the 2009 US preventive services task force breast cancer screening recommendation. Prev Med 2012; 55(5):485–7.

106. Yasmeen S, Romano PS, Tancredi DJ, et al. Screening mammography beliefs and recommendations: a web-based survey of primary care physicians. BMC Health Serv Res 2012;12:32, 6963–12-32.

107. Meissner HI, Klabunde CN, Han PK, et al. Breast cancer screening beliefs, recommendations and practices: primary care physicians in the United States. Cancer 2011;117(14):3101–11.

108. Centers for Disease Control and Prevention (CDC). Cancer screening—United States, 2010. MMWR Morb Mortal Wkly Rep 2012;61(3):41–5.

109. Older Americans 2012: key indicators of well-being. Available at: http://www.agingstats.gov/agingstatsdotnet/Main_Site/Data/2012_Documents/Docs/Entire Chartbook.pdf. Accessed November 18, 2013.

110. Schueler KM, Chu PW, Smith-Bindman R. Factors associated with mammography utilization: a systematic quantitative review of the literature. J Womens Health (Larchmt) 2008;17(9):1477–98.

111. Curry SJ, Byers T, Hewitt M, editors. Fulfilling the potential for cancer prevention and early detection. Washington, DC: National Academies Press; 2003.

112. Watson-Johnson LC, DeGroff A, Steele CB, et al. Mammography adherence: a qualitative study. J Womens Health (Larchmt) 2011;20(12):1887–94.

113. Meissner HI, Klabunde CN, Breen N, et al. Breast and colorectal cancer screening: U.S. primary care physicians' reports of barriers. Am J Prev Med 2012;43(6):584–9.

114. Taplin SH, Ichikawa L, Yood MU, et al. Reason for late-stage breast cancer: absence of screening or detection, or breakdown in follow-up? J Natl Cancer Inst 2004;96(20):1518–27.

115. Zapka J, Taplin SH, Price RA, et al. Factors in quality care—the case of follow-up to abnormal cancer screening tests—problems in the steps and interfaces of care. J Natl Cancer Inst Monogr 2010;2010(40):58–71.

116. Campbell RT, Li X, Dolecek TA, et al. Economic, racial and ethnic disparities in breast cancer in the US: towards a more comprehensive model. Health Place 2009;15(3):855–64.

117. Silber JH, Rosenbaum PR, Clark AS, et al. Characteristics associated with differences in survival among black and white women with breast cancer. JAMA 2013;310(4):389–97.

118. Levy AR, Bruen BK, Ku L. Health care reform and women's insurance coverage for breast and cervical cancer screening. Prev Chronic Dis 2012;9:E159.

119. Sarfaty M, Wender R, Smith R. Promoting cancer screening within the patient centered medical home. CA Cancer J Clin 2011;61(6):397–408.

120. Peek ME, Han JH. Disparities in screening mammography: current status, interventions and implications. J Gen Intern Med 2004;19(2):184–94.

121. Plescia M, Richardson LC, Joseph D. New roles for public health in cancer screening. CA Cancer J Clin 2012;62(4):217–9.

122. Kern LM, Barron Y, Dhopeshwarkar RV, et al. Electronic health records and ambulatory quality of care. J Gen Intern Med 2013;28(4):496–503.

Lung Cancer Screening with Low-Dose Computed Tomography for Primary Care Providers

Thomas B. Richards, MD[a],*, Mary C. White, ScD[a],
Ralph S. Caraballo, PhD[b]

KEYWORDS

- Lung neoplasms • Screening • Computed tomography • Primary health care
- Practice guidelines • Smoking cessation • Shared decision making

KEY POINTS

- The US Preventive Services Task Force recommends annual low-dose computed tomography (LDCT) screening for lung cancer for persons at high risk for lung cancer, based on the age and smoking history of the individual.
- Lung cancer screening with LDCT does not prevent lung cancer, nor does it eliminate the need to extend smoking cessation referral and support to current smokers screened for lung cancer.
- Several organizations have recommended that lung cancer screening with LDCT be conducted as part of structured, high-volume, high-quality programs by a multidisciplinary team skilled in the evaluation and treatment of lung cancer.
- It is important for primary care providers to know the resources available in their communities for lung cancer screening with LDCT and smoking cessation, and the key points to be communicated to patients for informed and shared decision-making discussion about lung cancer screening.

The findings and conclusions in this report are those of the authors and do not necessarily represent the official position of the Centers for Disease Control and Prevention.
Disclosures, Funding Sources, and Conflicts of Interest: None.
a Division of Cancer Prevention and Control, National Center for Chronic Disease Prevention and Health Promotion, Centers for Disease Control and Prevention, Building 107, F-76, 4770 Buford Highway Northeast, Atlanta, GA 30341-3717, USA; b Office of Smoking and Health, National Center for Chronic Disease Prevention and Health Promotion, Centers for Disease Control and Prevention, Building 107, F-79, 4770 Buford Highway Northeast, Atlanta, GA 30341-3717, USA
* Corresponding author. Epidemiology and Applied Research Branch, Division of Cancer Prevention and Control, National Center for Chronic Disease Prevention and Health Promotion, Centers for Disease Control and Prevention, Building 107, F-76, 4770 Buford Highway Northeast, Atlanta, GA 30341-3717.
E-mail address: TRichards@cdc.gov

POPULATION MEASURES OF LUNG CANCER
Occurrence

Each year in the United States 206,000 people are told that they have lung cancer, and 160,000 die of this disease.[1] Lung cancer represents 14% of all invasive cancers diagnosed each year and 28% of all cancer deaths in the United States population.[1] The overall 5-year relative survival of patients with lung cancer is less than 18%.[2] More than half of lung cancers have distant metastasis at the time of diagnosis, and the 5-year relative survival after distant metastasis is less than 5%.[2] The average life expectancy of a patient with lung cancer is shortened by about 14 years.[3]

Cost

The total national cost of lung cancer care in 2010 was estimated at more than US$12 billion, and the cost could grow to exceed $18 billion by the year 2020.[4] The deductibles and copays incurred by individual patients with lung cancer can exceed well over $1000 per month.[5] Lung cancer screening with low-dose computed tomography (LDCT) at the patient's own expense can result in decreased intention to undergo screening and a lower adherence to attend an annual follow-up.[6] Some health care facilities have developed initiatives to provide the initial examination for lung cancer screening with LDCT at no cost to the patient.[7] National estimates of additional annual health expenditures related to lung cancer screening are still in the early stages, make different assumptions, and have come to varying conclusions.[8–12] The costs of an initial LDCT examination for lung cancer screening have been advertised at $99 to $1000.[13] The additional costs associated with follow-up evaluation and the treatment of abnormalities can be substantial; the implementation of lung cancer screening with LDCT has been estimated to increase the annual national health care expenditures by $1.3 to $2.0 billion if the screening rates were to reach 50% to 75% among those eligible for screening.[11]

Patterns Across Age, Sex, and Time

During the period 2005 to 2009, the incidence of lung cancer in the United States was highest among those aged 75 years and older, and decreased with decreasing age.[14] In all age groups except persons younger than 44 years, incidence rates of lung cancer were higher among men than among women; this difference being greatest among those aged 75 years and older, and narrowed with decreasing age.[14] In men, age-adjusted death rates for lung cancer increased until 1990 and then began to decrease.[15,16] In women, age-adjusted death rates for lung cancer peaked in 2004 and have had a lower rate of decline than for men.[16] These trends in incidence and mortality are thought to reflect changes in smoking patterns over time.[17,18]

Disparities

Disparities exist in the incidence and death rates of lung cancer within the United States population by race, ethnicity, and geography. Among men, the incidence and death rates are highest among blacks than among other racial and ethnic groups.[1] Among women, the incidence and death rates are similar between whites and blacks and highest among whites in comparison with other groups.[1] At all ages for both men and women, Asian and Pacific Islanders and Hispanics have lower incidence and death rates than other groups.[1] Incidence of lung cancer varies between states,[14,19] and is highest in the South and lowest in the West.[20] Large geographic differences have been demonstrated in incidence rates of lung cancer for American Indian and Alaska Native populations, with the highest rates in the Plains and Alaska.[21] Research suggests that multiple factors may be associated with tobacco use, including socio-economic status, education, cultural beliefs, and environmental influences.[22–24] Differences in the prevalence of exposures to other carcinogens and risk factors may also explain some of the observed differences in incidence rates between whites and blacks.[25] In addition, differences in access to and the use of health care services, in addition to the quality of treatment, have been shown to contribute to disparities in outcomes of lung cancer.[26,27] In a recent study, fatalistic beliefs including the concern that radiation exposure from a computed tomography (CT) scan could cause lung cancer and anxiety related to CT scans were reported to be strongly associated with a decrease in the intention to undergo screening among black and Hispanic adults in comparison with nonminority adults.[28]

Histology

Lung cancer refers to a group of cancers that form in the lung; different types have traditionally been distinguished by the differences in the morphologic appearance observed under a light microscope. Genetic and genomic criteria are needed to better understand and predict the varying biologic behavior of the different types.[29] Often in public health statistics, nearly all lung cancer is presented as 2 categories: non–small cell carcinoma (85% of the total lung cancer cases) and small cell carcinoma (14%).[2] Non–small cell carcinomas are further classified as adenocarcinoma (41% of the total lung cancer cases), squamous cell and transitional cell carcinoma (21%), large-cell carcinoma (3%), and non–small cell not otherwise specified (20%).[2] Data from selected cancer registries in the 1960s and 1970s showed an increase in the rates of adenocarcinoma, and by the 1980s adenocarcinoma had become more common than squamous cell carcinoma among both men and women.[30] The incidence of small cell lung cancer has decreased over time; whereas 73% of cases of small cell lung cancer were initially in men, the male-to-female ratio is now 1:1.22.[31] Details on the histology of lung cancer are important considerations for its clinical management. For example, surgical resection is the primary treatment for stage I and II non–small cell lung cancer in patients with small surgical risk.[32] By contrast, localized-stage small cell lung cancer is treated with concurrent chemoradiotherapy.[33]

ETIOLOGY
Tobacco

Cigarette smoking is the major cause of lung cancer in the United States and worldwide.[34–36] During the period 2005 to 2009 in the United States, excluding deaths from second hand smoke, 84% of annual deaths from lung cancer in men and 76% in women were attributed to cigarette smoking.[35] Only a fraction of smokers develop lung cancer in their lifetime and lung cancer can develop in non-smokers, indicating that other factors in addition to smoking play a role in its development.[18,37,38] The most effective preventive measures are to never start smoking or to stop cigarette smoking as soon as possible. In 2012, 18% (42 million) of United States adults aged 18 years upward were current cigarette smokers.[39] The risk of lung cancer increases with both the duration and intensity of smoking,[34] but the number of years smoked is a stronger predictor of lung cancer than the number of cigarettes smoked per day.[40]

Over the course of a lifetime, the risk of developing lung cancer can be 20 times or greater for smokers than for lifetime nonsmokers.[34] Smokers who quit smoking continue to have a higher risk than lifetime nonsmokers of developing lung cancer, but this risk diminishes over time.[38,41] More than half of all adult current smokers have attempted to quit for at least 1 day in the past year.[42] Charts to demonstrate the harms of cigarette smoking have been developed for use by physicians to discuss these issues with patients.[43] The charts show the 10-year risks of dying of lung cancer considering age, sex, and smoking status (current smoker, former smoker, and lifetime nonsmoker). The charts are available online in several formats, and can be posted in clinic offices for easy reference or distributed among patients.[43]

Secondhand Smoke

Secondhand smoke is the term used to describe sidestream smoke (the smoke released from the burning end of a cigarette) and exhaled mainstream smoke (the smoke exhaled by the smoker). Secondhand smoke is a recognized cause of lung cancer; however, the secondhand smoke-attributable mortality for lung cancer is 4%.[35] The increase over the background risk of lung cancer among nonsmokers living with a smoker has been estimated to be 20% to 30%.[35] According to data from the National Health and Nutrition Examination Survey, during 2007 to 2008 approximately 88 million nonsmokers aged 3 years or older in the United States were exposed to secondhand smoke. The prevalence of exposure was higher for children (aged 3–11 years) and youth (aged 12–19 years) than for adults aged 20 years or older.[35] During 2005 to 2009 in the United States, 7330 deaths from lung cancer were attributed to exposure to secondhand smoke among nonsmokers.[35]

Radon

The US Environmental Protection Agency (EPA) publication "A Citizen's Guide to Radon" is an excellent resource for any questions about radon.[44] Selected highlights are as follows. Radon is a radioactive gas produced by the natural decay of uranium in soils, rocks, and water. Radon gas can seep into buildings through cracks in foundations, accumulate in indoor air, and thereby increase the risk of lung cancer for both smokers and nonsmokers.[45] In the United States, an estimated 1 in 15 American homes have high levels of radon. The EPA and the Surgeon General recommend testing all homes for radon. Test kits can be obtained from state radon programs, home improvement and hardware stores, and other sources.[44,46] Radon is measured in picocuries per liter of air (pCi/L). On average, radon levels are 0.4 pCi/L for outdoor air and 1.3 pCi/L for indoor air. The EPA recommends radon mitigation to 2 pCi/L or less if indoor air levels remain at least 4 pCi/L.[44] A certified or qualified radon contractor should design and install the radon-reduction system.[44] The design depends on the house, but a common example is a soil-suction system to prevent radon from entering the home, whereby a pipe system and fans are used to draw radon gas from below the home and vent it to the outside.[44]

Occupational Exposures

Many chemical and physical agents have been demonstrated to cause lung cancer among working populations. Some of the most frequently mentioned occupational lung carcinogens include asbestos, beryllium, cadmium, chloromethyl ethers, chromium (hexavalent, hereafter abbreviated VI), nickel, diesel exhaust, radon, and silica.[36,47] Industries with higher levels of exposure to lung carcinogens include mining, construction, manufacturing, agriculture, and certain service sectors. The number of adult workers in the United States exposed to carcinogens at work has been estimated to be many millions.[48] Tens of thousands of chemicals used in industries have never been evaluated for their carcinogenicity, and many of these chemicals are found in the general environment and consumer products.[48] Special occupational standards have been established for only a relatively small number of lung carcinogens, including asbestos, arsenic, chromium(VI), cadmium, and formaldehyde.[49]

These standards were established after lengthy regulatory proceedings that considered many factors in addition to the health risk, including the feasibility of controlling the exposures and limits in the monitoring technology.

Outdoor Air Pollution

The combustion of fossil fuels by motor vehicles and other sources releases fine particulate matter, diesel exhaust, and other pollutants into the atmosphere. A growing body of evidence links outdoor air pollution with increased rates of lung cancer in the general population.[50,51] In 2013, the International Agency for Research on Cancer (IARC), a special agency of the World Health Organization, classified outdoor air pollution as carcinogenic to humans and found sufficient evidence to conclude that exposure to outdoor air pollution causes lung cancer.[52] Particulate matter, a major component of outdoor air pollution, was evaluated separately and was also classified by the IARC as carcinogenic to humans. In 2007, 13.6% of the general United States population resided in counties that exceeded the air pollution standard for fine particles, and minority groups were more likely than whites to live in these areas.[53] In addition, an estimated 1.8 million tons of mobile sources of toxic emissions in the air were reported in 2005 in the United States; a Healthy People 2020 objective is to reduce this figure to 1 million tons.[54]

Additional Risk Factors

Several other factors are associated with the increased risk of lung cancer. Examples include family history of lung cancer; chronic obstructive lung disease; fibrotic lung disorders such as pneumoconiosis; and human immunodeficiency virus (HIV) infection.[36,55]

LUNG CANCER SCREENING TESTS
Computed Tomography Lung Examinations

LDCT tests (sometimes abbreviated as low-dose CT) can be used to screen individuals at high risk for lung cancer. The individual lies still on a table, and the LDCT scanner rotates around the individual as the table passes through the center of the scanner. The entire chest is scanned in about 7 to 15 seconds during a single breath-hold. The scanner may include more than 1 source of x-rays. The x-ray sources follow a path similar to a helix or spiral as they rotate around the patient (some publications use helix and others use spiral; these terms are interchangeable). Rows of detectors are used to capture the x-ray information corresponding to multiple cross sections (thin slices) of the lung. Computers can create images from the x-ray information and assemble the images into a series of 2-dimensional slices of the lung at very small intervals.

Additional evaluation is needed to confirm that lung cancer is present if an LDCT scan reveals a pulmonary nodule.[56–59] Pulmonary nodules with a low probability of cancer may be followed with repeat LDCT screening over a period of time for growth-rate evaluation.[13] For nodules with a moderate probability of lung cancer, higher-dose diagnostic LDCT scans are often used in combination with positron emission tomography scans to evaluate the possibility of cancer metastasis. Biopsies may also be obtained. Depending on the results, patients are further evaluated for treatment.

A national consensus has not yet been developed for a standardized reporting system for lung cancer screening with LDCT equivalent to the Breast Imaging Reporting and Data System for mammography reporting.[60] A Lung Reporting and Data System equivalent has been proposed.[7]

National Surveys of Practice Patterns

Recent national survey information on lung cancer screening is limited. In a national survey of 962 practicing primary care physicians in 2006/2007, 55% had ordered chest radiography for lung cancer screening and 22% had ordered LDCT scans.[61,62] In the 2010 National Health Interview Survey, 2.5% of adults reported undergoing chest radiography in the prior year to check for lung cancer, and 1.3% reported undergoing chest CT to check for lung cancer.[63]

National Lung Screening Trial

The National Lung Screening Trial (NLST) was a randomized controlled trial to compare the effects of helical LDCT and standard chest radiography on the death rates for lung cancer among individuals at high risk for lung cancer in the United States.[64,65] The NLST was conducted at 33 locations and enrolled 53,454 adults starting in 2002. Eligible participants were between 55 and 74 years of age at the time of randomization with a history of cigarette smoking of at least 30 pack-years, and former smokers if they had quit within the previous 15 years. Half of the participants were randomly assigned to lung cancer screening with LDCT, and the other half to screening with single-view posteroanterior chest radiography. Subjects were screened annually for 3 years. In 2011, the NLST reported a 20% reduction in mortality from lung cancer among individuals screened by LDCT when compared with individuals screened by chest radiography.[65] **Table 1** summarizes selected NLST benefits and harms. The benefits of lung LDCT screening for reducing deaths from lung cancer was greater among older, heavier smokers who greatly exceeded the minimum eligibility requirements for screening than among younger, less heavy smokers closer to the minimum eligibility requirements.[66,67] Two annual LDCT screenings resulted in a decrease in the number of advanced-stage cancers diagnosed and an increase in the number of early-stage lung cancers diagnosed.[68]

Cancer Intervention and Surveillance Modeling Network

The Cancer Intervention and Surveillance Modeling Network (CISNET) used data from the NLST and the Prostate, Lung, Colorectal, and Ovarian Cancer Screening trial to compare multiple scenarios of lung cancer screening.[69] All scenarios followed a cohort of 100,000 persons aged 45 to 90 years until death from any cause. Variations included the frequency of screening (annual, every 2 years, or every 3 years); age to begin screening (age 45, 50, 55, or 60 years); age to end screening (age 75, 80, or 85 years); minimum pack-years for screening eligibility (10, 20, 30, or 40 years); and maximum years since quitting for screening eligibility (10, 15, 20, or 25 years). Five models, developed by investigators at 5 different institutions, were used in the analyses, and estimates were averaged across the 5 models. CISNET analyses of the number of deaths from lung cancer included 7.5 years of follow-up compared with the 6.5 years in the NLST. With the additional year, the estimated lung cancer–specific reduction in mortality was 14%, rather than the 20% reduction reported in 2011 by the NLST. Annual screening resulted in the greatest reduction in mortality (11%–21% reduction), in comparison with biennial screening (6.5%–9.6% reduction) and triennial screening (≤6% reduction). The CISNET modelers concluded that the optimal balance of benefits and harms would be provided by starting annual screening at age 55 years, and ending screening at the age of 80 years for smokers with at least 30 pack-years and for former smokers no more than 15 years since quitting.[69] The CISNET identification code for this scenario was A55-80-30-15. **Table 2** summarizes selected benefits and harms for this scenario projected by CISNET.

Table 1
Selected benefits and harms of lung cancer screening reported by the National Lung Screening Trial for all 3 rounds, comparing low-dose computed tomography (LDCT) with chest radiography[a]

	LDCT	Chest Radiography
Participants		
No. of participants	26,722	26,732
Adherence to 3 rounds of screening	95%	93%
Person-years	144,103	143,368
Benefits		
Lung cancer deaths	356	443
Rate of death from lung cancer per 100,000 person-years	247	309
Relative reduction in mortality from lung cancer with LDCT	62/309 = 20%	—
Risk of Harms		
Percentage of tests classified as positive	24.2%	6.9%
Percent of positive results that were false positives	96.4%	94.5%
Rate of at least 1 complication after the most invasive screening related diagnostic procedure[b]	1.4%	1.6%
Percentage of positive screening tests associated with a major complication from invasive screening related diagnostic procedures[b] when:		
Lung cancer not diagnosed	0.06%	0.02%
Lung cancer diagnosed	11.2%	8.2%
Deaths within 60 d after the most invasive screening-related diagnostic procedure[b]	16	10

[a] The NLST conducted screening from August 2002 to September 2007, and followed up the participants through December 31, 2009. Analysis of the number of deaths from lung cancer includes deaths that occurred from the date of randomization through January 15, 2009 (6.5 years' follow-up).
[b] Invasive procedures include mediastinoscopy or mediastinotomy, thoracoscopy, or thoracotomy.
Data from National Lung Screening Trial Research Team, Aberle DR, Adams AM, et al. Reduced lung-cancer mortality with low-dose computed tomographic screening. N Engl J Med 2011; 365(5):395–409.

Overdiagnosis of lung cancer is defined as the detection of indolent lung cancer that would not have become clinically apparent.[70] Overdiagnosis is possible using lung cancer screening with LDCT, but estimates of the frequency have varied. The NLST Overdiagnosis Writing Team estimated the upper bound on the probability of overdiagnosis to be 18.5% (95% confidence interval 5.4%–30.6%) for cases identified by LDCT screening.[70] The CISNET modelers estimated overdiagnosis to be present in 9.9% of all screen-detected cases for scenario A55-80-30-15.[69]

European Studies

In Europe, several randomized controlled trials are in various stages of progress.[71–76] In general, compared with the NLST, the European trials have studied a smaller number of subjects and have used different screening intervals, numbers of rounds, and methods. For example, some of the European studies have used 3-dimensional scans in addition to 2-dimensional scans. Moreover, volume-doubling time is being used in

Table 2
Selected benefits and harms of lung cancer screening with annual low-dose computed tomography (LDCT) screening reported by the Cancer Intervention and Surveillance Modeling Network

Screening Scenario	
Scenario identification code	A55-80-30-15
Frequency of screening	Annual
Smoking requirement	Ever-smokers with at least 30 pack-years, and no more than 15 y since quitting for former smokers
Start screening at age	55 y
End screening at age	80 y
Study Cohort	
Cohort size	100,000 persons
Cohort age range	45–90 y
Proportion of cohort that receive screening[a]	19%
Benefits	
Lung cancer detected at an early stage (stage I or II)	50.5%
Lung cancer mortality reduction[b]	14.0%
Lung cancer deaths averted	521
Harms	
Total no. of screenings with LDCT	286,813
No. of overdiagnosed cases[c]	190
Overdiagnosis, % of all cases[c]	3.7%
Overdiagnosis, % of screening detected cases[c]	9.9%
No. of lung cancer deaths related to radiation exposure	24
LDCT scans per lung cancer death averted	550

[a] The Cancer Intervention and Surveillance Modeling Network (CISNET) assumed that only eligible persons (19%) in the cohort were screened, whereas the NLST screened almost all enrolled persons in the LDCT arm.
[b] CISNET analysis of the number of deaths from lung cancer included 7.5 years of follow-up compared with the 6.5 years of follow-up reported in the National Lung Screening Trial.
[c] Overdiagnosis refers to slow-growing or indolent lung cancers.
    Data from de Koning HJ, Meza R, Plevritis SK, et al. Benefits and harms of computed tomography lung cancer screening strategies: a comparative modeling study for the US Preventive Services Task Force. Ann Intern Med 2013; http://dx.doi.org/10.7326/M13-2316.

some European trials to assess change in nodule size over time between 2 scans.[77] The probability that a nodule is malignant is low if the volume-doubling time is 400 days or more.[77,78]

SCREENING RECOMMENDATIONS
Task Force Recommendation

In 2013, the US Preventive Services Task Force (Task Force) recommended "annual screening for lung cancer with low-dose computed tomography in adults ages 55 to 80 years who have a 30 pack-year smoking history and currently smoke or have quit within the past 15 years."[79,80] The Task Force also recommended that "screening should be discontinued once a person has not smoked for 15 years or develops a health problem that substantially limits life expectancy or the ability or willingness to have curative lung surgery."[79,80] Approximately 10 million people in the United States would qualify for lung cancer screening with LDCT based on these NLST age and smoking criteria.[63]

Recommendations of Others

Many organizations in the United States updated their recommendations on lung cancer screening following the 2011 NLST report (**Table 3**).[81–86] Although differences exist between organizations, many recommend eligibility criteria similar to those of NLST; they also recommend smoking cessation services or referral, and performance of screening in facilities with access to multispecialty expertise for follow-up management.

Table 3
Lung cancer screening recommendations

Organization	Groups Eligible for Screening	Year
American Association for Thoracic Surgery[81]	1. Age 55–79 y with ≥30 pack-year smoking history 2. Long-term lung cancer survivors who have completed 4 y of surveillance without recurrence, and who can tolerate lung cancer treatment to detect second primary lung cancer until the age of 79 y 3. Age 50–79 y with a 20 pack-year smoking history and additional comorbidity that produces a cumulative risk of developing lung cancer ≥5% in 5 y	2012
American Cancer Society[82]	Age 55–74 y with ≥30 pack-year smoking history, either currently smoking or have quit within the past 15 y, and who are in relatively good health	2013
American College of Chest Physicians[83]	Age 55–74 y with ≥30 pack-year smoking history and either continue to smoke or have quit within the past 15 y	2013
American College of Chest Physicians and American Society of Clinical Oncology[84]	Age 55–74 y with ≥30 pack-year smoking history and either continue to smoke or have quit within the past 15 y	2012
American Lung Association[85]	Age 55–74 y with ≥30 pack-year smoking history and no history of lung cancer	2012
National Comprehensive Cancer Network[86]	1. Age 55–74 y with ≥30 pack-year smoking history and smoking cessation <15 y 2. Age ≥50 y and ≥20 pack-year smoking history and 1 additional risk factor (other than secondhand smoke)[a]	2012
US Preventive Services Task Force[79,80]	Age 55–80 y with ≥30 pack-year smoking history and smoking cessation <15 y	2013

[a] Additional risk factors include cancer history, lung disease history, family history of lung cancer, radon exposure, occupational exposure, and history of chronic obstructive pulmonary disease or pulmonary fibrosis. Cancers with increased risk of developing new primary lung cancer include survivors of lung cancer, lymphomas, cancer of the head and neck, and smoking-related cancers. Occupational exposures identified as carcinogens targeting the lungs include silica, cadmium, asbestos, arsenic, beryllium, chromium(VI), diesel fumes, and nickel.

ORGANIZATIONAL CHARACTERISTICS THAT FACILITATE BEST PRACTICE
Structured Screening Program

In the section labeled "Other Considerations," the Task Force's 2013 recommendation statement encourages standardization of LDCT screening and the follow-up of abnormal findings, and the development of a registry to collect the data needed to enable continuous improvement in screening program quality over time.[80] Several organizations in the United States have recommended that lung cancer screening and follow-up be conducted as part of a structured, high-volume, high-quality program including a multidisciplinary team skilled in the evaluation and treatment of lung cancer (**Box 1**).[81–86] A national consensus on the standards for structured programs does not exist at present; depending on the elements required, the availability of lung cancer screening services with LDCT might be limited to larger, urban health care markets, where specialists are more likely to practice.[87]

The Lung Cancer Alliance has published a National Framework for Excellence in Lung Cancer Screening and Continuum of Care.[88] The principles of this framework include: clear information on eligibility and risks and benefits; compliance with standards for best practices from the National Comprehensive Cancer Network and the International Early Lung Action Program; a multidisciplinary team for a coordinated continuum of care; comprehensive smoking cessation; reporting results expeditiously to patients and physicians; participation in outcome data collection; and providing information on how screened individuals can advance research.

The American College of Radiology (ACR) offers a Computed Tomography accreditation program that includes evaluation of personnel qualifications, equipment specifications, and quality control.[89] A searchable list of locations with ACR CT accreditation is available on the ACR Web site.[90] A practice guideline for radiologists is being developed by the ACR and the Society of Thoracic Radiology.[91] The American Lung Association has recommended that hospitals and screening centers establish ethical policies for advertising and promoting lung cancer screening services with LDCT.[85]

Quality Control

In its "Clinician Fact Sheet," the Task Force states that the effectiveness of lung cancer screening depends on accurate interpretation of LDCT images and resolving most false-positive results without invasive procedures, in addition to limiting screening to people at high risk.[79] Consistent quality of LDCT images is critical to identifying abnormalities

---

Box 1
Structured lung cancer screening

Formal program

Access to a multidisciplinary clinical team and clinical resources to provide diagnosis, follow-up treatment, and long-term patient management related to lung screening

Patient eligibility criteria consistent with Task Force recommendations

Informed and shared decision-making discussions before initial screening

Smoking cessation program

American College of Radiology certification in computed tomography

Staff and resources for data collection to monitor program quality

Participation in American College of Radiology data registry program

and tracking changes in suspicious findings over time while avoiding excessive exposure.[92,93] Quality control and accreditation programs are needed to monitor the equipment performance and adherence to imaging protocols.[92,93] A centralized database may be helpful in identifying and flagging deviations from established protocols. In the NLST, quality assurance included a centralized review of a random sample of 1504 LDCT examinations. Quality defect rates ranged from 0% to 7.1%.[93]

Radiation Exposure and Dose

In the NLST, each LDCT resulted in an estimated effective dose of 1.5 millisievert (mSv) per examination.[64] In a 2013 survey of 15 academic medical centers in the United States, the average mean effective radiation dose for LDCT screening was reported as less than 1 mSv at 5 centers (33%), 1 to 2 mSv at 7 centers (47%), 2 to 3 mSv at 2 centers (13%); 1 respondent did not know the dose.[91]

At least 1 radiology journal no longer accepts research articles that describe radiation as "low dose" because improvement in LDCT technology continually decreases the amount of radiation exposure considered low dose.[94] As an alternative, the following measures were suggested: volume CT dose index, dose length product, a measure of patient dimensions (effective diameter), and size-specific dose estimate on a per-patient basis.[94]

Methods are needed to track both the amount of radiation exposure during an individual examination and the total cumulative dose received by an individual over time.[95] Development of a multidisciplinary committee to reduce the radiation dose, repeat rate, and variability in quality of the LDCT image at a medium-sized community hospital has been described.[96]

Follow-up of Abnormal Results

In the section titled "Other Considerations," the Task Force's 2013 recommendation statement supports the establishment of protocols for follow-up of abnormal results such as the clinical practice guidelines in oncology for lung cancer screening by the National Comprehensive Care Network.[59] In the NLST, an LDCT screening examination was considered positive for potential lung cancer if there were noncalcified pulmonary nodules with a long-axis diameter of 4 mm or more in the axial plane.[97] Approximately 27% of initial screening examinations were positive.[97] Several different groups have developed recommendations for the follow-up management of solid and subsolid nodules (subsolid nodules are common with peripheral adenocarcinoma).[56–59] Many nodules are benign, but it may take 1 to 2 years to rule out cancer. The nodule size is one of the key decision parameters in the follow-up management algorithms. To reduce the number of false positives, increasing the minimum nodule size for positive results to 7 to 8 mm has been suggested.[98] Research is ongoing to accurately estimate the probability of a lung nodule detected by LDCT screening being malignant.[56,99,100]

SMOKING CESSATION

Smoking prevention and cessation remain the fundamental strategies to drastically reduce the number of cases of lung cancer in the United States and elsewhere. Several studies conclusively show that smoking cessation lowers the risks for lung cancer among smokers.[34,35,101] However, the risk for lung cancer remains greater in former smokers than in lifetime nonsmokers.[101,102]

A small number of studies have been conducted to determine whether lung cancer screening with LDCT increases the chances of smoking cessation or changes perceptions about quitting.[103-108] The limited available data seem to indicate that patients who receive LDCT screening, similarly to those who do not, have other factors that may better predict smoking cessation. For smokers, the factors associated with nicotine dependence at the time of the LDCT screening such as the number of cigarettes smoked per day and the time smoking the first cigarette in the morning, as well as other factors such as having 1 or more smoking-related diseases (eg, emphysema, chronic pulmonary obstructive disease), are likely to be better predictors of quit attempts and smoking cessation than receiving LDCT screening. For former smokers, the time passed since they last smoked a cigarette and having 1 or more smoking-related diseases are likely to be better predictors of relapse than receiving LDCT screening.

Under "Other Considerations," the 2013 Task Force recommendation statement indicates that lung cancer screening with LDCT should not be viewed as an alternative to tobacco cessation, and current smokers should be informed of their continued risk for lung cancer and be offered cessation treatments before referral.[80] A potential area for future research might be whether the expanded use of lung cancer screening with LDCT in community practice will be associated with increased attention to smoking cessation messages given by health professionals; in 2010, only 48.3% of adult smokers had been advised by a health professional to quit.[42] A smoking cessation message provided in a clear, strong, and personalized manner by a health professional increases abstinence by current smokers.[109] Former smokers, particularly those who have recently quit, may also potentially benefit from counseling that acknowledges the patient's success and addresses any problems associated with cessation; emphasizes the importance of continued abstinence when they are referred for lung cancer screening with LDCT; and underscores the availability of support to resume abstinence if they relapse.[109]

Information is available for physicians and other health care practitioners on how to help their patients quit smoking. The US Public Health Services 2008 update of the Clinical Practice Guideline on Treating Tobacco Use and Dependence[109] (hereafter referred to as the 2008 Tobacco Use Guideline) provides guidance on intervening with smokers who want to quit or who have recently quit, and includes motivational messages for those not currently willing to make an attempt to quit. Effective treatments include individual, group, and telephone counseling, as well as 7 medications approved by the Food and Drug Administration. The effectiveness of the treatment increases with increasing intensity. Multiple counseling sessions are more effective than a brief single counseling session, and therapy combining counseling and medications is more effective than either component alone.

In addition to the proven strategies to encourage and support smoking cessation by health professionals, the 2008 Tobacco Use Guideline also points out that these strategies have not yet been fully implemented in health care settings, and that health care administrators, insurers, and purchasers have an important role to play in helping to ensure that tobacco use is systematically assessed and treated with evidence-based strategies at every clinical encounter.[109] Examples of potential interventions by the health care system include automated systems to identify smokers and an expanded insurance coverage of evidence-based treatment for tobacco use (both medication and counseling). The 2008 Tobacco Use Guideline also acknowledges that additional research would be helpful for specific population groups (eg, smokers who have low socioeconomic status and limited formal education).[109]

Quitting smoking at any age improves health, and reduces the risk of lung cancer and other diseases.[110,111] It is never too late to help patients to quit smoking. A Web site at the Centers for Disease Control and Prevention (http://www.cdc.gov/tobacco/campaign/tips/quit-smoking/) includes tips from former smokers and resources for smokers who are ready to quit, and the National Cancer Institute (NCI) Web site (www.smokefree.gov) includes practical cessation information as well as information on how to sign up for SmokefreeTXT, which is a mobile text-messaging program for help to quit smoking. In addition, the NCI has a toll-free number that connects smokers to their state quitline, which smokers can call to talk to a coach for help to quit smoking: 1-800-QUIT-NOW (1-800-784-8669) or, for assistance in Spanish, 1-855-DÉJELO-YA (1-855-335-3569) (**Box 2**).

INFORMED AND SHARED DECISION-MAKING DISCUSSIONS

In the section "Other Considerations," the 2013 Task Force recommendation statement indicates that the decision to begin screening should be made through a shared decision-making process whereby patients and providers discuss the potential benefits, harms, and uncertainties of screening.[80] In its "Clinician Fact Sheet," the Task Force provides potential discussion points for 3 patient scenarios: patients who fit all screening criteria; patients who are outside the screening criteria; and patients who fit all screening criteria but have a significant comorbid condition.[79]

Other organizations recommending lung cancer screening with LDCT also have suggested an informed and shared decision-making process before referral for screening.[81–86] Studies suggest that primary care providers need to tailor their approach to informed and shared decision making for each patient, for example by asking each patient for his or her input on the desired level of participation.[112,113] Patients vary in their preference for participation in the decision-making process, with some preferring an active or collaborative role and others favoring a passive role. A patient's preference may also change over time, and a mismatch between patients' preferred and actual roles is common.[112,113] A taxonomy has been proposed to categorize the harms that might occur during lung cancer screening with LDCT, including physical harms, psychological harms, financial strain, and opportunity costs.[114]

Box 2
Resources for smoking cessation

Resources for Patients

Anyone can reach the state tobacco quitline by calling 1-800-QUITNOW

Support for quitters

   http://www.smokefree.gov

   http://www.cdc.gov/tobacco/quit_smoking/index.htm

Tips from former smokers

   http://www.cdc.gov/tobacco/campaign/tips/index.html

Resources for Clinicians and Other Health Providers

Treating tobacco use and dependence

   http://www.ahrq.gov/professionals/clinicians-providers/guidelines-recommendations/
   tobacco/clinicians/presentations/2008update-overview/index.html

Charts that show the 10-year risks of dying from lung cancer

   http://jnci.oxfordjournals.org/content/100/12/845/suppl/DC1

Telephone quitlines

   http://www.cdc.gov/tobacco/quit_smoking/cessation/quitlines/index.htm

Higher-Risk Individuals

Tables 4 and **5** list selected examples of potential items for consideration during informed and shared decision-making discussions with patients, organized according to the Task Force's previously suggested "5 As" framework: assess, advise, agree, assist, and arrange.[115] One of the more important topics to be addressed is that lung cancer screening with LDCT may involve a process over an extended period of time, rather than a single scan.[83,116] For example, after a pulmonary nodule is identified, evaluation to determine whether the nodule is benign or malignant may require additional CT scans, more invasive procedures, additional cost, and follow-up for 1 to 2 years.[116] The informed and shared decision-making discussion needs to occur before referral to LDCT screening, because many patients might assume that they

Table 4
Selected examples of items to be considered in informed and shared decision-making discussions about screening for cancer with low-dose computed tomography (LDCT)

Steps	Components
Assess	*Availability:* Is an organized, high-volume, high-quality lung cancer screening program available with a multidisciplinary team skilled in lung cancer evaluation and treatment? *Eligibility:* Does the patient meet lung screening eligibility criteria? *Time:* Is time available for informed and shared decision-making discussions with the patient? *Knowledge:* What is the patient's level of knowledge about lung cancer and lung cancer screening? What is the patient's literacy level? *Preferences:* Does the patient prefer an active, shared, or passive role in the decision-making discussions?
Advise	*Purpose:* Annual LDCT screening can detect lung cancer at an early stage in asymptomatic high-risk individuals. Lung cancer screening should be thought of as a process rather than a single test *Smoking cessation:* Current smokers should STOP SMOKING. Screening should not be viewed as an alternative to smoking cessation. Avoiding cigarettes can lower the risk of lung cancer, emphysema, heart disease, and vascular disease *Benefits:* LDCT may reduce the risk of dying from lung cancer in heavy smokers. For individuals meeting the minimum eligibility requirements, benefits of screening are greater in individuals who have been heavier smokers *Harms:* There is a significant chance of false alarms (false positives) with LDCT screening. Repeat testing over 1–2 y may be required to evaluate if a screen detected abnormality increases in size. In some cases, an invasive procedure (eg, needle biopsy, bronchoscopy, or thoracotomy) is needed to determine whether the abnormality is lung cancer. Invasive diagnostic procedures may result in major complications, and are more common in patients who have lung cancer. Death within 60 d has occurred after an invasive diagnostic procedure, but is rare *Radiation exposure:* Provide estimated radiation exposure for your location with 1 LDCT lung screening scan, and the cumulative lifetime total radiation with repeat annual screening *Patient costs:* How much does the patient need to pay for a scan? What is the cost of patient copayments for follow-up consultations and procedures? *Scientific uncertainties:* Negative screening results do not absolutely rule out the chance for lung cancer incidence. LDCT will not detect all lung cancers or all lung cancers early, and not all patients who have a lung cancer detected by LDCT will avoid death from lung cancer *Research:* How can screened individuals donate images and biospecimens to advance research in the prevention, diagnosis, and treatment of lung cancer? *Alternatives:* LDCT is the only screening test shown to lower the chances of dying of lung cancer. Chest radiography should not be used for lung cancer screening

Table 5	
Informed and shared decision-making discussions	
Steps	**Components**
Agree	Provider needs to help individuals clarify their preferences and willingness to be screened
	Decide to screen with LDCT every year: Individual assigns higher value to potential benefits than to potential harms
	Decide against LDCT screening: Individual assigns higher value to potential harms than to the potential benefits
Assist	*Costs:* Help individuals determine if they have to pay for the initial LDCT scan and how much
	Referral: Provider identifies screening facilities with appropriate expertise, refers individual for screening, and informs individual how to schedule the screening test or that the screening clinic will contact the individual
Arrange	*Smoking cessation:* Provider should provide smoking cessation or refer current smokers to smoking cessation programs
	Results: How and when will the LDCT results be communicated to patients?
	Follow-up: When will the informed-shared decision-making process about LDCT screening be revisited in the future?
Update	*Preferences and decisions:* Assess any change over time in patient preferences and decisions before referral for the next annual LDCT screening
Document	*Documentation:* Clearly document the informed and shared decision-making process and decisions to safeguard against potential medicolegal consequences (eg, if a case of lung cancer is detected before a decision has been made about lung cancer screening; or if the individual has major complications from lung cancer screening). Documentation may potentially need to cover more than 1 visit (eg, initial discussion with patient, follow-up discussions between patient and support staff, and educational materials provided to patient)

have cancer when told that the LDCT scan has revealed a nodule.[116] Patients with significant comorbid conditions should be informed that they may be at greater risk for harm with screening,[79] and screening is not recommended if the comorbid conditions substantially limit life expectancy or the ability to undergo curative lung surgery.[80]

Lower-Risk Individuals

Primary care providers need to be prepared to answer questions about lung cancer screening with LDCT from individuals who do not meet the criteria for lung cancer screening with LDCT. Several examples include heavy smokers who are younger than the recommended age to begin screening, current or former smokers with fewer pack-years of smoking, individuals with other risk factors for lung cancer (eg, chronic obstructive lung disease), and healthy adults who have never smoked.[79] In its "Clinical Fact Sheet" scenarios, the Task Force recommends that health providers inform patients in lower risk categories about the potential harms of screening and that there is not enough evidence to recommend screening for individuals at lower risk for lung cancer.[79] The American Cancer Society also recommends informing individuals in lower risk categories that screening is not recommended at this time because there is too much uncertainty regarding the balance of benefits and harms (**Box 3**).[82]

HEALTH CARE CHANGES
Reimbursement for Grade A or B Preventive Services

The Patient Protection and Affordable Care Act requires most health insurance plans to cover preventive services at no additional cost to the patient if the Task Force

---

Box 3
Resources for patients about lung cancer screening

American Cancer Society. Patient Page. Testing for lung cancer in people at high risk. CA Cancer J Clin 2013;63(2):118–9. http://www.cancer.org/healthy/informationforhealthcareprofes sionals/acsguidelines/lungcancerscreeningguidelines/index

American Lung Association. Lung cancer CT screening for early detection. One pager. http://www.lung.org/lung-disease/lung-cancer/lung-cancer-screening-guidelines/lung-cancer-one-pager.pdf

American Lung Association. Provides guidance on lung cancer screening. Full Report. Appendix I. American Lung Association Toolkit. Making an individual decision to be screened. http://www.lung.org/lung-disease/lung-cancer/lung-cancer-screening-guidelines/

National Cancer Institute. Patient and physician guide: National Lung Screening Trial. http://www.cancer.gov/newscenter/qa/2002/NLSTstudyGuidePatientsPhysicians

National Cancer Institute. Lung cancer screening (PDQ). Patient version. http://www.cancer.gov/cancertopics/pdq/screening/lung/Patient/page1/AllPages

National Comprehensive Cancer Network. NCCN guidelines for patients. Lung cancer screening. Version 1. 2014. http://www.nccn.org/

National Framework for Excellence in Lung Cancer Screening and Continuum of Care. Lung Cancer Alliance. http://www.lungcanceralliance.org

US Preventive Services Task Force. Consumer fact sheet. Understanding Task Force recommendations. Screening for lung cancer. http://www.uspreventiveservicestaskforce.org/adultrec.htm

---

grades the preventive service recommendation as A (strongly recommended) or B (recommended).[117] Both tobacco cessation (graded A) and lung cancer screening with LDCT (graded B) would qualify for insurance coverage at no additional cost.

Patient-Centered Medical Home

The patient-centered medical home is a model to improve the delivery of primary care by greater involvement of the patient in care plans, coordinated and comprehensive team-based care, improved patient access to care after hours and by e-mail and phone, and a commitment to quality improvement and population health management.[118] In the context of lung cancer screening with LDCT, the primary care patient-centered medical home will remain important even if the primary care provider refers patients to a structured program that offers lung cancer screening and follow-up management. Several examples of potential activities for the primary care provider include identification of patients eligible for lung cancer screening with LDCT, informed and shared decision-making discussions with patients before referral, promotion of smoking cessation, management of comorbid conditions that are not addressed by specialists, and eliminating barriers to timely care.[119,120]

Electronic Health Records

If electronic health records (EHRs) include information on patient age and pack-years of smoking, EHRs may be used to identify individuals who meet the eligibility criteria for lung cancer screening with LDCT. Computer algorithms may be designed to use with EHRs to provide patients with cellphone reminders about the need to schedule their annual lung cancer screening with LDCT and the importance of smoking cessation.[121,122] An integrated system of EHRs may also facilitate the retrieval of information from multiple providers to evaluate the performance and quality of a lung cancer screening program with LDCT, notify the responsible clinicians about abnormal imaging results that need follow-up, and improve the early recognition of patients with lung cancer.[121,122]

Accountable Care Organizations

The Patient Protection and Affordable Care Act encourages groups of providers to collaborate, manage, and coordinate the care of patients through accountable care organizations (ACOs).[117] ACOs that meet quality performance standards are eligible to receive payments for shared savings. Bekelman and colleagues[123] have suggested that cancer specialists in larger, urban health care markets may want to develop Cancer Care Groups to provide guideline-concordant, patient-centered, coordinated care among cancer specialists and primary care providers. Activities related to lung cancer screening with LDCT would seem reasonable for ACOs to consider, especially if lung cancer screening with LDCT and follow-up is managed as part of a structured program with a multidisciplinary team.

SUMMARY

Annual LDCT screening for lung cancer cannot prevent lung cancer, but can reduce mortality from lung cancer in persons at high risk based on the age and smoking history of the individual. Lung cancer screening can supplement, but not replace, efforts to address the primary prevention of lung cancer through the control of tobacco and other known risk factors associated with lung cancer. Considerations for primary care providers may include the resources available in their communities for lung cancer screening with LDCT and for smoking cessation, and the key points that need to be addressed in the informed and shared decision-making discussions with patients. Lung cancer screening with LDCT is a rapidly evolving area. Examples of upcoming areas of potential importance may include the following: decisions from Centers for Medicare and Medicaid Services about reimbursement and billing codes; ACR recommendations on quality control and reporting of LDCT findings; results from additional analyses of the NLST data; results from European studies, especially on the use of volume-doubling time to evaluate whether pulmonary nodule sizes have changed over time; and whether a national consensus can be developed with standard algorithms for patient management.

REFERENCES

1. US Cancer Statistics Working Group. United States cancer statistics: 1999-2010 incidence and mortality web-based report. Atlanta (GA): US Department of Health and Human Services, Centers for Disease Control and Prevention and National Cancer Institute; 2013. Available at: http://www.cdc.gov/uscs. Accessed January 15, 2014.
2. Howlader N, Noone AM, Krapcho M, et al. SEER cancer statistics review, 1975-2010. Bethesda (MD): National Cancer Institute; 2013. Available at: http://seer.cancer.gov/csr/1975_2010/. Accessed January 15, 2014.
3. Liu PH, Wang JD, Keating NL. Expected years of life lost for six potentially preventable cancers in the United States. Prev Med 2013;56(5):309–13.
4. Mariotto AB, Yabroff KR, Shao Y, et al. Projections of the cost of cancer care in the United States: 2010-2020. J Natl Cancer Inst 2011;103(2):117–28.
5. Cipriano LE, Romanus D, Earle CC, et al. Lung cancer treatment costs, including patient responsibility, by disease stage and treatment modality, 1992 to 2003. Value Health 2011;14(1):41–52.

6. Wildstein KA, Faustini Y, Yip R, et al. Longitudinal predictors of adherence to annual follow-up in a lung cancer screening programme. J Med Screen 2011; 18(3):154–9.

7. McKee BJ, McKee AB, Flacke S, et al. Initial experience with a free, high-volume, low-dose CT lung cancer screening program. J Am Coll Radiol 2013;10(8):586–92.

8. Evans WK, Wolfson MC. Computed tomography screening for lung cancer without a smoking cessation program—not a cost-effective idea. J Thorac Oncol 2011;6(11):1781–3.

9. McMahon PM, Kong CY, Bouzan C, et al. Cost-effectiveness of computed tomography screening for lung cancer in the United States. J Thorac Oncol 2011;6(11):1841–8.

10. Pyenson BS, Sander MS, Jiang Y, et al. An actuarial analysis shows that offering lung cancer screening as an insurance benefit would save lives at relatively low cost. Health Aff (Millwood) 2012;31(4):770–9.

11. Goulart BH, Bensink ME, Mummy DG, et al. Lung cancer screening with low-dose computed tomography: costs, national expenditures, and cost-effectiveness. J Natl Compr Canc Netw 2012;10(2):267–75.

12. Villanti AC, Jiang Y, Abrams DB, et al. A cost-utility analysis of lung cancer screening and the additional benefits of incorporating smoking cessation interventions. PLoS One 2013;8(8):e71379.

13. Munden RF, Godoy MC. Lung cancer screening: state of the art. J Surg Oncol 2013;108(5):270–4.

14. Henley JS, Richards TB, Underwood MJ, et al. Lung cancer incidence trends among men and women—United States, 2005-2009. MMWR Morb Mortal Wkly Rep 2014;63(1):1–5.

15. Jemal A, Thun MJ, Ries LA, et al. Annual report to the nation on the status of cancer, 1975-2005, featuring trends in lung cancer, tobacco use, and tobacco control. J Natl Cancer Inst 2008;100(23):1672–94.

16. Edwards BK, Noone AM, Mariotto AB, et al. Annual report to the nation on the status of cancer, 1975-2010, featuring prevalence of comorbidity and impact on survival among persons with lung, colorectal, breast, or prostate cancer. Cancer 2013. [Epub ahead of print]. http://dx.doi.org/10.1002/cncr.28509.

17. Moolgavkar SH, Holford TR, Levy DT, et al. Impact of reduced tobacco smoking on lung cancer mortality in the United States during 1975-2000. J Natl Cancer Inst 2012;104(7):541–8.

18. Thun MJ, Carter BD, Feskanich D, et al. 50-year trends in smoking-related mortality in the United States. N Engl J Med 2013;368(4):351–64.

19. Henley SJ, Eheman CR, Richardson LC, et al. State-specific trends in lung cancer incidence and smoking—United States, 1999-2008. MMWR Morb Mortal Wkly Rep 2011;60(36):1243–7.

20. Underwood JM, Townsend JS, Tai E, et al. Racial and regional disparities in lung cancer incidence. Cancer 2012;118(7):1910–8.

21. Bliss A, Cobb N, Solomon T, et al. Lung cancer incidence among American Indians and Alaska Natives in the United States, 1999–2004. Cancer 2008; 113(Suppl 5):1168–78.

22. US Department of Health and Human Services. Tobacco use among US racial/ethnic minority groups—African Americans, American Indians and Alaska Natives, Asian Americans and Pacific Islanders, and Hispanicsa: report of the surgeon general. Atlanta (GA): US Department of Health and Human Services, Centers for Disease Control and Prevention, National Center for Chronic Disease Prevention and Health Promotion, Office on Smoking and Health; 1998.

23. Siahpush M, Singh GK, Jones PR, et al. Racial/ethnic and socioeconomic variations in duration of smoking: results from 2003, 2006, and 2007 Tobacco Use Supplement of the Current Population Survey. J Public Health (Oxf) 2010; 32(2):210–8.

24. Williams DR, Kontos EZ, Viswanath K, et al. Integrating multiple social statuses in health disparities research: the case of lung cancer. Health Serv Res 2012; 47(3 Pt 2):1255–77.

25. Etzel CJ, Kachroo S, Liu M, et al. Development and validation of a lung cancer risk prediction model for African-Americans. Cancer Prev Res (Phila) 2008;1(4): 255–65.

26. Slatore CG, Au DH, Gould MK, et al. An official American Thoracic Society systematic review: insurance status and disparities in lung cancer practices and outcomes. Am J Respir Crit Care Med 2010;182(9):1195–205.

27. Virgo KS, Little AG, Fedewa SA, et al. Safety-net burden hospitals and likelihood of curative-intent surgery for non-small cell lung cancer. J Am Coll Surg 2011; 213(5):633–43.

28. Jonnalagadda S, Bergamo C, Lin JJ, et al. Beliefs and attitudes about lung cancer screening among smokers. Lung Cancer 2012;77(3):526–31.

29. Travis WD, Brambilla E, Riely GJ. New pathologic classification of lung cancer: relevance for clinical practice and clinical trials. J Clin Oncol 2013;31(8): 992–1001.

30. Chen F, Cole P, Bina WF. Time trend and geographic patterns of lung adenocarcinoma in the United States, 1973-2002. Cancer Epidemiol Biomarkers Prev 2007;16(12):2724–9.

31. Govindan R, Page N, Morgensztern D, et al. Changing epidemiology of small-cell lung cancer in the United States over the last 30 years: analysis of the surveillance, epidemiologic, and end results database. J Clin Oncol 2006;24(28):4539–44.

32. Howington JA, Blum MG, Chang AC, et al. Treatment of stage I and II non-small cell lung cancer: diagnosis and management of lung cancer, 3rd ed. American College of Chest Physicians Evidence-Based Clinical Practice Guidelines. Chest 2013;143(Suppl 5):e278S–313S.

33. Jett JR, Schild SE, Kesler KA, et al. Treatment of small cell lung cancer: diagnosis and management of lung cancer, 3rd ed: American College of Chest Physicians Evidence-Based Clinical Practice Guidelines. Chest 2013;143(Suppl 5): e400S–19S.

34. US Department of Health and Human Services. The health consequences of smoking: a report of the surgeon general. Atlanta (GA): US Department of Health and Human Services, Centers for Disease Control and Prevention, National Center for Chronic Disease Prevention and Health Promotion, Office on Smoking and Health; 2004.

35. US Department of Health and Human Services. The health consequences of smoking: 50 years of progress. A report of the surgeon general. Atlanta (GA): US Department of Health and Human Services, Centers for Disease Control and Prevention, National Center for Chronic Disease Prevention and Health Promotion, Office on Smoking and Health; 2014.

36. Alberg AJ, Brock MV, Ford JG, et al. Epidemiology of lung cancer: diagnosis and management of lung cancer, 3rd ed: American College of Chest Physicians evidence-based clinical practice guidelines. Chest 2013;143(Suppl 5):e1S–29S.

37. Samet JM, Avila-Tang E, Boffetta P, et al. Lung cancer in never smokers: clinical epidemiology and environmental risk factors. Clin Cancer Res 2009;15(18): 5626–45.

38. Peto R, Darby S, Deo H, et al. Smoking, smoking cessation, and lung cancer in the UK since 1950: combination of national statistics with two case-control studies. BMJ 2000;321(7257):323–9.

39. Agaku IT, King BA, Dube SR. Current cigarette smoking among adults—United States, 2005-2012. MMWR Morb Mortal Wkly Rep 2014;63(2):29–34.

40. Flanders WD, Lally CA, Zhu BP, et al. Lung cancer mortality in relation to age, duration of smoking, and daily cigarette consumption: results from Cancer Prevention Study II. Cancer Res 2003;63(19):6556–62.

41. Ebbert JO, Yang P, Vachon CM, et al. Lung cancer risk reduction after smoking cessation: observations from a prospective cohort of women. J Clin Oncol 2003; 21(5):921–6.

42. Centers for Disease Control and Prevention (CDC). Quitting smoking among adults—United States, 2001-2010. MMWR Morb Mortal Wkly Rep 2011;60(44): 1513–9.

43. Woloshin S, Schwartz LM, Welch HG. The risk of death by age, sex, and smoking status in the United States: putting health risks in context. J Natl Cancer Inst 2008;100(12):845–53. Supplementary materials available at: http://jnci.oxford journals.org/content/100/12/845/suppl/DC1. Accessed January 15, 2014.

44. US Environmental Protection Agency. A citizen's guide to radon. The guide to protecting yourself and your family from radon. Available at: http://www.epa. gov/radon/pubs/citguide.html. Accessed January 15, 2014.

45. Committee on Health Effects of Exposure to Radon (BEIR VI). Health effects of exposure to Radon. Washington, DC: National Academy of Science; 1999.

46. Kansas State University, National Radon Program Services. Increasing public knowledge of radon and the need to test and fix homes. Available at: http:// sosradon.org/. Accessed January 15, 2014.

47. Field RW, Withers BL. Occupational and environmental causes of lung cancer. Clin Chest Med 2012;33(4):681–703.

48. President's Cancer Panel. Reducing environmental cancer risk. What we can do now. Bethesda (MD): US Department of Health and Human Services, National Institutes of Health, National Cancer Institute; 2010.

49. Occupational Safety and Health Administration. US Department of Labor. Carcinogens. OSHA standards. 2012. Available at: https://www.osha.gov/SLTC/ carcinogens/index.html. Accessed January 15, 2014.

50. Thurston GD, Bekkedal MY, Roberts EM, et al. Use of health information in air pollution health research: past successes and emerging needs. J Expo Sci Environ Epidemiol 2009;19(1):45–58.

51. Raaschou-Nielsen O, Andersen ZJ, Beelen R, et al. Air pollution and lung cancer incidence in 17 European cohorts: prospective analyses from the European Study of Cohorts for Air Pollution Effects (ESCAPE). Lancet Oncol 2013;14(9): 813–22.

52. eISBN 978-92-832-2161-6. ISSN 0300-5085. In: Straif K, Cohen A, Samet J, editors. International Agency for Research on Cancer scientific publication no. 161. Air pollution and cancer. Lyon (France): International Agency for Research on Cancer, World Health Organization; 2013.

53. Yip FY, Pearcy JN, Garbe PL, et al. Unhealthy air quality—United States, 2006-2009. MMWR Surveill Summ 2011;60(Suppl):28–32.

54. Healthy people 2020 objectives. Environmental health. Outdoor Air Quality EH-3.1. Reduce air toxic emissions to decrease the risk of adverse health effects caused by mobile, area, and major sources of airborne toxics. Available at: http://www.healthypeople.gov/2020/. Accessed January 15, 2014.

55. Winstone TA, Man SF, Hull M, et al. Epidemic of lung cancer in patients with HIV infection. Chest 2013;143(2):305–14.

56. Gould MK, Donington J, Lynch WR, et al. Evaluation of individuals with pulmonary nodules: when is it lung cancer? Diagnosis and management of lung cancer, 3rd ed: American College of Chest Physicians Evidence-Based Clinical Practice Guidelines. Chest 2013;143(Suppl 5):e93S–120S.

57. MacMahon H, Austin JH, Gamsu G, et al. Guidelines for management of small pulmonary nodules detected on CT scans: a statement from the Fleischner Society. Radiology 2005;237(2):395–400.

58. Naidich DP, Bankier AA, MacMahon H, et al. Recommendations for the management of subsolid pulmonary nodules detected at CT: a statement from the Fleischner Society. Radiology 2013;266(1):304–17.

59. National Comprehensive Cancer Network. NCCN clinical practice guidelines in oncology. Lung cancer screening. Version I. 2014. Available at: http://www.nccn.org/. Accessed January 15, 2014.

60. American College of Radiology. BI-RADS atlas. Available at: http://www.acr.org/Quality-Safety/Resources/BIRADS. Accessed January 15, 2014.

61. Klabunde CN, Marcus PM, Silvestri GA, et al. US primary care physicians' lung cancer screening beliefs and recommendations. Am J Prev Med 2010;39(5):411–20.

62. Klabunde CN, Marcus PM, Han PK, et al. Lung cancer screening practices of primary care physicians: results from a national survey. Ann Fam Med 2012; 10(2):102–10.

63. Doria-Rose VP, White MC, Klabunde CN, et al. Use of lung cancer screening tests in the United States: results from the 2010 National Health Interview Survey. Cancer Epidemiol Biomarkers Prev 2012;21(7):1049–59.

64. National Lung Screening Trial Research Team, Aberle DR, Berg CD, et al. The National Lung Screening Trial: overview and study design. Radiology 2011; 258(1):243–53.

65. National Lung Screening Trial Research Team, Aberle DR, Adams AM, et al. Reduced lung-cancer mortality with low-dose computed tomographic screening. N Engl J Med 2011;365(5):395–409.

66. Bach PB, Gould MK. When the average applies to no one: personalized decision making about potential benefits of lung cancer screening. Ann Intern Med 2012;157(8):571–3.

67. Kovalchik SA, Tammemagi M, Berg CD, et al. Targeting of low-dose CT screening according to the risk of lung-cancer death. N Engl J Med 2013; 369(3):245–54.

68. Aberle DR, DeMello S, Berg CD, et al. Results of the two incidence screenings in the National Lung Screening Trial. N Engl J Med 2013;369(10):920–31.

69. de Koning HJ, Meza R, Plevritis SK, et al. Benefits and harms of computed tomography lung cancer screening strategies: a comparative modeling study for the US Preventive Services Task Force. Ann Intern Med 2013. [Epub ahead of print]. http://dx.doi.org/10.7326/M13-2316.

70. Patz EF Jr, Pinsky P, Gatsonis C, et al. Overdiagnosis in low-dose computed tomography screening for lung cancer. JAMA Intern Med 2014;174(2):269–74.

71. Baldwin DR, Duffy SW, Wald NJ, et al. UK Lung Screen (UKLS) nodule management protocol: modelling of a single screen randomised controlled trial of low-dose CT screening for lung cancer. Thorax 2011;66(4):308–13.

72. Horeweg N, van der Aalst CM, Thunnissen E, et al. Characteristics of lung cancers detected by computer tomography screening in the randomized NELSON trial. Am J Respir Crit Care Med 2013;187(8):848–54.

73. Saghir Z, Dirksen A, Ashraf H, et al. CT screening for lung cancer brings forward early disease. The randomised Danish Lung Cancer Screening Trial: status after five annual screening rounds with low-dose CT. Thorax 2012;67(4):296–301.

74. Becker N, Motsch E, Gross ML, et al. Randomized study on early detection of lung cancer with MSCT in Germany: study design and results of the first screening round. J Cancer Res Clin Oncol 2012;138(9):1475–86.

75. Pastorino U, Rossi M, Rosato V, et al. Annual or biennial CT screening versus observation in heavy smokers: 5-year results of the MILD trial. Eur J Cancer Prev 2012;21(3):308–15.

76. Lopes Pegna A, Picozzi G, Mascalchi M, et al. Design, recruitment and baseline results of the ITALUNG trial for lung cancer screening with low-dose CT. Lung Cancer 2009;64:34–40.

77. van Klaveren RJ, Oudkerk M, Prokop M, et al. Management of lung nodules detected by volume CT scanning. N Engl J Med 2009;361(23):2221–9.

78. Henschke CI, Yankelevitz DF, Yip R, et al. Lung cancers diagnosed at annual CT screening: volume doubling times. Radiology 2012;263(2):578–83.

79. US Preventive Services Task Force. Screening for lung cancer. 2013. Available at: http://www.uspreventiveservicestaskforce.org/uspstf/uspslung.htm. Accessed January 15, 2014.

80. Moyer VA. Screening for lung cancer: US Preventive Services Task Force Recommendation statement. Ann Intern Med 2013. [Epub ahead of print]. http://dx.doi.org/10.7326/M13-2771.

81. Jaklitsch MT, Jacobson FL, Austin JH, et al. The American Association for Thoracic Surgery guidelines for lung cancer screening using low-dose computed tomography scans for lung cancer survivors and other high-risk groups. J Thorac Cardiovasc Surg 2012;144(1):33–8.

82. Smith RA, Manassaram-Baptiste D, Brooks D, et al. Cancer screening in the United States, 2014: a review of current American Cancer Society guidelines and current issues in cancer screening. CA Cancer J Clin 2014;64(1):30–51. http://dx.doi.org/10.3322/caac.21212.

83. Detterbeck FC, Mazzone PJ, Naidich DP, et al. Screening for lung cancer: diagnosis and management of lung cancer, 3rd ed: American College of Chest Physicians evidence-based clinical practice guidelines. Chest 2013;143(Suppl 5): e78S–92S.

84. Bach PB, Mirkin JN, Oliver TK, et al. Benefits and harms of CT screening for lung cancer: a systematic review. JAMA 2012;307(22):2418–29.

85. American Lung Association. Providing guidance on lung cancer screening to patients and physicians. 2012. Available at: http://www.lung.org/lung-disease/lung-cancer/lung-cancer-screening-guidelines/. Accessed January 15, 2014.

86. Wood DE, Eapen GA, Ettinger DS, et al. Lung cancer screening. J Natl Compr Canc Netw 2012;10(2):240–65.

87. Backhus LM, Hayanga AJ, Au D, et al. The effect of provider density on lung cancer survival among blacks and whites in the United States. J Thorac Oncol 2013;8(5):549–53.

88. Lung Cancer Alliance. National framework for excellence in lung cancer screening and continuum of care. Washington, DC: Lung Cancer Alliance; Available at: http://www.lungcanceralliance.org/get-information/am-i-at-risk/national-framework-for-lung-screening-excellence.html. Accessed January 15, 2014.

89. American College of Radiology. Computed tomography accreditation program. Available at: http://www.acr.org/Quality-Safety/Accreditation/CT. Accessed January 15, 2014.

90. American College of Radiology. Accredited facility search. Available at: http://www.acr.org/Quality-Safety/Accreditation/Accredited-Facility-Search. Accessed January 15, 2014.
91. Boiselle PM, White CS, Ravenel JG. Computed tomographic screening for lung cancer: current practice patterns at leading academic medical centers. JAMA Intern Med 2014;174(2):286–7.
92. Cagnon CH, Cody DD, McNitt-Gray MF, et al. Description and implementation of a quality control program in an imaging-based clinical trial. Acad Radiol 2006; 13:1431–41.
93. Gierada DS, Garg K, Nath H, et al. CT quality assurance in the lung screening study component of the National Lung Screening Trial: implications for multicenter imaging trials. AJR Am J Roentgenol 2009;193:419–24.
94. Bankier AA, Kressel HY. Through the looking glass revisited: the need for more meaning and less drama in the reporting of dose and dose reduction in CT. Radiology 2012;265(1):4–8.
95. Smith-Bindman R, Lipson J, Marcus R, et al. Radiation dose associated with common computed tomography examinations and the associated lifetime attributable risk of cancer. Arch Intern Med 2009;169(22):2078–86.
96. Siegelman JR, Gress DA. Radiology stewardship and quality improvement: the process and costs of implementing a CT radiation dose optimization committee in a medium-sized community hospital system. J Am Coll Radiol 2013;10(6): 416–22.
97. National Lung Screening Trial Research Team, Church TR, Black WC, et al. Results of initial low-dose computed tomographic screening for lung cancer. N Engl J Med 2013;368(21):1980–91.
98. Henschke CI, Yip R, Yankelevitz DF, et al. Definition of a positive test result in computed tomography screening for lung cancer. Ann Intern Med 2013; 158(4):246–52.
99. McWilliams A, Tammemagi MC, Mayo JR, et al. Probability of cancer in pulmonary nodules detected on first screening CT. N Engl J Med 2013;369(10):910–9.
100. Mehta HJ, Ravenel JG, Shaftman SR, et al. The utility of nodule volume in the context of malignancy prediction for small pulmonary nodules. Chest 2013. http://dx.doi.org/10.1378/chest.13-0708.
101. Hughes JR, Solomon LJ, Fingar JR, et al. The natural history of efforts to stop smoking: a prospective cohort study. Drug Alcohol Depend 2013;128(1–2): 171–4.
102. Alpert HR, Connolly GN, Biener L. A prospective cohort study challenging the effectiveness of population-based medical intervention for smoking cessation. Tob Control 2013;22(1):32–7.
103. Ashraf H, Tønnesen P, Holst Pedersen J, et al. Effect of CT screening on smoking habits at 1-year follow-up in the Danish Lung Cancer Screening Trial (DLCST). Thorax 2009;64(5):388–92.
104. Townsend CO, Clark MM, Jett JR, et al. Relation between smoking cessation and receiving results from three annual spiral chest computed tomography scans for lung carcinoma screening. Cancer 2005;103(10):2154–62.
105. Styn MA, Land SR, Perkins KA, et al. Smoking behavior 1 year after computed tomography screening for lung cancer: effect of physician referral for abnormal CT findings. Cancer Epidemiol Biomarkers Prev 2009;18(12):3484–9.
106. Park ER, Ostroff JS, Rakowski W, et al. Risk perceptions among participants undergoing lung cancer screening: baseline results from the National Lung Screening Trial. Ann Behav Med 2009;37(3):268–79.

107. Park ER, Gareen IF, Jain A, et al. Examining whether lung screening changes risk perceptions: National Lung Screening Trial participants at 1-year follow-up. Cancer 2013;119(7):1306–13.

108. Park ER, Streck JM, Gareen IF, et al. A qualitative study of lung cancer risk perceptions and smoking beliefs among National Lung Screening Trial Participants. Nicotine Tob Res 2014;16(2):166–73.

109. Fiore MC, Jaén CR, Baker TB, et al. Treating tobacco use and dependence: 2008 update. Clinical practice guideline. Rockville (MD): US Department of Health and Human Services, Public Health Service; 2008.

110. Piper ME, Kenford S, Fiore MC, et al. Smoking cessation and quality of life: changes in life satisfaction over 3 years following a quit attempt. Ann Behav Med 2012;43(2):262–70.

111. US Department of Health and Human Services. The health benefits of smoking cessation: a report of the surgeon general. Atlanta (GA): US Department of Health and Human Services, Public Health Services, Centers for Disease Control, Center for Chronic Disease Prevention and Health Promotion, Office on Smoking and Health; 1990. DHHS Publication No. (CDC) 90–8416.

112. Tariman JD, Berry DL, Cochrane B, et al. Preferred and actual participation roles during health care decision making in persons with cancer: a systematic review. Ann Oncol 2010;21(6):1145–51.

113. Singh JA, Sloan JA, Atherton PJ, et al. Preferred roles in treatment decision making among patients with cancer: a pooled analysis of studies using the Control Preferences Scale. Am J Manag Care 2010;16(9):688–96.

114. Harris RP, Sheridan SL, Lewis CL, et al. The harms of screening: a proposed taxonomy and application to lung cancer screening. JAMA Intern Med 2014; 174(2):281–5.

115. Sheridan SL, Harris RP, Woolf SH, et al. Shared decision making about screening and chemoprevention: a suggested approach from the US Preventive Services Task Force. Am J Prev Med 2004;26(1):56–66.

116. Soylemez Wiener R, Gould MK, Woloshin S, et al. What do you mean, a spot? A qualitative analysis of patients' reactions to discussions with their physicians about pulmonary nodules. Chest 2013;143(3):672–7.

117. Patient Protection and Affordable Care Act (Public Law 111-148). 2010. Available at: https://www.healthcare.gov/where-can-i-read-the-affordable-care-act/. Accessed January 15, 2014.

118. Peikes D, Genevro J, Scholle SH, et al. The patient-centered medical home: strategies to put patients at the center of primary care. AHRQ Pub No. 11-0029. Rockville (MD): Agency for Healthcare Research and Quality; 2011.

119. Hunnibell LS, Slatore CG, Ballard EA. Foundations for lung nodule management for nurse navigators. Clin J Oncol Nurs 2013;17(5):525–31.

120. Klabunde CN, Ambs A, Keating NL, et al. The role of primary care physicians in cancer care. J Gen Intern Med 2009;24(9):1029–36.

121. Singh H, Hirani K, Kadiyala H, et al. Characteristics and predictors of missed opportunities in lung cancer diagnosis: an electronic health record-based study. J Clin Oncol 2010;28(20):3307–15.

122. Cole-Lewis H, Kershaw T. Text messaging as a tool for behavior change in disease prevention and management. Epidemiol Rev 2010;32(1):56–69.

123. Bekelman JE, Kim M, Emanuel EJ. Toward accountable cancer care. JAMA Intern Med 2013;173(11):958–9.

Screening Strategies for Colorectal Cancer in Asymptomatic Adults

D. Kim Turgeon, MD[a], Mack T. Ruffin IV, MD, MPH[b],*

KEYWORDS

- Colon cancer • Rectal cancer • Screening • Surveillance • Primary care

KEY POINTS

- Early detection of colorectal cancer and preinvasive forms prevents death from this cancer.
- All adults aged 50 years and older are at risk for colorectal cancer, and should be engaged in a decision to be screened.
- For adults at average risk for colorectal cancer, there is no preferred screening method.
- Colorectal cancer screening methods include stool-based tests and imaging of the colon directly or indirectly.
- Average-risk adults need help in defining their preferred screening method.
- Family health history and personal health history can place a person at increased risk for colorectal cancer.
- Adults at increased risk for colorectal cancer should be counseled to undergo colonoscopy.
- Adenoma and other colorectal findings require surveillance to prevent early recurrence or progression to invasive colorectal cancer.
- New screening methods are under development, although whether they perform better than the currently available methods has yet to be proved.

SEVERITY AND EPIDEMIOLOGY OF COLORECTAL CANCER

Excluding skin cancers, colorectal cancer (CRC) is the third most common cancer in the United States for both men and women, accounting for approximately 9% of all

Conflicts of Interest: None.
Dr M.T. Ruffin was supported by the Max and Buena Lichter Research Professorship in Family Medicine.
[a] Division of Gastroenterology, Department of Internal Medicine, University of Michigan, 1500 East Medical Center Drive, Ann Arbor, MI 48109, USA; [b] Department of Family Medicine, University of Michigan, 1018 Fuller Street, Ann Arbor, MI 48104-1213, USA
* Corresponding author.
E-mail address: mruffin@med.umich.edu

http://dx.doi.org/10.1016/j.pop.2014.02.008
0095-4543/14/$ – see front matter © 2014 Elsevier Inc. All rights reserved.
primarycare.theclinics.com

cancer deaths, and is the leading cause of cancer deaths in nonsmokers.[1,2] Approximately 5% of the United States population is estimated to develop CRC within their lifetime (5.2% and 4.8% for men and women, respectively).[1] The risk of CRC increases with age; 90% of cases are in those older than 50 years.[3] Mortality rates for CRC in the United States have been declining for both men and women over the last 2 decades.[1] Incidence rates for CRC declined 4.1% per year between 2005 and 2009 among those 50 years or older (ie, the screened population) in the United States, yet increased 1.1% per year among those younger than 50 years.[3] The observed decrease in mortality and incidence most likely reflects prevention (by polyp removal), early detection, and improvements in treatment. Although the total number of CRC cases among those younger than 50 years is small, the increase in incidence in this unscreened population may reflect environmental and other risk factors such as smoking, diet, obesity, and diabetes. Smoking increases the risk for CRC, and this effect may be even greater in female smokers.[4] The incidence and death rates for CRC are highest among African Americans regardless of gender.[1] Incidence and death rates in African Americans have declined in recent years, but not as much as observed in whites.[1] Before 1989, white men had higher CRC incidence rates in comparison with African American men; rates between white and African American women were similar. However, since 1989 incidence rates have been higher for African Americans of both genders when compared with their white counterparts.[5] These disparities may reflect differences in underlying risk factors or environmental exposures (eg, diet, physical activity, obesity, history of tobacco use), differences in comorbid conditions, and differences in access to and receipt of quality health care.[1,3,5] For example, African Americans are less likely to be diagnosed with CRC at a localized stage when treatment is most successful,[5] and are less likely to receive standard therapy for CRC.[6]

SCREENING STRATEGIES AND SUPPORTING EVIDENCE

For early detection to reduce mortality from CRC, the disease must be found in the early stages when a cure is possible. These early stages include adenomatous polyps and noninvasive cancer. Theoretically, interruption of the adenoma-carcinoma sequence with polypectomy reduces the incidence of CRC by as much as 90%[7]; however, not all adenomatous polyps place patients at the same risk for polyp recurrence or progression to cancer.[8] Patients with advanced adenomas are at higher risk for recurrent advanced adenomas or progression to cancer.[8] Advanced adenoma is defined as an adenoma with significant villous features (>25%), size of 1.0 cm or more, high-grade dysplasia, or early invasive cancer.[9] These characteristics are often referred to as a screen-relevant neoplasia (SRN). Experts have advocated using the advanced adenoma as the principal target of screening, as its detection and removal enables the prevention of CRC.[9] Therefore, it is important to understand how well CRC screening strategies in patients detect advanced adenomatous polyps, noninvasive cancer, and late-stage cancer.

Several screening strategies exist for CRC, including the fecal occult blood test (FOBT), the stool DNA (sDNA) test, flexible sigmoidoscopy (FS), double-contrast barium enema (DCBE), computed tomographic colonography (CTC), and ocular colonoscopy (OC). A summary of commonly recommended CRC screening options for average-risk adults aged 50 years and older are summarized in **Table 1**. Routine screening is recommended for average-risk individuals starting at age 50.[10] However, these preventive strategies reach a limited percentage of the target population, for a variety of reasons. Approximately 58% to 65% of adults at average risk for CRC and older than 50 years are current for CRC screening with any of the nationally

Table 1
Summary of commonly recommended screening options for colorectal cancer for average-risk adults aged 50 years and older

Test	Interval[a]	Efficacy	Critical Details
Highly sensitive fecal occult blood test (FOBT)[b]	Annual	When used consistently and with proper technique over time—including proper follow-up when test results are positive—significant reductions in mortality and incidence have been observed	Two samples from each of 3 consecutive bowel movements collected at home Dietary and medication restrictions recommended during collection period Avoid aspirin and other nonsteroidal anti-inflammatory drugs, vitamin C, red meat, poultry, fish, and some raw vegetables A single sample of stool collected during a digital rectal examination is not acceptable
Fecal immunohistochemical test (FIT)	Annual	Though some report no clear patterns of superior performance between highly sensitive FOBT and FIT,[c] limited evidence suggests FIT may have superior sensitivity and specificity[d]	Only 1 stool sample collected at home No dietary or medication restrictions required A single sample of stool collected during a digital rectal examination is not acceptable
Flexible sigmoidoscopy	Every 5 y	More effective at detecting advanced adenoma and carcinoma than stool-based tests[e]	Does not require sedation or as extensive colonic preparation as colonoscopy Protective effect is limited to the portion of the colon examined
Double-contrast barium enema (DCBE)	Every 5 y	Sensitivity varies from 50% to 90% depending on polyp size and cancer stage[f]; recent evidence suggests using colonoscopy in lieu of DCBE[g]	Requires colonic preparation Does not require sedation
Colonoscopy	Every 10 y	All other forms of screening, if positive, require colonoscopy as a second procedure Colonoscopy with clearing of neoplasms by polypectomy has a significant impact on CRC incidence and, by extension, mortality	Requires extensive colonic preparation, sedation, and assistance of another person after procedure

[a] Interval between screening procedures if the test is normal.
[b] The American Cancer Society recommends discontinuing the use of older, lower-sensitivity versions of the guaiac test in favor of newer, high-sensitivity FOBT.[10]
[c] From Rabeneck and colleagues.[90]
[d] From Medical Advisory Secretariat,[91] Faivre and colleagues,[22] and Denters and colleagues.[23]
[e] From Littlejohn and colleagues.[92]
[f] From Winawer and colleagues.[28]
[g] From Maheswaren and Tighe[93] and Shariff and colleagues.[94]
Adapted from Levin B, Lieberman DA, McFarland B, et al. Screening and surveillance for the early detection of colorectal cancer and adenomatous polyps, 2008: a joint guideline from the American Cancer Society, the US Multi-Society Task Force on Colorectal Cancer, and the American College of Radiology. Gastroenterology 2008;134(5):1570–95.

recommended strategies.[11,12] As with all screening strategies, CRC screening requires attention to management of screen-positive and screen-negative patients to ensure adequate follow-up. Without such attention, the goal of the screening (ie, prevention of colon cancer) will not be met.

Target Population

In all adults the risk for CRC increases with age. Age 50 years is the point at which the prevalence of CRC becomes high enough that screening is feasible. Adults with a family history of early-onset CRC should be screened 10 years younger than the age of family member diagnosed with CRC. Screening is recommended for all asymptomatic adults aged 50 to 75 years. However, clinicians and patients need to understand that screened adults need to be able to undergo complete diagnostic evaluation of their colon if they screen positive. For example, one should not use stool cards to screen a patient with chronic obstructive lung disease who is physically unable to undergo an OC if the stool cards are positive.

Screening for CRC is recommended by most expert groups to stop at age 75 years.[10,13,14] For older adults with no CRC screening exposure, some recommend screening until age 80 years.[15]

Evidence that Screening Works

Stool blood tests

Stool blood tests fall into 2 categories based on the analyte detected: guaiac (FOBT) or immunochemical (fecal immunochemical test [FIT]). When performed for CRC screening, a positive result for either test requires a diagnostic evaluation with OC. A screening interval of 1 year is recommended for either test if negative. Several large randomized controlled trials (RCTs) have evaluated the efficacy of screening with FOBT.[16–20] The data have consistently demonstrated that screening with FOBT reduces the mortality from CRC. The reduction ranged from 33% for studies with annual screening in the Minnesota Colon Cancer Control Study[20] to 15% with biannual screening.[21] These differences in mortality reduction reflect the variability in the frequency and type of FOBT used among the different studies. FIT tests have been shown to be superior to FOBT in a population-based organized European screening program.[22,23] As noted by others, FITs have been slow to be adopted by American opinion leaders and United States CRC guidelines.[24] By contrast, the European Guidelines for Quality Assurance in Colorectal Cancer Screening and Diagnosis recommend FIT as the test of choice for population-based screening.[25] An advantage of FOBT and FIT screening is that they can be performed in privacy at home and are inexpensive; therefore, the compliance rates in the general population are likely to be higher than those for more invasive methods. The disadvantage is the social stigma of handling stool. The FITs require only a single sample of stool annually, compared with 3 stool samples for FOBT.

A positive stool test is any stool sample that is positive on the FOBT or FIT. A positive result should not be repeated for confirmation. A patient with a positive test needs a complete diagnostic evaluation of the colon. Ideally this would be an OC, but DCBE is an alternative approach.

Stool DNA

The sDNA test has recently been included as an option for CRC screening.[26] These tests look for known alterations in the adenoma-carcinoma sequence that may be shed into the stool. Because no single alteration is present in all CRC, a multitarget assay is needed to obtain adequate sensitivity. There is currently only one commercially available sDNA test in the United States.[27] This test, requiring an entire stool (minimum 30 g), is significantly more expensive than FOBT. sDNA testing, like FOBT and FIT, offers the advantage of privacy but the disadvantage of stool handling. Like FOBT and FIT, if the sDNA test is positive a diagnostic OC is recommended. As sDNA tests continue to evolve, positive result criteria must be clearly defined. Future sDNA tests may include FIT along with a panel of DNA. The appropriate interval for repeat testing has not been determined. At present, there is no sDNA test approved for clinical use.

Flexible sigmoidoscopy

FS examination covers only the distal colon, and allows the detection of colorectal neoplasia only in that visualized portion.[28] This screening modality has been advocated as being more convenient than OC, as the preparation (2 small enemas 1 hour before the examination) is considered less onerous to patients. However, the percentage of Medicare enrollees completing this procedure declined from 1998 to 2005,[29] largely because of the procedure's inability to detect abnormalities beyond the distal colon. A case-control study has shown that rigid sigmoidoscopy decreases the odds ratio (OR) of CRC mortality for tumors that are within reach of the scope.[30] Two other case-control studies have also suggested that screening sigmoidoscopy reduces CRC mortality.[31,32] Data from RCTs are lacking. In an attempt to improve its effectiveness, FS screening has been combined with FOBT. In an RCT of 12,479 patients from New York, the addition of FOBT testing lowered the mortality of CRC, and patients in the combined screening strategy had cancer detected at an earlier stage and survived longer.[19] One recent study of a single FS screen in patients between the ages 55 and 64 years reduced the incidence of CRC by 23% and mortality by 31%.[33]

A positive FS is visual observation of an SRN with or without pathologic confirmation. It is within the standard of care to visually confirm an SRN that warrants complete colonic evaluation and to stop the FS with further examination or biopsy of the lesion. Like OC, the operator needs to define the quality of the colonic preparation and define the depth of insertion. Preparation that limits visual inspection or incomplete insertion represents an incomplete screening study that should be repeated, or the patient should be referred for OC.

Double-contrast barium enema

The sensitivity of DCBE varies widely, from 50% to 80% for polyps smaller than 1 cm, 70% to 90% for polyps larger than 1 cm, and 55% to 85% for Dukes stage A and B colon cancers.[28] The sensitivity of DCBE for detecting cancers is lower than that of OC, as shown in a retrospective analysis of 2193 consecutive CRC cases.[34] DCBE has been combined with FS to improve sensitivity by better visualization of the rectosigmoid area. The sensitivity of this combined method was 97.6% for carcinoma and 99% for adenoma.[35] The patient experience (pain, comfort) with DCBE is significantly worse than that with FOBT, FS, or OC.[36] The disadvantage of this combined method is that it requires the individual to complete 2 preparations and 2 relatively uncomfortable screening tests unless logistics permit both procedures to be done on the same day. A positive DCBE consists of radiographic images suggestive of SRN. Patients with such images need complete diagnostic colonic evaluation with an OC. DCBE studies with stool or other bowel content that limits the screening should be repeated, or the patient should be referred for OC.

Computer tomographic colonoscopy

CTC, also referred to as virtual colonoscopy, is a minimally invasive imaging examination of the entire colon and rectum. There has not been a prospective RCT (nor is one anticipated) to evaluate the efficacy of CTC in reducing CRC mortality. It offers less risk to the patient than OC, but requires the same bowel preparation. CTC has some associated discomfort because sedation is not used and it also involves some radiation exposure. There have been several large prospective trials comparing CTC with OC in patients referred for OC. Cotton and colleagues[37] and Rockey and colleagues[38] found sensitivity for polyps (≥10 mm) of 55% and 59%, respectively. In 1233 asymptomatic adults, Pickhardt and colleagues[39] reported 93.8% sensitivity for polyps larger than 10 mm and 88.7% for polyps 6 mm or larger. Similar to DCBE, a positive CTC presents images suggestive of SRN and requires a complete diagnostic OC. A CTC with stool obscuring the images or poor-quality preparation should be repeated, or the patient should be referred for OC.

Ocular colonoscopy

OC provides the most complete visualization of the colon, and allows for the removal of polyps.[40] OC detected advanced colorectal neoplasms (adenomas ≥10 mm, villous adenomas, adenomas with high-grade dysplasia, invasive cancer) in 10.5% of 3121 predominantly male United States veterans.[41] Among patients with no adenomas distal to the splenic flexure, 2.7% had advanced proximal neoplasms. Patients with adenomas in the distal colon were more likely to have advanced proximal neoplasm than were patients with no distal adenomas (OR = 3.4, 90% confidence interval [CI] 1.8–6.5 vs OR = 2.6, 90% CI 1.7–4.1). One-half of those with advanced proximal neoplasm, however, had no distal adenomas. In a study of 1994 adults (≥50 years) who underwent an employer-sponsored OC screening program, 5.6% had advanced neoplasm.[42] Acceptability of OC includes risk for perforation (<1%, up to 2% if polypectomy or coagulation is performed), sedation-related adverse events (1%), preparation discomfort and inconvenience, cost, and access.

A positive OC is an SRN proved on histopathology. The referring clinician also needs to know whether the screening OC was adequate enough to be able to determine the timing of the next surveillance examination. The key quality markers are summarized in **Table 2**.

Patients at Increased Risk

Individuals at increased risk (above-average risk) should have individualized screening recommendations. Colonoscopy is recommended as the first-line test in these individuals. Individuals at increased risk are those with a family history of CRC (**Table 3**). Surveillance colonoscopy is recommended for those at increased risk attributable to: (1) a personal history of CRC; (2) a history of ulcerative or Crohn colitis; or (3) a personal history of adenoma (**Table 4**). Persons in whom an inherited CRC syndrome is suspected (eg, strong family history or ≥10 polyps) should be referred for genetic evaluation. There are a variety of genetic syndromes that significantly increase a patient's risk, but these are rare, and as such are not addressed in this article. For more details on CRC screening among those with inherited CRC syndrome, the authors recommend the National Comprehensive Cancer Network CRC screening guidelines, which can be accessed free at http://www.nccn.org/professionals/default.aspx. Of importance, a system developed to address average-risk and increased-risk individuals based on family and personal history covers 98% of the population.

HELPING PATIENTS DETERMINE THEIR PREFERRED SCREENING METHOD

No strong evidence favors one CRC screening method over another for reducing CRC mortality.[43] The US Preventive Services Task Force (USPSTF), the American Cancer

Table 2
Quality markers of colonoscopy

Quality Marker	Details
Colonic preparation[a]	Excellent, Good, Fair, Poor, Unsatisfactory
Cecal intubation[a]	Should be documented by at least 2 landmarks (appendiceal orifice, ileocecal valve [ICV], cecal sling, intubation of the terminal ileum)
Pathology	A letter should be sent after endoscopy to the patient and the referring physician with the actual histology of the polyps removed and recommended interval for the next follow-up examination
Withdrawal time[b]	Colonoscopy withdrawal times of >8 min are associated with higher adenoma detection rates[95]
Adenoma detection rate (ADR)[c]	Men: >25%; women: >15%[96]

[a] Quality markers that should be reported on the colonoscopy document. A copy of the endoscopy report should be given to the patient and sent to the referring physician. Adequate examination preparations for colorectal cancer surveillance are limited to Excellent and Good preps. Effective colonoscopists should be able to intubate the cecum in ≥90% of all cases and ≥95% when the indication is screening in a healthy adult.[97]

[b] Withdrawal time, the endoscopist's cecal intubation rate are not reported on an individual patient's colonoscopy report.

[c] The ADR is defined as the proportion of screening colonoscopies in which 1 or more adenomas are found. The endoscopy unit often calculates these statistics on their endoscopists, but the statistics are not on public record (although means and ranges for the unit may be on public record). ADR has been inversely associated with risk of interval colorectal cancer.[98] Future quality measures will probably include mean number of adenomas per procedure and serrated polyp detection rate.[96,99]

Table 3
Screening recommendations for persons at increased risk because of family history of colorectal cancer[a]

Family History	Age to Start Colonoscopy (y)	Surveillance Interval (y)
First-degree relative (FDR) <50 y or 2 FDR any age[b]	40, or 10 y before earliest diagnosis	Repeat every 3–5
FDR >50 y	50	Repeat every 5
Second-degree relative (SDR) <50 y[b]	50	Repeat every 5
Two or more SDR	50	Repeat every 7–8
SDR and 2 third-degree relatives (TDR)[b]	50	Repeat every 7–8
Grandparent >50 y	50	Repeat every 7–8
Aunt/uncle or TDR	50	Repeat every 10
FDR with history of advanced adenoma	50	Repeat every 7–8

First-degree relative: parents, full siblings, or children.
Second-degree relative: grandparents, grandchildren, aunts, uncles, nephews, nieces, or half-siblings.
Third-degree relative: first cousins, great-grandparents, or great-grandchildren.
[a] Colonoscopy recommended as the first line screening test.
[b] Consider inherited colorectal cancer syndrome.
Adapted from National Comprehensive Cancer Network. NCCN clinical practice guidelines in oncology for colorectal cancer screening. Version 2.2013. NCCN; 2013.

Table 4
Screening recommendations for persons at increased risk because of ulcerative colitis or Crohn colitis, history of adenomas and advanced adenomas, and personal history of colorectal cancer

Risk Factor	Age to Start Colonoscopy	Surveillance Intervals
Ulcerative colitis or Crohn colitis	8–10 y after onset of pancolitis; 12 y after onset of left-sided colitis	Repeat every 1–2 y with >40 random surveillance biopsies
History of adenomas	—	Repeat every 5 y
History of advanced adenomas	—	Repeat every 3 y
Personal history of colorectal cancer	—	At 1 y, then in 2–3 y if negative and 3–5 y if continues to be negative; if adenoma is found, repeat every 1–3 y

Adapted from National Comprehensive Cancer Network. NCCN clinical practice guidelines in oncology: colorectal cancer screening. Version 2.2013. NCCN; 2013.

Society, and the National Institutes of Health State-of-the-Science Conference recommend that CRC screening should be based on patient preferences so as to optimize the completion rate.[13,26,44] Patient preferences for CRC screening are highly variable and relate to the particular test characteristics of efficacy, sensitivity, cost, complexity, and possible harm.[45–55] Patient-preference clarification does not mean merely offering choices without guidance: when the information and options are not provided within the context of patients' preferences and values, patients' ability to make a decision may actually decrease.[56] Physicians are encouraged to incorporate patient values when discussing CRC screening and eliciting their screening choice, counseling patients to choose the test most congruous with their preferences and values.[43,57,58]

Implementing the recommendation to incorporate patient values and preferences into decision making on CRC screening is not simple; it takes time, effort, and skills. Shared decision making (SDM) is an approach that may facilitate this process. SDM recognizes the central role of the patient-physician relationship in helping patients make such decisions. However, SDM requires more time and resources than most physicians have for a single issue, especially when faced with multiple and sometimes competing agendas.[59–62] Moreover, physicians do not always correctly perceive and address those factors important to patients, and may not have the training and skills to provide for effective SDM.[63–65]

Detailed and explicit guidelines outlining how the primary care clinician should undertake SDM for CRC screening do not exist. However, in a report describing the USPSTF's position on SDM, Sheridan and colleagues[43] outline that decisions using SDM encompass the following 4 principles: (1) The patient understands the risk and seriousness of the condition; (2) the patient understands the preventive service, including its risks and benefits as well as alternatives and uncertainties; (3) the patient has evaluated his or her values regarding possible benefits and harms; and (4) the patient and clinician work together as partners, with each clarifying their knowledge and preferences for the decision.

The authors recommend for patients who are already participating in screening by a given method that clinicians confirm with the patient that it is their preferred method. If so, clinicians should implement a system to keep patients current with that method; if not, clinicians should discuss screening options in a manner consistent with the 4 principles described. Confirming a patient's preferred screening method could occur through the use of this single question:

There are several ways to screen for colorectal cancer, with no single method having a clear advantage over another. Last time you were screened using _____ [insert previous method here]. Would you like to continue with this method?

For patients who have not followed through on a previously agreed-upon screening method, the authors suggest discussing their barriers to screening and, when applicable, exploring alternative screening options that minimize identified barriers. For patients just becoming eligible for screening, clinicians should not assume there is a best screening test for the average-risk patient older than 50 years. When time does not allow for a detailed discussion of screening options, or if some screening options are not easily accessible in a given area, it is suggested that the discussion be narrowed to 2 options: stool testing or OC. As discussed next, decision aids can also be used to help patients make an informed screening choice. The authors recommend against simply assuming that the best test for the average-risk patient is OC. The best test is the one performed correctly and repeatedly, whether the interval is every year or once every 10 years.

Decision Aids

Decision aids are designed to help patients make informed and value-based decisions about health care when more than one medically reasonable test or treatment option exists. Such aids can help inform patients about CRC screening options and promote SDM.[66,67] Moreover, decision aids can help align patient values with screening options and decrease decisional conflict, and activate patient follow-through.[66,68,69] By helping to clarify patient preferences, decision aids can also help reduce health care costs by preventing unnecessary or unwanted care.[66,68]

Despite their promise, the use of decision aids in practice remains modest.[2,3,5,68–70] This lackluster uptake can be explained, in part, by clinical inertia, insufficient economic incentives, inadequate clinician training, and a poor match between available decision aids and the needs and demands of the clinical setting.[68,70,71] To overcome these barriers several strategies have been suggested, including training clinicians in SDM and decision-aid use; promoting decision-aid use via an in-house champion or thought leader; choosing/tailoring decision aids to match patients' needs (eg, literacy level, cultural orientation); support from clinic leadership advocating the use of decision aids (eg, committing resources to ensure decision aids are consistently available); integrating decision aids into clinical workflows; implementing reminder systems to trigger SDM and decision-aid use; linking SDM and decision aids to quality indicators (eg, patient satisfaction, improved screening rates); and implementing reward systems linked to SDM and effective use of decision aids.[66,72–75]

The USPSTF advocates the practice of SDM when helping patients decide on a given CRC screening modality, noting that discussions with patients about screening should not only incorporate information on test quality (eg, efficacy, benefits, and risks of screening options) but also on the availability of a given test within a given setting (eg, rural settings may often have poorer access to some screening tests in comparison with academic settings in suburban or urban environments). The resources for clinicians to facilitate this SDM are the usual paper and Web pages of information. To the authors' knowledge, there are currently no readily available, nonproprietary interactive tools patients can access that would allow them to arrive at a preferred screening option and then engage their clinician in an informed discussion. For more on the topic of SDM the reader is referred to the article "Prostate Cancer Screening" elsewhere in this issue, in which Ragsdale and colleagues discuss in detail a strategy to promote SDM with patients in the primary care setting (see their section on shared decision making).

SURVEILLANCE

As with all screening strategies, CRC screening involves surveillance of patients screened positive and treated. Surveillance involves serial colonic examination with OC. Blood and stool markers are being developed for surveillance, but none are ready for clinical use at the time of writing. The recommended interval of surveillance OC depends on the colonic disorder as summarized in **Table 5**. Quality of the baseline OC is associated with the risk of interval cancer development. It is not clear whether the risk for recurrence(s) continues to be elevated if the subsequent surveillance OC reveals no polyps or only low-risk adenomas.[76] The current recommendation is for patients with low-risk adenomas (≤ 2 tubular adenomas, ≤ 1 cm in size with low-grade dysplasia) at baseline followed by a normal OC at the first surveillance OC to move to OC every 10 years; the current recommendation is not to perform fecal blood testing for CRC screening in patients under OC surveillance.[76]

Care and attention to previous OC reports is required to avoid "polyp surveillance creep": the tendency to increase surveillance OC frequency in the absence of

Table 5
Recommended intervals for next colonoscopy based upon findings

Colonoscopy and Pathology Results	Recommended Surveillance Interval (y)
No polyps	10
<10 mm hyperplastic polyps in rectum or sigmoid area	10
1–2 tubular adenomas <10 mm	5–10
3–10 tubular adenomas	3
>10 adenomas	<3
≥1 tubular adenoma ≥10 mm	3
≥1 villous adenoma	3
Adenoma with high-grade dysplasia	3
Serrated lesions	
<10 mm with no dysplasia	5
≥10 mm	3
Any size serrated with dysplasia	3
Traditional serrated adenoma any size	3
Serrated polyposis syndrome[a]	1

[a] The World Health Organization defines serrated polyposis syndrome as one of the following: (1) at least 5 serrated polyps proximal to sigmoid with 2 or more ≥10 mm, (2) any serrated polyps proximal to sigmoid with family history of serrated polyposis syndrome, or (3) >20 serrated polyps of any size anywhere in the colon.

Adapted from Lieberman DA, Rex DK, Winawer SJ, et al. Guidelines for colonoscopy surveillance after screening and polypectomy: a consensus update by the US Multi-Society Task Force on Colorectal Cancer. Gastroenterology 2012;143(3):844–57.

high-quality evidence to do so. For example, patients may report a previous OC was abnormal with polyps (which would lead to a shorter interval for surveillance OC), whereas a clinician's review of the previous OC and pathology reports might find a normal OC with diverticulosis (which the patient confused with polyps) or only hyperplastic polyps (which had been reported to the patient as benign polyps without specifying histology). In these examples, early OC (ie, before the 10-year interval) could be avoided through attendance to previous OC and related reports.

GUIDELINES

In **Table 6** the range of screening procedures for CRC for adults age 50 years and older at average risk are summarized, along with the interval for each procedure.[76] These CRC screening procedures reflect the consensus of the USPSTF, the American College of Physicians, and the American Cancer Society, whose singular recommendations are outlined. Given time constraints and the multiple demands placed on the typical patient-clinician encounter, many primary care clinicians narrow the range of screening options down to stool test (ie, highly sensitive FOBT, FIT) or OC. Importantly there is not a preferred test for the average-risk adult; the best test for any given patient is the test that patients will complete correctly and repeatedly in accordance with the specified testing interval.

In patients with either CRC or adenomatous polyps in a first-degree relative before the age of 60 years or in 2 or more relatives at any age, the consensus is to recommend OC over the other screening options, and to begin screening at age 40 years or 10 years before the youngest case in the immediate family.[76] For a detailed overview of screening and surveillance recommendations for other high-risk populations, the reader is referred to the joint statement from the American Cancer Society, the US Multi-Society Task Force on Colorectal Cancer, and the American College of Radiology (available at http://onlinelibrary.wiley.com/doi/10.3322/CA.2007.0018/pdf).[26]

CURRENT PRACTICE PATTERNS

The 2006-2007 National Survey of Primary Care Physicians' Recommendations and Practices for Breast, Cervical, Colorectal, and Lung Cancer found that OC is now the most frequently recommended test and that most physicians do not recommend the full menu of test options recommended.[77] This same survey conducted in 1999-2000 had found that FOBT was the most frequently recommended test.[78] At present, few primary care clinicians in the United States perform sigmoidoscopy (<4%), and office systems for follow-up on CRC screening tests are lacking in most primary care practices.[77] It is interesting that despite the screening-attributable decline in CRC incidence and mortality over the last 2 decades, the 2006-2007 survey revealed that fewer physicians perceived CRC screening tests to be effective in comparison with the 1999-2000 survey.[77] These changes in attitude may reflect the attention on OC as the ideal screening test while acknowledging that not all patients have access or will accept OC.

Despite the steady but modest increase in CRC screening rates in the United States over the last 2 decades, the screening rate remains lower for CRC in comparison with those for breast, prostate, and cervical cancer. The 2005 National Health Interview Survey found that, after adjustment, having health care coverage and a usual source of health care were the strongest correlates for use of a CRC screening test. The most commonly reported reasons for not having CRC screening were "never thought about it" and "doctor did not order it."[79] The coming changes in our health care system may help clinicians eliminate these as reasons for not being screened.

Table 6
Guidelines for screening from the United States Preventive Services Task Force, the American College of Physicians, and American Cancer Society

Organization	Recommendations	Evidence Grade[a]
United States Preventive Services Task Force (USPSTF)[b]	Age 50–75 y: Screen with high-sensitivity fecal occult blood test (FOBT), sigmoidoscopy, or colonoscopy	A
	Age 76–85 y: Do not screen routinely	C
	Age 85 y and older: Do not screen	D
	For all populations: Evidence is insufficient to assess the benefits and harms of screening with computed tomographic colonography and fecal DNA testing	I
	Screening tests: High-sensitivity FOBT, sigmoidoscopy with FOBT, and colonoscopy are effective in decreasing colorectal cancer mortality. The risks and benefits of these screening methods vary. Colonoscopy and flexible sigmoidoscopy (to a lesser degree) entail possible serious complications	
	Screening intervals	
	• Annual screening with high-sensitivity FOBT	
	• Sigmoidoscopy every 5 y, with high-sensitivity FOBT every 3 y	
	• Screening colonoscopy every 10 y	
	Implementation	
	• Focus on strategies that maximize the number of individuals who get screened	
	• Practice shared decision making; discussions with patients should incorporate information on test quality and availability	
	• Individuals with a personal history of cancer or adenomatous polyps are followed by a surveillance regimen, and screening guidelines are not applicable	
	Relevant recommendations: Recommends against the use of aspirin or nonsteroidal anti-inflammatory drugs for the primary prevention of colorectal cancer	
American College of Physicians guidance statements[c]	1. Clinicians perform individualized assessment of risk for colorectal cancer in all adults	
	2. Clinicians screen for colorectal cancer in average-risk adults starting at the age of 50 y, and in high-risk adults starting at the age of 40 y or 10 y younger than the age at which the youngest affected relative was diagnosed with colorectal cancer	
	3. Use a stool-based test, flexible sigmoidoscopy, or optical colonoscopy as a screening test in patients who are at average risk; Recommends using optical colonoscopy as a screening test in patients who are at high risk; Clinicians should select the test based on the benefits and harms of the screening test, availability of the screening test, and patient preferences	
	4. Clinicians stop screening for colorectal cancer in adults older than 75 y or in adults with a life expectancy of less than 10 y	

American Cancer Society[d]	FOBT with at least 50% test sensitivity for cancer, or fecal immunochemical test with at least 50% test sensitivity for cancer, or...	• Annual, starting at age 50 y • Testing at home with adherence to manufacturer's recommendation for collection techniques and number of samples • FOBT with the single stool sample collected on the clinician's fingertip during a digital rectal examination in the health care setting is not recommended • Guaiac-based toilet-bowl FOBT tests are not recommended • In comparison with guaiac-based tests for the detection of occult blood, immunochemical tests are more patient-friendly, and are likely to be equal or better in sensitivity and specificity • There is no justification for repeating FOBT in response to an initial positive finding
	Stool DNA test, or...	• Interval uncertain, starting at age 50 y
	Flexible sigmoidoscopy (FS), or...	• Every 5 y, starting at age 50 y • FS can be performed alone, or consideration can be given to combining FS performed every 5 y with a highly sensitive guaiac-based FOBT or fecal immunohistochemical test performed annually
	Double-contrast barium enema, or...	• Every 5 y, starting at age 50 y
	Colonoscopy	• Every 10 y, starting at age 50 y
	Computed tomographic colonography	• Every 5 y, starting at age 50 y

a Grade A: The USPSTF recommends the service. There is high certainty that the net benefit is substantial; Grade C: Clinicians may provide this service to selected patients depending on individual circumstances. However, for most individuals without signs or symptoms there is likely to be only a small benefit from this service; Grade D: The USPSTF recommends against the service. There is moderate or high certainty that the service has no net benefit or that the harms outweigh the benefits; I Statement: The USPSTF concludes that the current evidence is insufficient to assess the balance of benefits and harms of the service. Evidence is lacking, of poor quality, or conflicting, and the balance of benefits and harms cannot be determined.

b From USPSTF.[13]

c From Qaseem and colleagues.[14]

d From Smith and colleagues.[10]

IMPACT OF CHANGES WITHIN HEALTH CARE
Affordable Care Act

Findings from the 2010 wave of the Behavioral Risk Factor Surveillance System indicate that only about 65% of United States adults aged 50 to 75 years are up to date with CRC screening.[80] Among those without health insurance the rate decreases to 36%, and for those without a regular care provider the rate drops even further, to 32%.[80] While Medicare has ensured coverage of OC to most Americans age 65 years and older since July 2001, the Patient Protection and Affordable Care Act (PPACA) assures that most other Americans will similarly have access to affordable CRC screening. With the exception of a small number of grandfathered health plans (ie, those plans created before March 2010 and have since not had major changes to their provisions), the PPACA requires self-funded and commercial health insurance policies to cover CRC cancer screening tests at no out-of-pocket cost to patients.[81] This coverage includes OC with polypectomy, which the Centers for Medicaid and Medicare Services recently clarified as an integral part of OC screening and not subject to cost sharing.[82] This ruling makes clear that both screening for CRC and removal of polyps will be fully covered by the PPACA.

Although the PPACA is a positive development for the prevention and early detection of CRC, it remains to be seen whether the United States health care system will successfully meet the future demand. The Department of Health and Human Services estimates that the physician supply will increase by only 7% in the next 10 years while the Census Bureau projects a 36% growth in the number of Americans older than 65. According to the Association of American Medical Colleges, the result will be approximately 45,000 too few primary care physicians.[83] To address this anticipated shortfall, health care providers, administrators, and policy experts need to identify innovative strategies to ensure adequate access to CRC screening that do not rely on the physician workforce. Several options that may warrant investigation include expanding both the role and the number of mid-level providers (eg, nurse practitioners and physician assistants); creating certificate programs that enable sub–mid-level providers (eg, nurses, specialized therapists, health educators) to provide most preventive services; establishing prevention-oriented health care sites that specialize in the provision of preventive services, where most services are provided by nonphysicians; expanding services provided by pharmacists to include noninvasive preventive health care; and exploring payment models that allow the use of nontraditional clinical venues (eg, telemedicine and group-based care).

Electronic Health Records

As clinicians complete the migration to electronic health records (EHRs), several new tools can easily be added to a practice's operation to facilitate CRC screening. EHRs can be searched for past screening tests and thus determine if a patient is current based on criteria established by the practice. With a valid database and criteria for current recommendations on CRC screening, the EHR can be programmed to prompt or remind office staff, patients, and/or clinicians about the need for CRC screening tests. Automated reminder messages are sent to patients' email, phone, or home to remind them about screening for CRC. Patients using their health portal are able to consult a personal to-do list that includes referral to screening for CRC. Ideally patients are able to select this item and determine which test they want to complete, or engage in an online education session to help them determine their preferred method. A request for the CRC screening test is sent directly to the patient's primary care clinician. The clinician's staff then arranges the test, confirms with the patient, and educates the patient about the preparation. This process is completed without the clinician ever being seen. Such lean processes will allow the limited number of primary care clinicians to serve more patients. In addition, the EHR is able to generate a list of patients not current in their screening for CRC. The clinician's staff can then reach out to these patients to assist in determining which screening CRC test the patient would prefer, and facilitate the test being completed. Better access to past records afforded by a comprehensive EHR also makes it easier for the clinician to prevent polyp surveillance creep. Although the research to date has shown no consistent association between EHRs, clinical decision support, and better quality,[84] specific features of an EHR system may have a positive impact on quality.[85] When implementing a new EHR system, care should be taken to ensure its specific features will improve the functionality of the medical practice rather than merely satisfying generic meaningful-use criteria.[85]

Patient-Centered Medical Home

Given the burden of cancer, the patient-centered medical home (PCMH) model has to address cancer screening and surveillance, including CRC. The features of PCMH expected to improve cancer screening are better patient access and communication, health risk assessment, periodic preventive health examinations, patient registries, tracking of screening orders and completion, feedback screening performance, and payment reform.[86,87] Of practices examined to date, most lack systematic organization to provide such care.[88] Relationship-centered aspects of PCMH are more highly correlated with delivery of preventive services in community primary care practices than with information technology resources.[89] As with EHR research, the transformation of practices into PCMH is at too early a stage to demonstrate any impact, especially given the lack of significant payment reform.

Accountable Care Organizations

If health systems are organized into units accountable for the care of defined populations with payment metrics that reward achievable goals for CRC screening, some of the innovative approaches discussed herein will be considered and funded by these organizations. These changes will require much better data systems, communication with patients and their primary clinical care team, and coordination with the clinical team providing the screening test. Knierim and colleagues article "Organizing Your Practice for Screening and Secondary Prevention among Adults" elsewhere in this issue presents a more thorough discussion on accountable care organizations.

SUMMARY AND DISCUSSION

As one of the most common cancers affecting the United States population, the cost of CRC in terms of its human suffering and economic burden is great. However, with early detection using a variety of screening strategies, CRC morbidity and mortality can be significantly reduced. The typical process for CRC screening within the primary care setting is often both inefficient and ineffective, and is susceptible to individual and systematic errors: it relies on patients having access to health care and to a primary care clinician; it relies on the primary care clinician using SDM and making an appropriate screening recommendation; it relies on the patient agreeing to complete the recommended procedure and actually following through with it; and it relies on the primary care clinician confirming the results, and assuring that the next screening test or surveillance is done at the appropriate time. Suffice to say, this is not a simple process. To improve efficiencies, primary care clinicians need to establish written procedures to ensure that their office infrastructure, staff, and EHRs are optimized so that patients needing CRC screening are successfully screened and appropriately monitored. To ensure effectiveness clinicians need to regularly review their performance, and promptly address shortfalls as soon as they are identified. Given expectations that the demand for preventive care will increase as the PPACA is implemented, it is incumbent on the primary care clinician to take the requisite steps to prepare the practice to meet the emergent need. With a coordinated and systematic approach to CRC screening and surveillance, not only will suffering from CRC be reduced but the quality and efficient delivery of health care will improve.

REFERENCES

1. Siegel R, Naishadham D, Jemal A. Cancer statistics, 2013. CA Cancer J Clin 2013;63(1):11–30.
2. Centers for Disease Control and Prevention (CDC). Vital signs: colorectal cancer screening among adults aged 50-75 years—United States, 2008. MMWR Morb Mortal Wkly Rep 2010;59(26):808–12.
3. American Cancer Society. Colorectal cancer facts & figures 2011-2013. Atlanta (GA): American Cancer Society; 2011.
4. Parajuli R, Bjerkaas E, Tverdal A, et al. The increased risk of colon cancer due to cigarette smoking may be greater in women than men. Cancer Epidemiol Biomarkers Prev 2013;22(5):862–71.
5. Desantis C, Naishadham D, Jemal A. Cancer statistics for African Americans, 2013. CA Cancer J Clin 2013;63(3):151–66.
6. Gross CP, Smith BD, Wolf E, et al. Racial disparities in cancer therapy: did the gap narrow between 1992 and 2002? Cancer 2008;112(4):900–8.
7. Winawer SJ, Zauber AG, O'Brien MJ, et al. Randomized comparison of surveillance intervals after colonoscopic removal of newly diagnosed adenomatous polyps. The National Polyp Study Workgroup [see comments]. N Engl J Med 1993;328(13):901–6.
8. Saini SD, Kim HM, Schoenfeld P. Incidence of advanced adenomas at surveillance colonoscopy in patients with a personal history of colon adenomas: a meta-analysis and systematic review. Gastrointest Endosc 2006;64(4):614–26.
9. Winawer SJ, Zauber AG. The advanced adenoma as the primary target of screening. Gastrointest Endosc Clin N Am 2002;12(1):1–9, v.
10. Smith RA, Brooks D, Cokkinides V, et al. Cancer screening in the United States, 2013: a review of current American Cancer Society guidelines, current issues in cancer screening, and new guidance on cervical cancer screening and lung cancer screening. CA Cancer J Clin 2013;63(2):88–105.
11. Rim SH, Joseph DA, Steele CB, et al. Colorectal cancer screening—United States, 2002, 2004, 2006, and 2008. MMWR Surveill Summ 2011;60(Suppl):42–6.
12. Centers for Disease Control and Prevention (CDC). Cancer screening—United States, 2010. MMWR Morb Mortal Wkly Rep 2012;61(3):41–5.
13. U.S. Preventive Services Task Force. Screening for colorectal cancer: U.S. Preventive Services Task Force recommendation statement. Ann Intern Med 2008; 149(9):627–37.
14. Qaseem A, Denberg TD, Hopkins RH Jr, et al. Screening for colorectal cancer: a guidance statement from the American College of Physicians. Ann Intern Med 2012;156(5):378–86.
15. Kaiser Permanente Care Management Institute. Colorectal cancer screening clinical practice guidelines. National Guideline Clearinghouse 2006. Available

at: http://www.guideline.gov/popups/printView.aspx?id=14345.   Accessed November 25, 2013.

16. Kewenter J, Bjork S, Haglind E, et al. Screening and rescreening for colorectal cancer. A controlled trial of fecal occult blood testing in 27,700 subjects. Cancer 1988;62(3):645–51.

17. Hardcastle JD, Thomas WM, Chamberlain J, et al. Randomised, controlled trial of faecal occult blood screening for colorectal cancer. Results for first 107,349 subjects. Lancet 1989;1(8648):1160–4.

18. Kronborg O, Fenger C, Olsen J, et al. Randomised study of screening for colorectal cancer with faecal-occult-blood test. Lancet 1996;348(9040): 1467–71.

19. Winawer SJ, Flehinger BJ, Schottenfeld D, et al. Screening for colorectal cancer with fecal occult blood testing and sigmoidoscopy. J Natl Cancer Inst 1993; 85(16):1311–8.

20. Mandel JS, Bond JH, Church TR, et al. Reducing mortality from colorectal cancer by screening for fecal occult blood. Minnesota Colon Cancer Control Study. N Engl J Med 1993;328(19):1365–71 [published erratum appears in N Engl J Med 1993;329(9):672. See comments].

21. Robinson MH, Marks CG, Farrands PA, et al. Screening for colorectal cancer with an immunological faecal occult blood test: 2-year follow-up. Br J Surg 1996;83(4):500–1.

22. Faivre J, Dancourt V, Denis B, et al. Comparison between a guaiac and three immunochemical faecal occult blood tests in screening for colorectal cancer. Eur J Cancer 2012;48(16):2969–76.

23. Denters MJ, Deutekom M, Bossuyt PM, et al. Lower risk of advanced neoplasia among patients with a previous negative result from a fecal test for colorectal cancer. Gastroenterology 2012;142(3):497–504.

24. Allison JE, Fraser CG, Halloran SP, et al. Comparing fecal immunochemical tests: improved standardization is needed. Gastroenterology 2012;142(3): 422–4.

25. European Colorectal Cancer Screening Guidelines Working Group, von Karsa L, Patnick J, et al. European guidelines for quality assurance in colorectal cancer screening and diagnosis: overview and introduction to the full supplement publication. Endoscopy 2013;45(1):51–9.

26. Levin B, Lieberman DA, McFarland B, et al. Screening and surveillance for the early detection of colorectal cancer and adenomatous polyps, 2008: a joint guideline from the American Cancer Society, the US Multi-Society Task Force on Colorectal Cancer, and the American College of Radiology. Gastroenterology 2008;134(5):1570–95.

27. Tagore KS, Lawson MJ, Yucaitis JA, et al. Sensitivity and specificity of a stool DNA multitarget assay panel for the detection of advanced colorectal neoplasia. Clin Colorectal Cancer 2003;3(1):47–53.

28. Winawer SJ, Fletcher RH, Miller L, et al. Colorectal cancer screening: clinical guidelines and rationale. Gastroenterology 1997;112(2):594–642.

29. Schenck AP, Peacock SC, Klabunde CN, et al. Trends in colorectal cancer test use in the Medicare population, 1998-2005. Am J Prev Med 2009;37(1):1–7.

30. Selby JV, Friedman GD, Quesenberry CP, et al. A case-control study of screening sigmoidoscopy and mortality from colorectal cancer. N Engl J Med 1992;326(10):653–7.

31. Newcomb PA, Norfleet RG, Storer BE, et al. Screening sigmoidoscopy and colorectal cancer mortality. J Natl Cancer Inst 1992;84(20):1572–5.

32. Muller A, Sonnenberg A. Protection by endoscopy against death from colorectal cancer. A case-control study among veterans. Arch Intern Med 1995;155(16): 1741–8.

33. Atkin WS, Edwards R, Kralj-Hans I, et al. Once-only flexible sigmoidoscopy screening in prevention of colorectal cancer: a multicentre randomised controlled trial. Lancet 2010;375(9726):1624–33.

34. Rex D. Barium enema and colon cancer screening: finally a study. Am J Gastro-enterol 1997;92(9):1570–2.

35. Faivre J, Bader JP, Bertario L, et al. Mass screening for colorectal cancer: State-ment of the European groups for colorectal cancer screening. Eur J Cancer Prev 1995;4(5):437–9.

36. Taylor SA, Halligan S, Saunders BP, et al. Acceptance by patients of multidetec-tor CT colonography compared with barium enema examinations, flexible sigmoidoscopy, and colonoscopy. AJR Am J Roentgenol 2003;181(4):913–21.

37. Cotton PB, Durkalski VL, Pineau BC, et al. Computed tomographic colonogra-phy (virtual colonoscopy): a multicenter comparison with standard colonoscopy for detection of colorectal neoplasia. JAMA 2004;291(14):1713–9.

38. Rockey DC, Paulson E, Niedzwiecki D, et al. Analysis of air contrast barium enema, computed tomographic colonography, and colonoscopy: prospective comparison. Lancet 2005;365(9456):305–11.

39. Pickhardt P, Choi J, Hwang I, et al. Computed tomographic virtual colonoscopy to screen for colorectal neoplasia in asymptomatic adults. N Engl J Med 2003; 349(23):2191–200.

40. Nelson DB, McQuaid KR, Bond JH, et al. Procedural success and complica-tions of large-scale screening colonoscopy. Gastrointest Endosc 2002;55(3): 307–14.

41. Lieberman DA, Weiss DG, Bond JH, et al. Use of colonoscopy to screen asymp-tomatic adults for colorectal cancer. Veterans Affairs Cooperative Study Group 380. N Engl J Med 2000;343(3):162–8.

42. Imperiale TF, Wagner DR, Lin CY, et al. Results of screening colonoscopy among persons 40 to 49 years of age. N Engl J Med 2002;346(23):1781–5.

43. Sheridan SL, Harris RP, Woolf SH. Shared decision making about screening and chemoprevention: a suggested approach from the U.S. Preventive Services Task Force. Am J Prev Med 2004;26(1):56–66.

44. Steinwachs D, Allen JD, Barlow WE, et al. NIH state-of-the-science conference statement: enhancing use and quality of colorectal cancer screening. NIH Con-sens State Sci Statements 2010;27(1):1–31.

45. Van Ness MM, Chobanian SJ, Winters C Jr, et al. A study of patient acceptance of double-contrast barium enema and colonoscopy. Which procedure is preferred by patients? Arch Intern Med 1987;147(12):2175–6.

46. Dominitz JA, Provenzale D. Patient preferences and quality of life associated with colorectal cancer screening. Am J Gastroenterol 1997;92(12):2171–8.

47. Leard LE, Savides TJ, Ganiats TG. Patient preferences for colorectal cancer screening. J Fam Pract 1997;45(3):211–8.

48. Pignone M, Bucholtz D, Harris R. Patient preferences for colon cancer screening. J Gen Intern Med 1999;14(7):432–7.

49. Wolf AM, Schorling JB. Does informed consent alter elderly patients' prefer-ences for colorectal cancer screening? Results of a randomized trial. J Gen Intern Med 2000;15(1):24–30.

50. Sheikh RA, Kapre S, Calof OM, et al. Screening preferences for colorectal can-cer: a patient demographic study. South Med J 2004;97(3):224–30.

51. Nelson RL, Schwartz A. A survey of individual preference for colorectal cancer screening technique. BMC Cancer 2004;4(1):76.
52. Frew E, Wolstenholme J, Whynes D. Mass population screening for colorectal cancer: factors influencing subjects' choice of screening test. J Health Serv Res Policy 2001;6(2):85–91.
53. Frew E, Wolstenholme JL, Whynes DK. Willingness-to-pay for colorectal cancer screening. Eur J Cancer 2001;37(14):1746–51.
54. Frew EJ, Wolstenholme JL, Whynes DK. Comparing willingness-to-pay: bidding game format versus open-ended and payment scale formats. Health Policy 2004;68(3):289–98.
55. Frew EJ, Wolstenholme JL, Whynes DK. Eliciting relative preferences for two methods of colorectal cancer screening. Eur J Cancer Care (Engl) 2005;14(2):124–31.
56. Iyengar SS, Lepper MR. When choice is demotivating: can one desire too much of a good thing? J Pers Soc Psychol 2000;79(6):995–1006.
57. Ling BS, Moskowitz MA, Wachs D, et al. Attitudes toward colorectal cancer screening tests. J Gen Intern Med 2001;16(12):822–30.
58. Briss P, Rimer B, Reilley B, et al. Promoting informed decisions about cancer screening in communities and healthcare systems. Am J Prev Med 2004;26(1): 67–80.
59. Jaen CR, Stange KC, Nutting PA. Competing demands of primary care: a model for the delivery of clinical preventive services. J Fam Pract 1994;38(2):166–71.
60. Flocke SA, Frank SH, Wenger DA. Addressing multiple problems in the family practice office visit. J Fam Pract 2001;50(3):211–6.
61. Elwyn G, Edwards A, Kinnersley P. Shared decision-making in primary care: the neglected second half of the consultation. Br J Gen Pract 1999;49(443):477–82.
62. Edwards A, Elwyn G. Inside the black box of shared decision making: distinguishing between the process of involvement and who makes the decision. Health Expect 2006;9(4):307–20.
63. McQueen A, Bartholomew LK, Greisinger AJ, et al. Behind closed doors: physician-patient discussions about colorectal cancer screening. J Gen Intern Med 2009;24(11):1228–35.
64. Schroy PC 3rd, Mylvaganam S, Davidson P. Provider perspectives on the utility of a colorectal cancer screening decision aid for facilitating shared decision making. Health Expect 2014;17(1):27–35.
65. Elston Lafata J, Divine G, Moon C, et al. Patient-physician colorectal cancer screening discussions and screening use. Am J Prev Med 2007;31(3):202–9.
66. Stacey D, Bennett CL, Barry MJ, et al. Decision aids for people facing health treatment or screening decisions. Cochrane Database Syst Rev 2011;(10):CD001431.
67. Schroy PC 3rd, Emmons K, Peters E, et al. The impact of a novel computer-based decision aid on shared decision making for colorectal cancer screening: a randomized trial. Med Decis Making 2011;31(1):93–107.
68. O'Connor AM, Wennberg JE, Legare F, et al. Toward the 'tipping point': decision aids and informed patient choice. Health Aff 2007;26(3):716–25.
69. Jimbo M, Rana GK, Hawley S, et al. What is lacking in current decision aids on cancer screening? CA Cancer J Clin 2013;63(3):193–214.
70. Lin GA, Halley M, Rendle KA, et al. An effort to spread decision aids in five California primary care practices yielded low distribution, highlighting hurdles. Health Aff 2013;32(2):311–20.
71. Hsu C, Liss DT, Westbrook EO, et al. Incorporating patient decision aids into standard clinical practice in an integrated delivery system. Med Decis Making 2013;33(1):85–97.

72. O'Donnell S, Cranney A, Jacobsen MJ, et al. Understanding and overcoming the barriers of implementing patient decision aids in clinical practice. J Eval Clin Pract 2006;12(2):174–81.

73. Silvia KA, Sepucha KR. Decision aids in routine practice: lessons from the breast cancer initiative. Health Expect 2006;9(3):255–64.

74. Legare F, Ratte S, Gravel K, et al. Barriers and facilitators to implementing shared decision-making in clinical practice: update of a systematic review of health professionals' perceptions. Patient Educ Couns 2008;73(3):526–35.

75. Elwyn G, Laitner S, Coulter A, et al. Implementing shared decision making in the NHS. BMJ 2010;341:c5146.

76. Levin B, Lieberman DA, McFarland B, et al. Screening and surveillance for the early detection of colorectal cancer and adenomatous polyps, 2008: a joint guideline from the American Cancer Society, the US Multi-Society Task Force on Colorectal Cancer, and the American College of Radiology. CA Cancer J Clin 2008;58(3):130–60.

77. Klabunde CN, Lanier D, Nadel MR, et al. Colorectal cancer screening by primary care physicians: recommendations and practices, 2006-2007. Am J Prev Med 2009;37(1):8–16.

78. Klabunde CN, Frame PS, Meadow A, et al. A national survey of primary care physicians' colorectal cancer screening recommendations and practices. Prev Med 2003;36(3):352–62.

79. Shapiro JA, Seeff LC, Thompson TD, et al. Colorectal cancer test use from the 2005 National Health Interview Survey. Cancer Epidemiol Biomarkers Prev 2008;17(7):1623–30.

80. Joseph DA, King JB, Miller JW, et al. Prevalence of colorectal cancer screening among adults—Behavioral Risk Factor Surveillance System, United States, 2010. MMWR Morb Mortal Wkly Rep 2012;61(Suppl):51–6.

81. H.R. 3590 Patient Protection and Affordable Care Act. Washington, DC: One Hundred Eleventh Congress of the United States of America; 2010. p. 1–906.

82. US Department of Labor, Employee Benefits Security Administration. FAQs about Affordable Care Act Implementation Part XII. Washington, DC: United States Department of Labor; 2013.

83. Projected supply and demands, physicians 2008-2020. 2008. Available at: https://www.aamc.org/advocacy/campaigns_and_coalitions/fixdocshortage/. Accessed November 25, 2013.

84. Romano MJ, Stafford RS. Electronic health records and clinical decision support systems: impact on national ambulatory care quality. Arch Intern Med 2011;171(10):897–903.

85. Poon EG, Wright A, Simon SR, et al. Relationship between use of electronic health record features and health care quality: results of a statewide survey. Med Care 2010;48(3):203–9.

86. Sarfaty M, Myers RE, Harris DM, et al. Variation in colorectal cancer screening steps in primary care: basis for practice improvement. Am J Med Qual 2012;27(6):458–66.

87. Sarfaty M, Wender R, Smith R. Promoting cancer screening within the patient centered medical home. CA Cancer J Clin 2011;61(6):397–408.

88. Sarfaty M, Stello B, Johnson M, et al. Colorectal cancer screening in the framework of the medical home model: findings from focus groups and interviews. Am J Med Qual 2013;28(5):422–8.

89. Ferrante JM, Balasubramanian BA, Hudson SV, et al. Principles of the patient-centered medical home and preventive services delivery. Ann Fam Med 2010;8(2):108–16.

90. Rabeneck L, Rumble RB, Thompson F, et al. Fecal immunochemical tests compared with guaiac fecal occult blood tests for population-based colorectal cancer screening. Can J Gastroenterol 2012;26(3):131–47.
91. Health Quality Ontario. Fecal occult blood test for colorectal cancer screening: an evidence-based analysis. Ont Health Technol Assess Ser 2009;9(10):1–40.
92. Littlejohn C, Hilton S, Macfarlane GJ, et al. Systematic review and meta-analysis of the evidence for flexible sigmoidoscopy as a screening method for the prevention of colorectal cancer. Br J Surg 2012;99(11):1488–500.
93. Maheswaran T, Tighe R. Colorectal cancer rates following a barium enema or colonoscopy. Gut 2011;60(Suppl 1):A69–70.
94. Shariff MK, Sheikh K, Carroll NR, et al. Colorectal cancer detection: time to abandon barium enema? Frontline Gastroenterol 2011;2(2):105–9.
95. Barclay RL, Vicari JJ, Greenlaw RL. Effect of a time-dependent colonoscopic withdrawal protocol on adenoma detection during screening colonoscopy. Clin Gastroenterol Hepatol 2008;6(10):1091–8.
96. Anderson JC, Butterly LF, Goodrich M, et al. Differences in detection rates of adenomas and serrated polyps in screening versus surveillance colonoscopies, based on the new hampshire colonoscopy registry. Clin Gastroenterol Hepatol 2013;11(10):1308–12.
97. Rex DK, Petrini JL, Baron TH, et al. Quality indicators for colonoscopy. Am J Gastroenterol 2006;101(4):873–85.
98. Kaminski MF, Regula J, Kraszewska E, et al. Quality indicators for colonoscopy and the risk of interval cancer. N Engl J Med 2010;362(19):1795–803.
99. Albert D, Weinberg J, Kakkaer A, et al. Reliability of adenoma detection rate is based on procedural volume. Gastrointest Endosc 2013;77(3):376–80.

Prostate Cancer Screening

John W. Ragsdale III, MD*, Brian Halstater, MD,
Viviana Martinez-Bianchi, MD

KEYWORDS

- Screening • Prostate cancer • Prostate-specific antigen • PSA
- Digital rectal examination • DRE

KEY POINTS

- The US Preventive Services Task Force recommends against prostate-specific antigen (PSA)-based screening for prostate cancer (Pca) in men of all ages, because evidence suggests that the potential harms of screening outweigh potential benefits.
- The case for Pca screening requires a paradigm shift, one that emphasizes the risks of screening over the risks of undetected cancer.
- For patients who express an interest in Pca screening, primary care providers must use a shared decision-making process, helping patients weigh individual risk factors (eg, age, life expectancy, family history, black race) against probable harms and possible benefits.
- Although there are race-based differences for Pca incidence and mortality, there is insufficient evidence to selectively recommend PSA-based screening based on a patient's race.
- New models of care informed by the Patient Protection and Affordable Care Act, such as accountable care organizations, patient-centered medical homes, and team-based primary care, are poised to assist clinicians in providing recommended preventive care.
- Electronic health records offer a potential means to provide higher quality care at lower cost.

INTRODUCTION

After skin cancer, prostate cancer (Pca) is the most common cancer in men in the United States.[1] The National Institutes of Health projected that there would be roughly 240,000 new diagnoses and 30,000 deaths from Pca in 2013.[2] Despite a relatively high prevalence of approximately 15%, the lifetime risk of dying from Pca is fairly low (less than 3%), suggesting that conservative management is appropriate for most patients.[3] Conservative management is further warranted given evidence the potential risks of prostate-specific antigen (PSA)-based screening outweigh potential benefits.[4] Primary care providers must understand changes in Pca screening guidelines to effectively communicate and promote informed decision making.

Conflict of Interest: None.
Department of Community and Family Medicine, Duke Family Medicine Center, Duke University, 2100 Erwin Drive, Durham, NC 27710, USA
* Corresponding author.
E-mail address: john.ragsdale@duke.edu

0095-4543/14/$ – see front matter © 2014 Elsevier Inc. All rights reserved.

EPIDEMIOLOGY

More than 2.5 million men in the United States are living with Pca.[1] Pca incidence rates decreased, on average, about 2% per year between 2001 and 2010; Pca mortality decreased even more quickly, on average about 3% per year, over the same 10-year period.[5] As shown in **Table 1**, there remains considerable variation in both Pca incidence and mortality when examined by race. The incidence of Pca is substantially higher for blacks when compared with whites, at 192.9 and 115.6 cases per 100,000 men, respectively. Mortality is also substantially higher for blacks when compared with whites, at 48.2 and 20.1 deaths per 100,000 men, respectively.[6]

The literature suggests that several factors likely contribute to these race-based differences, including biological explanations, differences in screening behavior and access to health care, the pattern of care, and the quality of treatment.[7] Even in health care sites such as the US Veterans Administration (in which race-based differences in access, screening, and treatment of Pca are minimized), black men with Pca are more likely than their white counterparts to present with higher-risk disease characteristics, such as greater PSA levels, higher clinical Gleason scores, and more advanced disease at a younger age.[8] Compared with white men, black men also have higher odds of complications with prostate surgery, including an increased need for blood transfusions, longer lengths of stay, and greater inpatient mortality.[9] Research investigating race-based disparities in the pattern of Pca care show that blacks are less likely to receive surgical and radiation treatment, and are more likely to have not chosen a definitive therapy or to have chosen no treatment at all.

A review of epidemiologic studies published over the 39-year period between 1970 and 2008[10] showed no race-based differences in associations between Pca and tobacco use, alcohol intake, and family history of Pca; a modest positive association between height and Pca risk for whites only; and no clear pattern of association with weight, body mass index, physical activity, dietary factors, sexual behavior, sexually transmitted infections, occupational history, and other health conditions (eg, diabetes and high blood pressure). Another review,[11] focusing largely on social determinants of health, suggested that multiple factors likely contribute to black-white differences in Pca, including poorer access to health care and other resources, lower socioeconomic status, cultural and behavioral factors, and ineffective partnerships between patients and clinicians. However, the relative contribution of these factors to mortality is not clear, because biological measures such as Gleason score and PSA (not race) are the most salient predictors of mortality.[12]

Table 1 Age-adjusted[a] rates of Pca incidence and mortality by race (2010)		
Race/Ethnicity	Incidence per 100,000 Men	Mortalities per 100,000 Men
All races	126.1	21.8
American Indian/Alaska native	66.8	15.2
Asian/Pacific Islander	63.7	9.5
Black	192.9	48.2
Hispanic	104.8	18.2
White	115.6	20.8

[a] Age-adjusted to the 2000 US standard population.

Data from Centers for Disease Control and Prevention. US cancer statistics: 2010 cancer types grouped by race and ethnicity. Available at: http://apps.nccd.cdc.gov/uscs/cancersbyraceandethnicity.aspx. Accessed January 4, 2014.

Although evidence suggests that the most common alterations in gene expression associated with Pca do not vary significantly by race/ethnicity, several metastasis-related genes have been found to be more highly expressed in tumors from black patients when compared with white patients. Researchers hypothesize that the causes for these differences are multifactorial (environmental, or genetic), noting that the gene signature in tumors of black patients could be associated with viral involvement.[13] Although a recent meta-analysis indicated that BRCA1 mutations do not increase Pca risk,[14] some BRCA2 mutations may.[15] Evidence suggests that BRCA1 and BRCA2 mutations have comparable prevalence among white, black, Asian, and Hispanic populations. Although between-group differences in the spectrum of mutations have been observed, the significance of differences remains unknown.[16] The potential benefits of screening for Pca in men carrying BRCA-related mutations is not known.[17]

Family history of Pca is an established risk factor for men of any race. Men with a family history of a first-degree relative with Pca are at increased risk for the disease compared with those without an affected first-degree relative (**Table 2**).[18] As with those carrying BRCA-related mutations, current evidence cannot satisfactorily determine whether the benefits of Pca screening outweigh the risks among those with a family history of the disease; likewise, there is insufficient evidence to selectively recommend PSA-based screening based on a patient's race.[4]

THE EFFICACY OF THE DIGITAL RECTAL EXAMINATION AND PSA-BASED SCREENING

Two screening modalities have commonly been used to detect Pca: digital rectal examination (DRE) and PSA assay.[19]

DRE

Despite its use as a screening tool for many years, a careful evaluation of DRE remains wanting.[20] Research published in the late 1980s showed that of 4160 DREs performed on 2131 men older than 45 years, 144 prostate biopsies were performed and 36 malignant tumors were identified. Researchers concluded that DRE may not add significant benefit over conventional medical care.[21] Although inexpensive, easy to perform, and relatively noninvasive, the effectiveness of DRE is contingent on the experience and skill of the examiner. Since the advent of widely available PSA assays in the late 1980s, DRE by itself is seldom considered as a screening tool.[20]

Table 2
Relative risk of Pca based on family history

Risk Group	Relative Risk for Pca
Brother(s) with Pca; diagnosed at any age	3.14
Father with Pca; diagnosed at any age	2.35
1 affected FDR; diagnosed at any age	2.48
≥2 affected FDRs; diagnosed at any age	4.39
Second-degree relative(s); diagnosed at any age	2.52
Affected FDR(s); diagnosed <65 y	2.87
Affected FDR(s); diagnosed ≥65 y	1.92

Abbreviation: FDR, first-degree relative.

Adapted from National Cancer Institute at the National Institutes of Health. Genetics of prostate cancer (PDQ). Available at: http://www.cancer.gov/cancertopics/pdq/genetics/prostate/Health Professional/#Reference1.21. Accessed January 4, 2014.

PSA-Based Screening

As noted by the National Cancer Institute, "There is no PSA value below which a man can be assured that he has no risk of prostate cancer." Although several methods intended to improve the performance of PSA-based screening have been studied (including Pca gene 3 [PCA3], complexed PSA and percent-free PSA, ultrasensitive PSA assay, PSA density, PSA density of the transition zone, age-adjusted PSA, PSA velocity, altering PSA cutoff level, and frequency of screening), evidence shows that none is demonstrably better than total serum PSA.[20]

Over the past several years, the approach to Pca screening has shifted, because new findings indicate that the potential benefits from PSA testing are small.[22–25] For example, the Prostate Cancer Intervention vs Observation Trial concluded that among men with clinically localized Pca that had been diagnosed after PSA testing, radical prostatectomy did not reduce all-cause or prostate cancer mortality, compared with observation, through at least 12 years of follow-up.[26] Similarly, the European Randomized Study of Screening for Prostate Cancer concluded that to prevent a single death from Pca at 11 years of follow-up, more than 1050 men would need to be screened and 37 cancers would need to be detected.[27] In addition, the Prostate, Lung, Colorectal, and Ovarian Cancer Screening Trial concluded that after 13 years of follow-up, there was no mortality benefit for organized annual PSA screening versus opportunistic PSA screening.[28]

POSSIBLE BENEFITS AND EXPECTED HARMS OF PSA-BASED SCREENING AND SUBSEQUENT TREATMENT
Screening

As described by the US Preventive Services Task Force (USPSTF)[25] and others,[22,24] PSA-based screening for Pca sets in motion a clinical path leading to overdiagnosis and overtreatment of most patients who screen positive. **Box 1** summarizes the expected harms, as well as the possible benefits. The USPSTF asserts the following:

> There is convincing evidence that PSA-based screening leads to substantial overdiagnosis of prostate tumors. The amount of overdiagnosis of prostate cancer is of important concern because a man with cancer that would remain asymptomatic for the remainder of his life cannot benefit from screening or treatment. There is a high propensity for physicians and patients to elect to treat most cases of screen-detected cancer, given our current inability to distinguish tumors that will remain indolent from those destined to be lethal. Thus, many men are being subjected to the harms of treatment of prostate cancer that will never become symptomatic. Even for men whose screen-detected cancer would otherwise have been later identified without screening, most experience the same outcome and are, therefore, subjected to the harms of treatment for a much longer period of time. There is convincing evidence that PSA-based screening for prostate cancer results in considerable overtreatment and its associated harms.[29]

Potential harms from the most common forms of Pca treatment include erectile dysfunction, urinary and fecal incontinence, and systemic injury. These harms must be weighed against the likelihood of a lifesaving intervention of only 1 in (approximately) 1000.

A recent study examining the perspectives of primary care providers on discontinuing Pca screening found that most clinicians considered both the patients' age and life expectancy when making decisions about Pca screening, although nearly two-thirds of clinicians noted difficultly in gauging life expectancy. The most commonly cited barriers to not performing Pca screening were patients' expectations and time constraints.

Box 1
Expected harms and possible benefits from PSA-based screening for Pca

Expected harms

- False-positive results. About 100 to 120 of every 1000 men screened receive a false-positive test. Most positive tests result in biopsy and can cause worry and anxiety. Up to one-third of men undergoing biopsy experience fever, infection, bleeding, urinary problems, and pain that they consider a moderate or major problem. One percent are hospitalized for complications.

- Overdiagnosis. In most cases, Pca does not grow or cause symptoms. If it does grow, it usually grows so slowly that it is not likely to cause health problems during a man's lifetime. Currently, it is not possible to reliably distinguish indolent from aggressive cancers. Many cancers diagnosed would have remained asymptomatic for life and do not require treatment.

- Overtreatment. Because of the uncertainty about which cancers need to be treated, 90% of men with Pca found by PSA choose to receive treatment. Many of these men cannot benefit from treatment, because their cancer does not grow or cause health problems. Harms of treatment include:

  1. Erectile dysfunction from surgery, radiation therapy, or hormone therapy (29 men affected per 1000 men screened)

  2. Urinary incontinence from radiation therapy or surgery (18 men affected per 1000 men screened)

  3. A small risk of death and serious complications from surgery:
     - 2 serious cardiovascular events per 1000 men screened
     - 1 case of pulmonary embolus or deep venous thrombosis per 1000 men screened
     - 1 perioperative death every 3000 men screened

Possible benefits

In an unscreened population, about 5 of every 1000 men die from Pca after 10 years. Results of several large trials have shown that, at best, PSA screening may help 1 man in 1000 avoid death from Pca after at least 10 years. Most likely, the number helped is even smaller. This observation means that with PSA screening, 4 or 5 of every 1000 men die from Pca after 10 years.

Adapted from US Preventive Services Task Force. Talking with your patients about screening for prostate cancer. 2012. Available at: http://www.uspreventiveservicestaskforce.org/prostate cancerscreening/prostatecancerscript.pdf. Accessed January 5, 2014.

Concerns about malpractice were noted as a barrier by more than half of respondents, and more than a quarter indicated a concern that their patients would think they were trying to cut costs. Researchers concluded that barriers may be mitigated, in part, through the practice of shared decision making within patient-centered medical homes (PCMHs).[30] Both shared decision making and PCMH are described in more detail later.

PCA SCREENING RECOMMENDATIONS

Screening recommendations for Pca from the USPSTF, American College of Physicians (ACP), the American Urological Association (AUA), and the American Cancer Society (ACS) are outlined in **Table 3**.

SHARED DECISION MAKING

Given the recent shift against Pca screening, primary care providers play an important role in helping patients make informed decisions about Pca screening; however, many

Table 3
Screening for Pca

Organization	Recommendations, Guidance Statements, and Clinical Considerations	Evidence Grade

USPSTF[a]	Recommends against PSA-based screening for Pca in the general US population, regardless of age; this recommendation does not apply to the use of the PSA test for surveillance after diagnosis or treatment of Pca
	
	In cases in which men request screening, the USPSTF suggests the following:
	  The decision to initiate or continue PSA screening should reflect an explicit understanding of the possible benefits and harms and respect patients' preferences
	  Physicians should not offer or order PSA screening unless they are prepared to engage in shared decision making, which enables an informed choice by patients
	  Patients requesting PSA screening should be provided with the opportunity to make informed choices to be screened, which reflect their values about specific benefits and harms
	UPSTF Recommendation Summary Sheet: Talking with Patients About Screening for Prostate Cancer[31]: http://www.uspreventive servicestaskforce.org/prostatecancerscreening/prostatecancerscript.pdf
		D[b]

ACP[c]	Men aged 50–69 y:
	  Clinicians inform patient about the limited potential benefits and substantial harms of screening for Pca
	  Base the decision to screen for Pca using the PSA test on the following criteria: (1) the risk for Pca, (2) a discussion of the benefits and harms of screening, (3) the patient's general health and life expectancy, and (4) patient preferences
	  Clinicians should not screen for Pca using the PSA test in patients who do not express a clear preference for screening
	Men aged <50 y, >69 y, or with a life expectancy <10–15 y:
	  Clinicians should not screen for Pca using the PSA test in men at average risk
	  Some men still prefer to be screened, because they may put more value on the possible small benefit and less value on the harms.
	  In these cases, use shared decision making and document the conversation as it relates to the following points:
	  Pca screening with the PSA test is controversial
	  The chances of harm from screening with the PSA test outweigh the chances of benefit
	  Most Pca is slow growing and does not cause death
	  Most men who choose not to have PSA testing are not diagnosed with Pca and die of something else
	  Patients who choose PSA testing are more likely than those who decline testing to be diagnosed with Pca	

	The PSA test often does not distinguish between serious cancer and nonserious cancer; men with markedly increased PSA levels (>10 μg/L) may have a reduced chance of dying from Pca by having surgical treatment	
	There are many potential harms of screening	
	The PSA test is not just a blood test; it is a test that can open the door to more testing and treatment that may cause harm	
	Recommendations about screening may change over time; men are welcome to change their minds at any time by asking for screening that they have previously declined or discontinue screening that they have previously requested	
	ACP Guidance Statement: Screening for Prostate Cancer: http://annals.org/article.aspx?articleID=1676183&atab=7	
AUA[d]	Men aged <40 y:	
	Recommends against PSA screening	C[e]
	Men aged 40–54 y at average risk	
	Does not recommend routine screening	C[e]
	Men aged 55–69 y	
	Recommends shared decision making and proceeding with PSA screening based on a man's values and preferences	B[f]
	Men aged >70 y, or with a life expectancy <10–15 y	
	Does not recommend routine PSA screening	C[e]
	To reduce the harms of screening, a routine screening interval of ≥ 2 y may be preferred over annual screening in those men who have participated in shared decision making and decided on screening	C[e]
	Shared decision making between clinicians and men is a strategy for making health care decisions when there is more than 1 medically reasonable option. Shared decision making includes the following characteristics:	
	Involvement of both the clinician and patient in the decision-making process	
	Bilateral sharing of information	
	Joint participation in the decision-making process	
	Reaching agreement on the management strategy to implement	
	Decision aids may help facilitate shared decision making (eg, http://www.asco.org/sites/www.asco.org/files/psa_pco_decision_aid_71612.pdf[32])	
	AUA Guideline on Early Detection of Prostate Cancer: http://www.auanet.org/education/guidelines/prostate-cancer-detection.cfm	

(continued on next page)

Table 3
(continued)

Organization	Recommendations, Guidance Statements, and Clinical Considerations	Evidence Grade
ACS[g]	Pca screening should not occur without an informed decision-making process	
	Men aged ≥50 y at average risk	
	Recommends that asymptomatic men who have a ≥10-year life expectancy make an informed decision with their health care provider about screening after receiving information about the uncertainties, risks, and potential benefits	
	Men at higher risk (including black men and those with first-degree relative diagnosed with Pca before age 65 y) aged 40–49 y	
	Recommends men make an informed decision with their health care provider about screening after receiving information about the uncertainties, risks, and potential benefits	
	Men with <10-year life expectancy	
	Recommends not offering Pca screening	
	Men should either receive this information directly from their health care providers or be referred to reliable and culturally appropriate sources	
	Patient decision aids are helpful in preparing men to make a decision whether to be tested	
	For men who choose to be screened for Pca after considering the possible benefits and risks:	
	Screening is recommended with PSA with or without DRE	
	Screening should be conducted yearly for men whose PSA level is ≥2.5 ng/mL	
	For men whose PSA is <2.5 ng/mL, screening intervals can be extended to every 2 y	
	A PSA level of ≥4.0 ng/mL historically has been used to recommend referral for further evaluation or biopsy, which remains a reasonable approach for men at average risk for Pca	
	For PSA levels between 2.5 ng/mL and 4.0 ng/mL, health care providers should consider an individualized risk assessment that incorporates other risk factors for Pca, particularly for high-grade cancer, which may be used to recommend a biopsy	
	ACS Guideline for the Early Detection of Prostate Cancer: http://mr.crossref.org/iPage?doi=10.3322%2Fcaac.20066	
Additional guidelines/ resources	National Comprehensive Cancer Network, Prostate Cancer Early Detection (version 2.2012)[33]: http://www.nccn.org/professionals/physician_gls/pdf/prostate_detection.pdf (registration is required to access the guidelines)	
	European Association of Urology[34]: http://www.uroweb.org/gls/pdf/09_Prostate_Cancer_LR.pdf	
	UK National Health Service[35]: http://www.nhs.uk/Conditions/Cancer-of-the-prostate/Pages/Prevention.aspx	

[a] Adapted from the USPSTF.[4]
[b] Evidence grade D: the USPSTF concludes that there is moderate or high certainty that the service has no net benefit or that the harms outweigh the benefits.
[c] Adapted from the ACP.[36]
[d] Adapted from the AUA.[22]
[e] Evidence grade C: the AUA concludes that strength of evidence in support of the intervention is low.
[f] Evidence grade B: the AUA concludes that strength of evidence in support of the intervention is moderate.
[g] Adapted from the ACS.[37]

US men describe not having engaged in shared decision making with their clinician when making decisions about Pca screening.[38] The decision to undergo Pca screening must involve an explicit discussion between patient and clinician of the possible benefits weighed against expected harms.

Shared decision making is a technique to help guide a clinical decision by taking into account patient preferences, health literacy, clinical science, available resources, expected benefits, and potential harms. Because it relates to Pca screening, the primary care provider must communicate to patients that the best available evidence does not support routine Pca screening, and that any future testing or intervention is likely to result in more harm than good. Unlike most cancer screening guidelines, which recommend screening unless the patient opts out, Pca screening should not be performed unless the patient opts in. Clinicians must not strive to talk men out of screening if they make an informed decision to be screened; rather, clinicians must clearly communicate the subsequent risks associated with screening, assess patients' understanding of these risks, and document the shared decision-making process in the patients' electronic health record (EHR). For patients who decline screening, future discussions about screening should occur if a patient's risk profile changes, when/if a patient raises the topic themselves, or at an agreed interval reflecting the patient's informed preference (in such cases, this interval should be documented in the patient's EHR). Clinicians must strive to not talk men into screening if they make an informed decision not to be screened.

As highlighted in **Table 3**, the USPSTF, ACP, AUA, and ACS all endorse shared decision making as an essential component of Pca screening. One strategy to assist in shared decision making is through the Elwyn model. There are 3 major steps to the Elwyn model: choice talk, option talk, and decision talk. The purpose of choice talk is to convey to the patient that more than 1 reasonable treatment option exists; option talk includes a more detailed discussion about the various treatment options; and decision talk solicits patients' preferences and values in light of choices and options.[39] **Box 2** outlines several key aspects of choice talk, option talk, and decision talk, and provides examples that are specific to Pca.

DECISION AIDS: ANOTHER TOOL FOR SHARED DECISION MAKING

Decision aids (tools that provide patients with unbiased, evidence-based information about available treatment options) can improve patients' ability to make educated, value-based decisions about care when more than 1 medically reasonable test or treatment option exists. Decision aids can help to improve patients' health literacy, clarify preferences, improve decision making, align values with treatment options, stimulate shared decision making, and promote follow-through. By helping patients identify health care preferences, decision aids can also reduce health care costs by preventing unwanted or unnecessary care.[40–42]

There are many decision aids available to help men make health care choices relating to Pca screening (see Lin and colleagues[40] for a review on the topic). In addition to the tool developed by the American Society for Clinical Oncology and referenced by the AUA in its guidelines on early detection of Pca (see **Table 3**), Thompson and colleagues developed a prostate risk calculator (available at http://deb.uthscsa.edu/URORiskCalc/Pages/calcs.jsp),[43] which generates risk percentages based on an individual patient's Pca risk. Because of its simplicity, the tool could be used within the context of the clinical encounter as a resource to help patients and clinicians make informed Pca screening decisions.[44]

Box 2
The Elwyn model for shared decision making in Pca screening: choice talk, option talk, and decision talk

Choice talk

- Assessing knowledge: "Now that you are 50 years old it is time to discuss prostate cancer screening"

- Offering a choice: "There are some new guidelines regarding prostate cancer screening, and I'd like to discuss them with you"

- Justifying the choice: "There are potential risks and benefits to screening, and I am here to help you sort through them"

- Checking reaction: "This is a lot to take in, shall we continue?"

- Postponing closure (if necessary): "I can see you still have concerns, and we don't need to make a decision today. My goal is to help you make a decision that is best for you. Would you like me to describe the screening options in more detail? Please interrupt me if you have questions or concerns"

Option talk

- Checking knowledge: "What have you heard about prostate cancer screening?"

- Listing options: provide options in writing

- Describing options (including harms and benefits): engage patient in dialogue and explore their preferences and values

- Providing decision support: consider the use of decision aids (eg, http://www.asco.org/sites/www.asco.org/files/psa_pco_decision_aid_71612.pdf[32])

- Providing summary (and assessing for understanding): review the list of options and ask the patient to describe back to you in their own words

Decision talk

- Focusing on patient preferences and values: solicit the patient's point of view

- Eliciting patient preference: help facilitate the conversation by offering guidance; do not rush a decision

- Decision making: ask the patient if they have reached a decision; if not, ask what you can do to help

- Offering review: confirm decisions and make sure that you understand the patient's concerns, preferences, and values

Adapted from Elwyn G, Frosch D, Thomson R, et al. Shared decision making: a model for clinical practice. J Gen Intern Med 2012;27(10):1361–7.

FUTURE OF SCREENING

The potential benefits of Pca screening do not outweigh the probable harms. What is needed are universal screening tool(s) that have both high specificity and high sensitivity (thus, maximizing true positives and true negatives), or an acceptably precise algorithm that correctly identifies those men at risk for developing aggressive forms of Pca. Further studies involving genetic markers, as well as studies of the interaction between genetics and the environment, may provide improved understanding of who to screen, and among those screening positive, who has indolent versus aggressive disease.[13,45]

As current PSA-based screening guidelines are put into practice, continued surveillance will be necessary to assess how changes in screening practice affect Pca outcomes (including outcomes related to undertreatment and overtreatment) among populations with varying demographic backgrounds.

HEALTH CARE DELIVERY SYSTEMS AND PCA SCREENING
Patient Protection and the Affordable Care Act

The Patient Protection and Affordable Care Act (ACA) puts considerable emphasis on USPSTF recommendations, requiring most insurers to provide recommended preventive services at no additional cost to patients. Because the USPSTF does not recommend Pca screening, the Secretary of the Department of Health and Human Services is authorized to deny reimbursement from Medicare for PSA testing.[46] Currently, Medicare covers 1 DRE and 1 PSA-based test per year for male enrollees aged 50 years and older.[47] Given the USPSTF position that patients requesting Pca screening should be provided with the opportunity to make an informed value-based choice, it seems unlikely that reimbursement for PSA testing will be stopped anytime soon; however, limiting payment would result in less screening and a subsequent reduction in overdiagnosis and overtreatment. Observed savings could then be allocated to other screening programs or treatments with proven efficacy. Policies that limit reimbursement may be worth debating, because they have the potential not only to improve patient outcomes (ie, reducing overdiagnosis and overtreatment) but to decrease health care costs.

EHR

EHRs have the potential to improve the delivery of preventive[48] and ambulatory[49] health care, including care related to Pca screening. For example, EHRs can be tailored to offer reminders or prompts about the need to discuss current recommendations (ie, not to screen), help facilitate shared decision making among those who wish to pursue screening, and help identify patients at higher risk for Pca based on factors such as age, life expectancy, race, and family history. Reflecting the patient's informed preference, EHRs could also be used to indicate timing for future discussions about screening, as well as document key components of shared decision making. For patients who choose to be screened, EHRs can be used to automatically flag patients who screen positive and require follow-up.[50]

PCMH

The Agency for Healthcare Research and Quality defines a PCMH "not simply as a place but as a model of the organization of primary care that delivers the core functions of primary health care[;]" that is, care that is patient-centered, comprehensive, coordinated, enables patient access, and provides a dedicated systems-based approach to quality and safety.[51] Emerging evidence suggests that the PCMH model delivers higher quality care at the same or lower cost than standard care and with increased patient satisfaction[52]; moreover, evidence suggests that patients who receive care in an established PCMH are more likely to undergo cancer screening and to follow the recommendations of their clinician.[53]

Capitalizing on the strengths of each team member, a team-based approach to Pca screening could help to promote several important principles related to the PCMH. In a team-based approach, front office staff could provide men older than 50 years with information about Pca screening when checking in for their appointment (eg, a brochure that outlines the limited possible benefits against the many expected harms). After taking the patient to the examination room, the medical assistant or nurse could ask the patient if they have any questions and provide information (patient education) as needed. The medical assistant or nurse could then document the conversation in the patient's EHR, including the need for follow-up conversation with the clinician, when applicable. For patients who express an interest in screening, the medical assistant or nurse could provide a decision aid (see **Table 3**), documenting its use in the EHR. Clinicians, then, could use the decision aid as a tool to facilitate shared decision making and record the outcome in the patient's EHR. For those choosing to be screened, follow-up tests/care could be coordinated within the medical home and its affiliated clinics, with staff arranging subsequent appointments with the team's preferred provider(s) or the provider of the patient's choosing. Alerts within the EHR could notify the team of test results; if test results remain outstanding, a care manager (or office staff or medical assistant) could follow up with laboratories or other clinics/departments to gather and enter findings into the EHR. At each stage of the screening/testing process, the clinician (or nurse or medical assistant) should confirm that the patient understands the risks of each test/procedure and provide an opportunity for the patient to discontinue the screening/testing process.

Although the specific processes for a team-based approach to Pca screening vary by setting, the key to ensuring an effective team process is careful planning, thoughtful reflection on how things are going, and reworking the care process as needed until it operates smoothly. Team members should continuously strive to ensure that patients are making informed decisions and receiving the right care, at the right time, and in the right care setting(s), and that the process of care is supported and recorded through the use of appropriate technology, which maximizes both quality and efficiency.

Accountable Care Organization

As defined by the Centers for Medicare and Medicaid Services, accountable care organizations (ACOs) are groups of hospitals, doctors, and other clinicians who work together to give high-quality and coordinated care to a population of patients, with the goal of avoiding unnecessary care or duplication of services. When ACOs successfully deliver high-quality care in a cost-effective manner, those providing the care share in the savings (for more about ACOs, see http://www.cms.gov/Medicare/Medicare-Fee-for-Service-Payment/ACO/index.html?redirect=/aco/).[54]   Although Pca screening is not an explicit quality performance measure that ACOs must meet for shared savings, the process for screening (ie, shared decision making) is.[55]

Among the most significant barriers described by clinicians to implementing shared decision making are time constraints.[56] ACOs may help to reduce this barrier: as described by Berwick,[57] coordinated care through an ACO "is meant to allow providers to break away from the tyranny of the 15-minute visit, instill a renewed sense of collegiality, and return to the type of medicine that patients and families want. For patients, coordinated care means more 'quality time' with their physician and care team...and more collaboration in leading a healthy life." Although the verdict is still out on whether ACOs gives primary care providers more time to engage in shared decision making, emerging evidence suggests that patients are more likely to receive education (a key component of shared decision making) if their provider received primarily capitated payment.[58]

SUMMARY

Universal screening for Pca is no longer recommended, because the potential harms associated with screening (overdiagnosis, overtreatment, and subsequent complications) outweigh the potential benefits. For those patients continuing to express an interest in Pca screening, primary care providers must engage the patient in shared decision making, helping them weigh individual risk factors (eg, age, life expectancy, family history, black race) against harms and benefits. New models of care informed by the ACA, such as ACOs, PCMHs, and team-based primary care, are poised to assist clinicians in providing recommended preventive care. In the case of Pca, screening is not recommended, and effective communication through shared decision making can help patients make informed decisions reflecting their preferences and values.

ACKNOWLEDGMENTS

The authors thank Cameron Shultz, PhD, MSW and Mack Ruffin IV, MD, MPH for their significant contribution in the development and writing of this article.

REFERENCES

1. American Cancer Society. Prostate cancer. 2013. Available at: http://www.cancer.org/cancer/prostatecancer/detailedguide/prostate-cancer-key-statistics. Accessed January 4, 2014.
2. National Cancer Institute at the National Institutes of Health. Prostate cancer. Available at: http://www.cancer.gov/cancertopics/types/prostate. Accessed January 4, 2014.
3. American Cancer Society. Lifetime risk of developing or dying from cancer. 2013. Available at: http://www.cancer.org/cancer/cancerbasics/lifetime-probability-of-developing-or-dying-from-cancer. Accessed January 4, 2014.
4. US Preventive Services Task Force. Screening for prostate cancer. 2012. Available at: http://www.uspreventiveservicestaskforce.org/prostatecancerscreening.htm. Accessed January 4, 2014.
5. National Cancer Institute. SEER cancer statistics factsheets: prostate cancer. Available at: http://seer.cancer.gov/statfacts/html/prost.html.
6. Centers for Disease Control and Prevention. US cancer statistics: 2010 cancer types grouped by race and ethnicity. Available at: http://apps.nccd.cdc.gov/uscs/cancersbyraceandethnicity.aspx. Accessed January 4, 2014.
7. Barocas DA, Penson DF. Racial variation in the pattern and quality of care for prostate cancer in the USA: mind the gap. BJU Int 2010;106(3):322–8.
8. Hudson MA, Luo S, Chrusciel T, et al. Do racial disparities exist in the use of prostate cancer screening and detection tools in veterans? Urol Oncol 2014; 32(1):34.e9–18.
9. Barocas DA, Gray DT, Fowke JH, et al. Racial variation in the quality of surgical care for prostate cancer. J Urol 2012;188(4):1279–85.
10. Mordukhovich I, Reiter PL, Backes DM, et al. A review of African American-white differences in risk factors for cancer: prostate cancer. Cancer Causes Control 2011;22(3):341–57.
11. Dimah K, Dimah A. Prostate cancer among African American men: a review of empirical literature. J Afr Am Stud 2003;7(1):20.
12. Koscuiszka M, Hatcher D, Christos PJ, et al. Impact of race on survival in patients with clinically nonmetastatic prostate cancer who deferred primary treatment. Cancer 2012;118(12):3145–52.
13. Wallace TA, Prueitt RL, Yi M, et al. Tumor immunobiological differences in prostate cancer between African-American and European-American men. Cancer Res 2008;68(3):927–36.

14. Fachal L, Gómez-Caamaño A, Celeiro-Muñoz C, et al. BRCA1 mutations do not increase prostate cancer risk: results from a meta-analysis including new data. Prostate 2011;71(16):1768–79.

15. Levy-Lahad E, Friedman E. Cancer risks among BRCA1 and BRCA2 mutation carriers. Br J Cancer 2007;96(1):11–5.

16. Kurian AW. BRCA1 and BRCA2 mutations across race and ethnicity: distribution and clinical implications. Curr Opin Obstet Gynecol 2010;22(1):72–8.

17. National Cancer Institute at the National Institutes of Health. BRCA1 and BRCA2: cancer risk and genetic testing. Available at: http://www.cancer.gov/cancertopics/factsheet/Risk/BRCA. Accessed January 4, 2014.

18. National Cancer Institute at the National Institutes of Health. Genetics of prostate cancer (PDQ). Available at: http://www.cancer.gov/cancertopics/pdq/genetics/prostate/HealthProfessional/#Reference1.21. Accessed January 4, 2014.

19. Centers for Disease Control and Prevention. Prostate cancer: what screening tests are there? 2013. Available at: http://www.cdc.gov/cancer/prostate/basic_info/screening.htm. Accessed January 5, 2014.

20. National Cancer Institute at the National Institutes of Health. Prostate cancer screening (PDQ). Available at: http://www.cancer.gov/cancertopics/pdq/screening/prostate/HealthProfessional/page3#Reference3.10. Accessed January 5, 2014.

21. Chodak GW, Keller P, Schoenberg HW. Assessment of screening for prostate cancer using the digital rectal examination. J Urol 1989;141(5):1136–8.

22. Carter HB, Albertsen PC, Barry MJ, et al. Early detection of prostate cancer: AUA guideline. 2013. Available at: http://www.auanet.org/common/pdf/education/clinical-guidance/Prostate-Cancer-Detection.pdf. Accessed January 5, 2014.

23. Heidenreich A, Bastian PJ, Bellmunt J, et al. EAU guidelines on prostate cancer. Part 1: screening, diagnosis, and local treatment with curative intent–update 2013. Eur Urol 2014;65(1):124–37.

24. Djulbegovic M, Beyth RJ, Neuberger MM, et al. Screening for prostate cancer: systematic review and meta-analysis of randomised controlled trials. BMJ 2010; 341:c4543.

25. Chou R, Croswell JM, Dana T, et al. Screening for prostate cancer: a review of the evidence for the US Preventive Services Task Force. Ann Intern Med 2011; 155(11):762–71.

26. Wilt TJ, Brawer MK, Barry MJ, et al. The Prostate cancer Intervention Versus Observation Trial: VA/NCI/AHRQ Cooperative Studies Program #407 (PIVOT): design and baseline results of a randomized controlled trial comparing radical prostatectomy to watchful waiting for men with clinically localized prostate cancer. Contemp Clin Trials 2009;30(1):81–7.

27. Schroder FH, Hugosson J, Roobol MJ, et al. Screening and prostate-cancer mortality in a randomized European study. N Engl J Med 2009;360(13): 1320–8.

28. Pinsky PF, Parnes HL, Andriole G. Mortality and complications after prostate biopsy in the Prostate, Lung, Colorectal and Ovarian Cancer Screening (PLCO) trial. BJU Int 2013. [Epub ahead of print].

29. US Preventive Services Task Force. Screening for prostate cancer: US Preventive Services Task Force recommendation statement. 2012. Available at: http://www.uspreventiveservicestaskforce.org/prostatecancerscreening/prostatefinalrs.htm. Accessed January 5, 2014.

30. Pollack CE, Platz EA, Bhavsar NA, et al. Primary care providers' perspectives on discontinuing prostate cancer screening. Cancer 2012;118(22):5518–24.

31. US Preventive Services Task Force. Talking with your patients about screening for prostate cancer. 2012. Available at: http://www.uspreventiveservicestaskforce.org/prostatecancerscreening/prostatecancerscript.pdf. Accessed January 5, 2014.

32. American Society of Clinical Oncology. ASCO guidelines: decision aid tool–prostate cancer screening with PSA testing. Available at: http://www.asco.org/sites/www.asco.org/files/psa_pco_decision_aid_71612.pdf. Accessed January 5, 2014.

33. National Comprehensive Cancer Network. NCCN clinical practice guidelines in oncology (NCCN guidelines): prostate cancer early detection (version 2.2012). Available at: http://www.nccn.org/professionals/physician_gls/pdf/prostate_detection.pdf. Accessed January 5, 2014.

34. Heidenreich A, Bastian PJ, Bellmunt J, et al. Guidelines on prostate cancer. 2013. Available at: http://www.uroweb.org/gls/pdf/09_Prostate_Cancer_LR.pdf. Accessed January 5, 2014.

35. National Health Service. Prostate cancer–PSA screening. 2012. Available at: http://www.nhs.uk/Conditions/Cancer-of-the-prostate/Pages/Prevention.aspx. Accessed January 5, 2014.

36. Qaseem A, Barry MJ, Denberg TD, et al. Screening for prostate cancer: a guidance statement from the Clinical Guidelines Committee of the American College of Physicians. Ann Intern Med 2013;158(10):761–9.

37. Wolf AM, Wender RC, Etzioni RB, et al. American Cancer Society guideline for the early detection of prostate cancer: update 2010. CA Cancer J Clin 2010; 60(2):70–98.

38. Han PK, Kobrin S, Breen N, et al. National evidence on the use of shared decision making in prostate-specific antigen screening. Ann Fam Med 2013;11(4): 306–14.

39. Elwyn G, Frosch D, Thomson R, et al. Shared decision making: a model for clinical practice. J Gen Intern Med 2012;27(10):1361–7.

40. Lin GA, Aaronson DS, Knight SJ, et al. Patient decision aids for prostate cancer treatment: a systematic review of the literature. CA Cancer J Clin 2009;59(6): 379–90.

41. O'Connor AM, Wennberg JE, Legare F, et al. Toward the 'tipping point': decision aids and informed patient choice. Health Aff (Millwood) 2007;26(3):716–25.

42. Stacey D, Bennett CL, Barry MJ, et al. Decision aids for people facing health treatment or screening decisions. Cochrane Database Syst Rev 2011;(10):CD001431.

43. University of Texas Health Science Center San Antonio. Individualized risk assessment of prostate cancer (PCPTRC 2.0). Available at: http://deb.uthscsa.edu/URORiskCalc/Pages/calcs.jsp. Accessed January 5, 2014.

44. Thompson IM, Ankerst DP, Chi C, et al. Assessing prostate cancer risk: results from the Prostate Cancer Prevention Trial. J Natl Cancer Inst 2006;98(8):529–34.

45. Rollins G. The next generation of prostate cancer diagnostics: are molecular tests ready? Clinical Laboratory News 2013;39(6). Available at: http://www.aacc.org/publications/cln/2013/june/Pages/Prostate-Cancer.aspx#. Accessed January 5, 2014.

46. Garg V, Gu NY, Borrego ME, et al. A literature review of cost-effectiveness analyses of prostate-specific antigen test in prostate cancer screening. Expert Rev Pharmacoecon Outcomes Res 2013;13(3):327–42.

47. American Cancer Society. Medicare coverage for cancer prevention and early detection. 2013. Available at: http://www.cancer.org/healthy/findcancerearly/cancerscreeningguidelines/medicare-coverage-for-cancer-prevention-and-early-detection. Accessed January 5, 2014.

48. De Leon SF, Shih SC. Tracking the delivery of prevention-oriented care among primary care providers who have adopted electronic health records. J Am Med Inform Assoc 2011;18(Suppl 1):i91–5.

49. Romano MJ, Stafford RS. Electronic health records and clinical decision support systems: impact on national ambulatory care quality. Arch Intern Med 2011; 171(10):897–903.

50. Murphy DR, Laxmisan A, Reis BA, et al. Electronic health record-based triggers to detect potential delays in cancer diagnosis. BMJ Qual Saf 2013;23(1):8–16.

51. Agency for Healthcare Research and Quality. Patient centered medical home resource center. Available at: http://pcmh.ahrq.gov/page/defining. Accessed March 18, 2014.

52. Shortell SM, Gillies R, Wu F. United States innovations in healthcare delivery. Public Health Reviews 2010;32(1):190–212.

53. Sarfaty M, Wender R, Smith R. Promoting cancer screening within the patient centered medical home. CA Cancer J Clin 2011;61(6):397–408.

54. Centers for Medicare and Medicaid Services. Accountable care organizations. 2013. Available at: http://www.cms.gov/Medicare/Medicare-Fee-for-Service-Payment/ACO/index.html?redirect=/aco/%20last%20accessed%209/4/2013. Accessed January 7, 2014.

55. Centers for Medicare and Medicaid Services. Accountable care organization 2013 program analysis: quality performance standards narrative measure specifications. 2012. Available at: http://www.cms.gov/Medicare/Medicare-Fee-for-Service-Payment/sharedsavingsprogram/Downloads/ACO-Narrative Measures-Specs.pdf. Accessed January 7, 2014.

56. Legare F, Ratte S, Gravel K, et al. Barriers and facilitators to implementing shared decision-making in clinical practice: update of a systematic review of health professionals' perceptions. Patient Educ Couns 2008;73(3):526–35.

57. Berwick DM. Making good on ACOs' promise–the final rule for the Medicare shared savings program. N Engl J Med 2011;365(19):1753–6.

58. Pearson WS, King DE, Richards C. Capitated payments to primary care providers and the delivery of patient education. J Am Board Fam Med 2013; 26(4):350–5.

Screening Strategies for Cardiovascular Disease in Asymptomatic Adults

Margaret L. Wallace, PharmD, BCACP*, Jason A. Ricco, MD, MPH, Bruce Barrett, MD, PhD

KEYWORDS

- Cardiovascular disease screening • Primary care • Evidence-based
- General-risk adult population

KEY POINTS

- Assessment of risk factors (eg, age, smoking, hypertension, family history) is key in determining the need for additional screening.
- Use of risk assessment tools, such as the Pooled Cohort Equations or Framingham in a United States population or Systematic Coronary Risk Evaluation or Prospective Cardiovascular Münster in a European population, improves the estimation of individual risk; however, these tools do not perform as well in Latinos or Asian Americans.
- Guidelines recommend assessment of risk factors, including lipid levels, every 4 to 6 years in adults 20 to 79 years of age without evidence of atherosclerotic cardiovascular disease (ASCVD), including the estimation of 10-year risk for ASCVD in those individuals aged 40 to 79 years.
- Abdominal aortic ultrasound is recommended one time in men aged 65 to 75 years who have ever smoked.
- There is insufficient evidence to recommend the use of lipoprotein (a), homocysteine, carotid intima-media thickness, or electrocardiography in a general-risk, asymptomatic, adult population.
- If risk-based decisions are uncertain after quantitative risk assessment, some guidelines suggest that family history, high-sensitivity C-reactive protein, or a coronary artery calcium score may be considered to further inform decision making.
- Cardiovascular disease results from a complex interplay of multiple genetic, environmental, and behavioral factors. Genetic screening is not recommended.

Conflict of Interest: None.

Drs M.L. Wallace and J.A. Ricco are supported by a National Research Service Award (T32HP10010) from the Health Resources and Services Administration to the University of Wisconsin Department of Family Medicine. Dr B. Barrett is supported by a Midcareer Investigator Award in Patient-Oriented Research and Mentoring (K24AT006543) from NIH NCCAM.

Department of Family Medicine, University of Wisconsin, 1100 Delaplaine Court, Madison, WI 53715, USA

* Corresponding author.

E-mail address: Margaret.Wallace@fammed.wisc.edu

0095-4543/14/$ – see front matter © 2014 Elsevier Inc. All rights reserved.

EPIDEMIOLOGY AND RISK FACTORS

Heart disease is the leading cause of death in the United States,[1] with heart attack and stroke accounting for about a third of all US deaths.[2] Cardiovascular diseases (CVDs) are also a leading cause of disability, with more than 4 million reporting a related disability in the United States.[2] The total cost of CVDs in the United States was estimated at $444 billion in 2010.[2] This number is expected to increase significantly as the US population ages.[2] Abdominal aortic aneurisms (AAA) affect 5% to 10% of men aged 65 to 79 years, and mortality following rupture of an abdominal aneurism is very high.[3]

Risk factors for CVD include family history, hypertension (HTN), dyslipidemia, smoking history, and diabetes mellitus. Smoking is associated with a 3- to 5-fold increase in the risk of AAA and AAA mortality.[4] Although most people with CVD have at least one conventional risk factor, it is important to know that almost 15% of men and 10% of women with CVD do not have any of the conventional risk factors.[5]

The risk for CVD varies across different populations, including race/ethnicity, age, and sex. Although a leading cause of death in the United States as a whole, heart disease has a higher prevalence, morbidity, and mortality in African Americans.[6,7] The reasons for these disparities have been debated. Risk factors, such as smoking, HTN, diabetes mellitus, and physical inactivity, are more common in African Americans; however, nondisease factors, such as genetic differences, health behaviors, and social factors, also play a role.[6] Race and ethnicity often correlate with social conditions or a person's environment, including education level, access to health care, and socioeconomic status. Lower socioeconomic status is linked to calorie-rich and nutrient-poor diets, which increases the risk of developing CVD.[8]

As the main point of contact within the health care system for most individuals, primary care providers play a critical role in the detection and management of risk factors for the primary prevention of CVD.

GLOBAL RISK ASSESSMENT TOOLS

Although evaluating cardiac risk is crucial for both determining the need for preventive treatment as well as specifying treatment intensity,[9–11] research suggests that health care providers tend to be poor estimators of patients' CVD risk.[12] The relative risk reduction from a given treatment tends to be constant across populations.[13] For example, if a treatment produces a relative risk reduction of approximately 30%, an individual with a baseline risk of 10% would have an absolute risk reduction of 3%. However, an individual with a baseline risk of 20% would have an absolute risk reduction of 6%. Thus, risk assessment is critical because the absolute risk reduction observed from treatment is a function of an individual's baseline risk, and treatment benefits may not outweigh treatment harms (which are likely constant) in low-risk individuals.

A variety of screening tools exist to help providers estimate the risk of a first cardiovascular event in adult patients,[12] including the Pooled Cohort Equations,[14] Framingham Risk Score (FRS), QRISK2 (version 2 of the QRISK CVD risk algorithm), Assessing Cardiovascular Risk using Scottish Intercollegiate Guidelines Network, Systematic Coronary Risk Evaluation (SCORE), Prospective Cardiovascular Münster (PROCAM), and United Kingdom Prospective Diabetes Study (UKPDS). Each tool is derived from a different sample and has associated advantages and disadvantages. As delineated in **Table 1**, consideration of unique characteristics and the source population is useful in guiding the selection of an appropriate risk assessment tool for a particular patient.

Table 1
Commonly used externally validated risk prediction models

Model	Outcome	Number of External Evaluations	Source Populations	Online Tool
Pooled Cohort Equations[33]	Nonfatal MI, CHD death, fatal and nonfatal stroke	—	Atherosclerosis Risk in Communities Study • United States • Aged 45–64 y • Men and women • Whites and African American[34] Cardiovascular Health Study • United States • Aged 65 y and older • Men and women[35] Coronary Artery Risk Development in Young Adults Study • United States • Aged 18–30 y • Men and women • White and African American[36] Framingham Heart Study • United States • Aged 30–62 y • 55% women • Primarily white Framingham Offspring Study • United States • Aged <10–70 y • 52% female • Primarily white[37]	http://my.americanheart.org/ professional/StatementsGuidelines/ PreventionGuidelines/Prevention- Guidelines_UCM_457698_ SubHomePage.jsp

(continued on next page)

Table 1
(continued)

Model	Outcome	Number of External Evaluations	Source Populations	Online Tool
1991 Framingham Risk Score Model	CVD	26	Framingham Heart Study • United States • Aged 30–62 y • 55% women • Primarily white Framingham Offspring Study • United States • Aged <10–70 y • 52% female • Primarily white[37]	http://reference.medscape.com/calculator/framingham-coronary-risk-ldl
1998 Framingham Risk Score Model	Total CHD (ie, angina, MI, sudden CHD death, cardiac procedure)	24	Framingham Heart Study, Framingham Offspring Study[38] • United States • Aged 30–74 y • 53% women • Primarily white[37]	
Framingham Risk Score Adult Treatment Panel III	Hard CHD (ie, sudden CHD death or MI)	16	Framingham Heart Study • United States • Aged 30–62 y • 55% women • Primarily white Framingham Offspring Study • United States • Aged <10–70 y • 52% female • Primarily white[37] *Excludes people with diabetes*	http://cvdrisk.nhlbi.nih.gov/calculator.asp

PROCAM	Hard CHD (ie, sudden CHD death or MI)	11	PROCAM[39] • Germany • Aged 35–65 y • White *Excludes women*	http://www.chd-taskforce.de/procam_interactive.html
SCORE	CVD mortality	11	SCORE[40] • Finland, Russia, Norway, United Kingdom, Denmark, Sweden, Belgium, Germany, Italy, France, Spain • Aged 19–80 y • Pooled dataset from cohort studies in 12 European countries; most of the cohorts were population-based; some occupational cohorts were included to increase representation from lower-risk areas	Access from the European Society of Cardiology

Abbreviations: CHD, coronary heart disease; MI, myocardial infarction.

Data from Matheny M, McPheeters M, Glasser A, et al. Systematic review of cardiovascular disease risk assessment tools. Evidence Synthesis No. 85. Rockville (MD): AHRQ Publication; 2011.

DESCRIPTION OF COMMONLY USED SCREENING METHODS
Blood Pressure Measurement

HTN is a common, preventable risk factor for the development of CVD and death.[15] Individuals with HTN have a much higher risk of stroke, myocardial infarction, heart failure, peripheral vascular disease, and AAA than those without HTN.[16] Office blood pressure measurement with an appropriately sized upper arm cuff is the standard screening test for HTN. In practice, errors may occur in measuring blood pressure as a result of instrument, observer, or patient factors. Factors leading to error include issues with the manometer, stethoscope, poorly fitting cuffs for the patient's arm size, trouble hearing Korotkoff sounds, inattention on the part of the observer, rapid release of air from the blood pressure cuff, and many more.[16] Precision in identifying those with HTN improves with the number of blood pressure measurements taken.[16]

When performed properly, office blood pressure measurement is highly correlated with the intra-arterial measurement and is predictive of cardiovascular risk.[16] The relationship between blood pressure and cardiovascular risk is continuous.[17] Individual blood pressure measurements tend to be variable; thus, HTN diagnosis should be made after at least 2 elevated readings taken on at least 2 visits.[17]

Blood Tests

Dyslipidemia is considered a major risk factor for the development of CVD. Lipid-lowering therapies, especially statins, are widely used in the primary and secondary prevention of CVD.[9] There are known associations between elevations in total cholesterol, low-density lipoproteins (LDL), and triglycerides as well as reductions in high-density lipoproteins (HDL) and CVD. Fasting lipid profiles including these 4 lipid biomarkers are widely used in screening and decision making in contemporary medicine. In recent years, some have also advocated for measuring elevations in lipoprotein (a).[18]

Inflammation seems to play an important role in the development of atherosclerosis. C-reactive protein (CRP) is a biomarker that increases in response to inflammation in the body. An elevated CRP level has been suggested as a potential nontraditional risk factor to use in estimating risk for those without known CVD.[19]

Homocysteine first became of interest in the prediction of CVD after observing that most children with genetic homocystinuria die of premature vascular disease. Severe homocysteine elevations can be the result of genetic mutations causing enzyme abnormalities. Insufficient consumption of folate, vitamin B_6, and vitamin B_{12}—vitamins that play a large role in homocysteine metabolism—accounts for most homocysteine elevations in the United States.[20]

Imaging

A variety of imaging tools have been studied and are increasingly used in practice to screen for CVD, including coronary artery calcium (CAC) obtained by computed tomography (CT), carotid artery ultrasound, and abdominal aorta ultrasound. CAC and carotid artery imaging are both used as markers of atherosclerosis,[21,22] although the interpretation of the 2 modalities differs in prediction of specific cardiovascular risk.[23]

Carotid intima-media thickness (cIMT) reflects primarily hypertensive medial hypertrophy, which is more predictive of stroke than myocardial infarction and is weakly associated with traditional cardiovascular risk factors.[23] Alternatively, carotid plaque area is more predictive of myocardial infarction than stroke and is often associated with traditional risk factors.[23] CAC scores predict cardiovascular events in asymptomatic adults[24] as well as both cardiovascular events and all-cause mortality in people with type 2 diabetes.[25] Screening for abdominal aneurism is conducted using ultrasonography to detect asymptomatic aneurisms for which surgery may reduce the risk of future rupture.[3]

Electrocardiography

Electrocardiography (ECG) has been used since the late 1800s in the diagnosis of CVD. ECG is frequently used to detect cardiac irregularities such as ventricular hypertrophy or conduction system delays. ECG abnormalities are associated with an increased risk of coronary heart disease (CHD) events[26] and mortality.[27]

Genetic Screening

Family history plays an important role in assessing the risk of CVD. In most cases, multiple genetic changes, which individually do not result in disease, are working together with environment and behavior to cause disease. Genetic screening is not yet sophisticated enough to detect this complex interplay between genes. However, some less common inherited heart diseases are caused by one or a few genetic changes that work to cause disease. Examples of these include familial hyperlipidemia, some forms of hypertrophic and dilated cardiomyopathy, arrhythmogenic right ventricular cardiomyopathy, long-QT syndrome, and Brugada syndrome. Genetic testing can help determine which relatives are at risk for developing a condition but cannot predict whether it will develop or its severity.[28]

EVIDENCE FOR RISK ASSESSMENT AND SCREENING
Global Risk Assessment

An impressive body of research demonstrates that the treatment of some cardiovascular risk factors reduces the rate of cardiovascular events. Numerous risk prediction models have been developed, but relatively few have been externally validated. An evidence review from the US Preventive Services Task Force (USPSTF) identified 17 risk prediction models that were validated in a population other than the one in which the model was developed. Risk prediction models are considered general population first-outcome incidence calculators, meaning they are intended to assess the individual risk of a first CVD event in a general-risk population.[12]

US models (ie, Framingham) validated in nationally representative US cohorts performed well in white and black populations but performed poorly among Hispanics and people of Asian descent living in the United States.[12,29,30] Social, cultural, and ethnic differences seem to influence CHD risk; thus, models are more likely to perform well in populations resembling the source population.[12,30] Models that excluded diabetes mellitus performed well in a general population. There are currently no externally validated models for use in a diabetic population in the United States.[12] US models had mixed performance when tested in European cohorts: US models underpredicted risk in European cohorts from high-risk populations (eg, people with diabetes) and overpredicted risk in the general population.[12]

More recently, the American College of Cardiology and the American Heart Association (ACC/AHA) have jointly developed new Pooled Cohort Equations in 2013 to estimate both the 10-year and lifetime risks for developing a first atherosclerotic cardiovascular disease (ASCVD) event, defined as CHD death, nonfatal myocardial infarction, and fatal or nonfatal stroke.[14] Participants from several large cohort studies were ultimately included for analysis and equation development, including participants in the ARIC (Atherosclerosis Risk in Communities) study,[22] Cardiovascular

Health Study,[21] and the CARDIA (Coronary Artery Risk Development in Young Adults) study,[31] in combination with data from the Framingham Study cohorts. The Pooled Cohort Equations include age, total and HDL cholesterol, systolic blood pressure (treated or untreated), diabetes, and current smoking status as statistically warranted variables and are only validated for use in African American and non-Hispanic white men and women because of insufficient data from the pooled cohorts for other racial/ethnic groups.[14]

In general, US models, such as the Pooled Cohorts Equations or FRS, should be used for screening in the United States, whereas European models, such as SCORE or PRO-CAM, should be used in European patients. Recognize that these models have significant limitations when used in populations that do not resemble the source population with regard to social, cultural, and ethnic characteristics. A major concern of the new Pooled Cohort Equations is that it systematically overestimated risks by roughly 75% to 150% based on its performance in 5 external validation cohorts. It is thought that this is caused by the use of cohort data from studies conducted more than 2 decades ago that do not necessarily reflect current levels of morbidity or improvements in overall health and health care since that time.[32] This conclusion suggests the need for routinely performing new external validation studies for any of these risk assessment models in contemporary cohorts to maintain model predictive value. Outcomes and cohort characteristics of several validated risk prediction models are described in **Table 1**.

Blood Pressure

Although there have been no randomized controlled trials (RCTs) evaluating the direct effect of screening for HTN on CVD event rates, trials evaluating HTN treatment demonstrated improved outcomes in the treatment of patients who were enrolled as a result of elevated blood pressures detected in screening.[16] Additionally, no studies have evaluated the relative effectiveness of selective versus universal blood pressure screening or the optimal frequency for blood pressure screening.[16] Although no direct evidence for HTN screening exists, indirect evidence supports screening adults for HTN because it is an important risk factor for CVD events and is reliably detected through office blood pressure screening. Additionally, treatment with lifestyle and pharmacologic therapy can effectively reduce blood pressure and CVD events.[16]

Lipids

Lipid screening in individuals with known CHD has been widely supported for some time. The benefits of lipid screening in a general risk population are relatively unknown because there have been no RCTs evaluating the direct effect of screening on CVD event rates. Because there is growing evidence demonstrating that statins reduce rates of CVD events in both intermediate- and high-risk individuals, dyslipidemia is considered a modifiable risk factor and lipids have become a target for CVD screening.[41] Nevertheless, there has not been clear consensus on whom, how, and when to screen for dyslipidemia for primary prevention of CHD.[42,43]

Because the absolute benefit of treating dyslipidemia is a function of baseline risk, a 10% baseline risk of events has been commonly used as a threshold for producing a meaningful difference in CVD outcomes given the significant drop-off in effectiveness for reducing CVD events in individuals with lower than a 10-year risk.[41,44] A 2008 USPSTF evidence review demonstrated that no combination of FRS ATP-III (Adult Treatment Panel III) risk factors in men aged 18 to 35 years or women younger than 40 years would result in a 10-year risk of cardiovascular events greater than 10% in nonsmokers or those without a history of HTN or diabetes mellitus. This finding means that limiting screening in men aged 18 to 35 years or women younger than 40 years to those with a smoking, HTN, or diabetes history will sufficiently identify those most likely to benefit from treating dyslipidemia.[43]

In 2013, the ACC/AHA released new guidelines for both cardiovascular risk assessment and treatment of cholesterol with statins that defined the threshold for 10-year risk at 7.5% rather than 10.0% as previously defined by ATP-III.[14,45] This risk threshold was based on data from both primary prevention statin RCTs and meta-analyses of statin RCTs included in the 2013 Cochrane review on statins for primary prevention of CVD that suggested that the ASCVD risk reduction benefit clearly outweighed the risks of statin therapy at a 7.5% or more 10-year risk threshold.[41,45,46] However, this redefinition of low ASCVD risk was met with controversy based on conflicting evidence for statin benefits in low-risk individuals as well as the methodology for setting the new threshold.[47–50] Indeed, the meta-analysis performed by the Cholesterol Treatment Trialists' (CTT) collaborators showed a 20% decrease in major vascular events for roughly every 40 mg/dL reduction in LDL cholesterol with statin treatment in low-risk individuals (the most significant finding for the meta-analysis of the 27 RCTs). However, 35% of the major vascular events were actually coronary revascularization procedures and not hard cardiovascular end points.[46,49]

Additionally, data from the CTT meta-analyses do not demonstrate that statins have a significant effect on overall mortality among low-risk individuals; the CTT collaborators did not consider the effect of statins on serious adverse effects despite having access to patient-level data.[49] Regardless of whether the threshold for low ASCVD 10-year risk is less than 7.5% or less than 10.0%, more research is currently needed to determine whether statin treatment in low-risk individuals actually provides a net benefit when taking into account the potential risks and harms of treatment. Future studies addressing this may very well influence the 10-year risk cutoff for risk assessment and more accurately determine whom and when to screen for dyslipidemia.

Screening for lipid disorders is recommended by both the ATP-III's and the USPSTF's guidelines. There are no trials that evaluate the effect of screening for triglycerides on clinical end points in individuals who would not otherwise qualify for lipid-lowering therapy. Although triglycerides seem to be a significant predictor when used as the sole predictor of CHD events, this association is reduced or eliminated when adjusting for other variables, such as those included in the FRS.[43] According to a 2001 evidence synthesis from the USPSTF, a Framingham-based algorithm that incorporates total cholesterol and HDL is the most accurate approach for predicting CHD events.[42] The updated 2013 risk assessment guidelines from the ACC/AHA retain both total and HDL cholesterol as statistically significant variables in the new Pooled Cohort Equations.[14] **Table 2** displays the reliability and accuracy, patient acceptance, and provider feasibility of different lipid screening strategies.

Evidence from epidemiologic studies and RCTs supports the use of CHD risk equivalents (ie, peripheral artery disease, AAA, carotid artery disease, and diabetes)[9] in targeting individuals who may benefit from lipid-lowering therapy.[43] There is not sufficient evidence to inform the recommended frequency of lipid screening in asymptomatic adults, although ATP-III suggests once every 5 years and the ACC/AHA's 2013 guidelines recommend risk factor assessment (including total and HDL cholesterol) every 4 to 6 years among adults.[14,42,43]

Lipoprotein (a)

There is insufficient evidence that using lipoprotein (a) improves risk stratification in asymptomatic adults compared with traditional risk factors alone.[51,52] A plasma lipoprotein (a) level of 30 mg/dL or greater is associated with an increased risk of CVD. There is little correlation between lipoprotein (a) and traditional CHD risk factors,

Table 2
Features of different lipid screening strategies for adults

Test	Reliability	Accuracy	Patient Acceptability	Feasibility for Providers
Nonfasting TC	Intermediate	Lower	Higher	Higher
Nonfasting TC/HDL	Lower	Intermediate	Higher	Intermediate
LDL/HDL ratio requires fasting TC, HDL, triglycerides	Higher	Intermediate	Lower	Intermediate
Nonfasting TC + HDL and NCEP guidelines	Intermediate	Intermediate	Intermediate	Lower
Nonfasting TC + HDL with calculation of Framingham risk	Intermediate	Higher	Intermediate	Lower

Abbreviations: NCEP, National Cholesterol Education Program; TC, total cholesterol.

From Helfand M, Carson S. Screening for lipid disorders in adults: selective update of 2001 US Preventive Services Task Force Review. Evidence synthesis no. 49. Rockville (MD): AHRQ Publication; 2008.

and studies have not evaluated the additive value of lipoprotein (a) with traditional risk factors in predicting CHD.[52]

CRP

Several studies have reported associations of CRP with CVD event rates; nevertheless, there is insufficient evidence that using CRP to stratify risk in asymptomatic adults leads to a reduction in CHD.[52] Adjusting for all Framingham risk factors in the evaluation of CRP, a meta-analysis of 10 studies of good quality from the USPSTF's 2009 evidence review found an increased relative risk (1.58; confidence interval [CI] 1.37–1.83) for those with high CRP (>3.0 mg/L) compared with those with low CRP (<1.0 mg/L). The included studies did not directly assess the impact of adding CRP to the assessment of FRS to reclassify individuals at intermediate risk. Several studies have evaluated the impact of CRP in reclassifying intermediate-risk individuals as high risk; however, the results of these studies are imprecise and conflicting and are not able to quantify how many people would be reclassified.[53]

Homocysteine

Homocysteine levels are positively associated with CVD and can be lowered by folic acid and other nutrients[54]; however, there is no evidence that screening with a homocysteine level in asymptomatic adults leads to a reduction in the prevalence of CHD events. An increase in homocysteine by 5 μmol/L was associated with a small increase in relative risk for total CHD (1.18; CI 1.10–1.26) when those with known CHD were excluded from the cohort. Administering folic acid can result in a reduction in homocysteine, though 2 large randomized trials, Health Outcomes Prevention (HOPE) trial and the Norwegian Vitamin Trial (NORVIT), testing whether folic acid can result in a decrease in myocardial infarction or recurrent CVD events were both negative.[55,56] The HOPE trial demonstrated a decreased relative risk of stroke from decreasing homocysteine with folic acid[56]; however, this was not confirmed in the NORVIT trial.[55] The Swiss Heart Study, which included 553 individuals following successful angioplasty of at least one coronary stenosis, demonstrated decreased relative risk of myocardial infarction or repeat revascularization after percutaneous coronary intervention with the use of homocysteine-lowering therapy.[57] These effects have not been confirmed in other studies.[52]

CAC Score

There is insufficient evidence that screening using a CAC score in asymptomatic adults leads to a reduction in the rate of CHD events.[51,52] A meta-analysis of 3 good-quality population-based cohort studies demonstrated increased relative risk for coronary events as the CAC score increased. Adjusted for other Framingham risk factors, the CAC score demonstrated the ability to better predict individuals at an increased risk over the estimated 10-year risk using FRS alone. Nevertheless, it is important to know that older studies overestimated the independent effect of CAC scores and that no studies have shown that CAC screening leads to better outcomes.[52]

A population-based cohort study from Rotterdam, Netherlands evaluated the utility of using 12 newer risk factors with standard risk factors. This study found that relative to the other emerging risk factors, the CAC score contributed significantly to the standard risk factors to predict CHD risk. However, these results are from a primarily white, European population and did not assess whether CAC screening results in better clinical outcomes.[58]

A cost-effectiveness modeling analysis of CAC score screening in an intermediate-risk population was conducted based on the Rotterdam study. In this analysis, CAC score screening in men just met a commonly used threshold for cost-effectiveness. Because of its retrospective nature, however, many assumptions were made. Sensitivity analysis demonstrated that by altering these assumptions, CAC screening was no longer cost-effective. In women, CAC screening was not cost-effective, even when using assumptions that generally favor CAC screening.[59]

cIMT

A USPSTF's 2009 evidence synthesis evaluating emerging risk factors for CHD found 3 cohort studies evaluating the potential utility of cIMT in screenings. However, these studies had serious limitations, such as including patients with known CAD, symptomatic peripheral vascular disease, or not reporting CHD events as end points. Although cIMT is predictive of some CVD events after adjusting for traditional risk factors, there is not consensus on examination technique or standards for interpreting the cIMT measures. The studies included in the analysis had differing methods for evaluating cIMT, making the synthesis of results unreliable.[51,52] A cohort study published following the USPSTF's 2009 report demonstrated similarly modest improvements in CHD risk prediction.[58]

Ultrasound of Abdominal Aorta

A Cochrane review evaluating ultrasound screening of asymptomatic adults for AAA identified 4 studies with 127891 men and 9342 women randomly assigned to receive ultrasound screening or no screening.[3] Only one trial included women. None of the trials were conducted in the United States (2 were in the United Kingdom, one in Denmark, and one in Australia). In 3 of these trials, screening was associated with a reduction in death from AAA in men aged 65 to 83 years (odds ratio [OR] 0.60; range 0.47–0.78). There was no reduction in mortality among women. Three to 5 years following the screening, all-cause mortality was not significantly different between the screened and unscreened groups. Screened men were more likely to have undergone surgery for AAA than men who were not screened (OR 2.03; range 1.59–2.59).

Screening among men aged 65 to 74 years seems to be cost-effective, but there is no evidence related to life expectancy, complications from surgery, or quality of life.[3]

In 2005, the USPSTF also completed an evidence synthesis. This synthesis included the same 4 trials identified in the Cochrane review; however, the USPSTF's review focused on answering questions related to screening in a high-risk population, repeat screening in individuals without AAA on initial screening, harms associated with AAA screening, and harms associated with repairing AAAs 5.5 cm or greater in diameter.[4] Age, smoking, family history, coronary artery disease, hypercholesterolemia, and cerebrovascular disease are risk factors for AAA. Only one trial evaluated mortality from AAA in different age groups. Invitation to screen was associated with significantly reduced mortality in men aged 65 to 75 years (OR 0.19, CI 0.04–0.89) and increased mortality in older men.[4] The researchers of the USPSTF's evidence syntheses developed a model to evaluate the impact of selectively screening those with a history of smoking. This model demonstrated that invitation to screen men aged 65 to 74 years with a lifetime history of smoking 100 or more cigarettes accounts for 89% of the expected reduction in mortality from screening all men aged 65 to 74 years.[4] However, limiting screening to current smokers was too restrictive and resulted in many missed AAAs. Population screening strategies based on coronary artery disease, hypercholesterolemia, and cerebrovascular disease do not perform better than approaches using age, sex, and smoking history in identifying high-risk populations for screening.[4]

Repeat screening in men with a negative AAA ultrasound at 65 years of age does not seem to be advantageous. In men with negative AAA screening at 65 years of age, the incidence of new AAA was low in 10 years of periodic AAA screening. When AAAs were found in follow-up screening, they were most commonly less than 4.0 cm and did not have a significant risk of rupture.[4] Ultrasonography is not associated with any physical harm in adults. Participants with positive ultrasonography compared with negative ultrasonography had slightly more anxiety and lower mental and physical health scores initially but soon returned to normal within 6 weeks of screening. Elective AAA repair has risks and is associated with significant morbidity and mortality. Outcomes are improved in hospitals conducting more AAA repairs and when repairs are done by experienced vascular surgeons.[4]

ECG

The USPSTF published an evidence synthesis evaluating the use of ECG in screening asymptomatic adults in 2011.[60] There were no RCTs or prospective cohort studies evaluating clinical outcomes following screening versus no screening in asymptomatic adults. No studies assessed the improved accuracy of stratifying cardiovascular risk by using traditional risk factors plus resting or stress ECG compared with traditional risk factors alone. A pooled analysis including 63 prospective cohort studies demonstrated that ST-segment or T-wave abnormalities, left ventricular hypertrophy, bundle branch block, or left-axis deviation on resting ECG or ST-segment depression with exercise, failure to reach maximum target heart rate, or low exercise capacity on exercise ECG are associated with an increased risk of a cardiovascular event after adjusting for traditional risk factors.[60]

Genetic Screening

Although most CVD results from a complex interaction of genetic and environmental influence, thereby precluding effective genetic screening, familial hypercholesterolemia (FH) is a monogenic disease that can be identified with genetic testing. The rate of FH varies greatly by region and ethnicity and responds well to treatment.[61] Genetic screening in family members of people with known FH demonstrated cost-effectiveness in analysis from the Netherlands. This type of screening allows detection of FH before it is symptomatic.[62] A second cost-effectiveness analysis in the United Kingdom demonstrated superiority of DNA testing in family members of people with known or probable FH followed by LDL testing in individuals in which a genetic mutation was not identified.[63] Importantly, these studies used a cascade design, meaning all first-degree relatives of those with known or probable FH are tested rather than general population-based genetic screening, which is not recommended.

CVD PREVENTION AND SCREENING RECOMMENDATIONS

Evidence-based research has allowed for the development of clinical practice guidelines as professional recommendations to guide clinical and health policy decision making. The USPSTF, the ACC/AHA, and other organizations have provided assessments of the current evidence for CVD prevention and screening through professional recommendations. The USPSTF is an independent group of 16 US experts in prevention and evidence-based medicine from the fields of preventive medicine and primary care assembled to provide recommendations based on scientific evidence reviews on a variety of clinical preventive medicine services.[64] The USPSTF provides recommendations for services when benefits clearly outweigh the harms, with a focus on health and quality of life. The USPSTF assigns a grade definition (A, B, C, D, or I) based on the strength of evidence and net benefit, and grade A and B services have clear benefit and should be offered to patients.[65]

The ACC and AHA have jointly produced guidelines for CVD since 1980, with experts in the subjects under consideration providing recommendations based on a thorough evidence review. The experts rank supporting evidence for recommendations according to previously established methodology, with level A evidence coming from multiple randomized clinical trials, level B evidence derived from a single randomized trial or nonrandomized studies, and level C evidence largely based on consensus opinion, case studies, or standard of care. In 2010, the ACC/AHA published a clinical guideline for assessing CVD risk in asymptomatic adults, addressing many of the screening strategies discussed in this article.[66] The ACC/AHA's updated 2013 guideline for assessing cardiovascular risk focuses mainly on the new model for global risk assessment, the Pooled Cohort Equations.[14]

The Joint National Committee on Prevention, Detection, Evaluation, and Treatment of High Blood Pressure (JNC) was established to provide an evidence-based approach to the prevention and management of HTN.[67] JNC is made up of a panel of experts; the most recent set of guidelines, JNC8, was published in 2013 focusing on the treatment of HTN in adults.[15] The National Heart, Lung, and Blood Institute established the National Cholesterol Education Program (NCEP) in 1985 with the goal of reducing CVD morbidity and mortality by lowering the percent of Americans with high cholesterol. As part of its educational efforts, NCEP has published a series of 3 clinical practice guidelines for cholesterol management beginning in 1988.[68] The most recent version, published in 2002 and updated in 2004, The Third Report of the Expert Panel on Detection, Evaluation, and Treatment of High Blood Cholesterol in Adults (ATP-III) was drafted by expert panel members, including representative experts from both ACC and AHA.[44,68] **Table 3** provides a summary of guidelines and recommendations for various screening strategies from these organizations.

CURRENT PRACTICE PATTERNS

Data documenting the current practice patterns for CVD screening using the newest testing modalities are limited. Health system reports and observational data provide

Table 3
Summary of guidelines

Screening	USPSTF's Guideline (Evidence Grade)[a]	ACC Foundation/AHA's Guideline (Evidence Grade)[b]	Other Guidelines
Global Risk Assessment	—	The race- and sex-specific Pooled Cohort Equations should be used in non-Hispanic African Americans and non-Hispanic whites 40–79 y of age (B) Use of the sex-specific Pooled Cohort Equations for non-Hispanic whites may be considered when estimating risk in patients from populations other than African Americans and non-Hispanic whites (C) It is reasonable to assess traditional ASCVD risk factors (age, sex, total and HDL cholesterol, systolic blood pressure, use of antihypertensive therapy, diabetes, and current smoking) every 4–6 y in adults 20–79 y of age who are free from ASCVD (B) Assessing 30-y or lifetime ASCVD risk based on traditional risk factors may be considered in adults 20–59 y of age without ASCVD and who are not at high short-term risk (C)[33]	—
Genetic Screening	—	Genotype testing for CHD risk assessment in asymptomatic adults is not recommended (B)[66]	National Institute for Health and Clinical Excellence: Recommends cascade screening with both cholesterol and DNA testing for the diagnosis of FH[69]
Blood Pressure	Recommends screening for high blood pressure in adults aged 18 y and older (A)[70]	Blood pressure screening is not specifically addressed; however, blood pressure is included in the Pooled Cohort Equation recommended for estimating risk[33]	Joint National Committee on Prevention, Detection, Evaluation, and Treatment of High Blood Pressure: Blood pressure screening is not specifically addressed[15]

Blood Tests

Lipids	Strongly recommends FLP screening men aged 35 y and older for lipid disorders (A) Recommends FLP screening men aged 20 to 35 y for lipid disorders if they have additional risks, such as smoking, HTN, or diabetes (B) Strongly recommends FLP screening women aged 45 y and older (A) Recommends FLP screening women aged 20 to 45 y for lipid disorders if they are at increased risk for coronary heart disease, such as smoking, HTN, or diabetes (B) No recommendation for or against routine screening for lipid disorders in men aged 20 to 35 y or in women aged 20 y and older who are not at increased risk for CHD (C)[71]	Measurement of lipid parameters beyond a standard FLP (total cholesterol, HDL, LDL, triglycerides) are not recommended in asymptomatic adults (C)[66]	NCEP ATP-III: Recommends a complete FLP (total cholesterol, LDL, HDL, and triglycerides) as the preferred initial test, rather than screening for total cholesterol and HDL alone Recommends screening all adults aged 20 y and older every 5 y or more frequently with a borderline result[44]
High-Sensitivity CRP	Current evidence is insufficient to the balance of benefits and harms of using nontraditional risk factors to screen asymptomatic men and women with no history of CHD to prevent CHD events (I)[72]	If, after quantitative risk assessment, a risk-based treatment decision is uncertain, assessment of high-sensitivity CRP may be considered to inform treatment decision making (B)[33]	ACPM: Does not recommend routine screening of the general adult population using high-sensitivity CRP[73] NCEP ATP-III: Does not recommend routine measurement of inflammatory markers for the purpose of modifying LDL cholesterol goals in primary prevention[44]
Homocysteine	Current evidence is insufficient to the balance of benefits and harms of using nontraditional risk factors to screen asymptomatic men and women with no history of CHD to prevent CHD events (I)[72]	Not addressed	NCEP ATP-III: Does not recommend routine measurement of homocysteine as part of risk assessment to modify LDL-cholesterol goals for primary prevention[44]

(continued on next page)

Table 3
(continued)

Screening	USPSTF's Guideline (Evidence Grade)[a]	ACC Foundation/AHA's Guideline (Evidence Grade)[b]	Other Guidelines
Imaging			
CAC Score	Current evidence is insufficient to the balance of benefits and harms of using nontraditional risk factors to screen asymptomatic men and women with no history of CHD to prevent CHD events (I)[72]	If, after quantitative risk assessment, a risk-based treatment decision is uncertain, assessment of CAC score may be considered to inform treatment decision making (B)[33]	NCEP ATP-III: Does not recommend indiscriminate screening for CAC in asymptomatic persons, particularly in persons without multiple risk factors Measurement of CAC is an option for advanced risk assessment in appropriately selected persons[44] ACPM: Does not recommend routine screening of the general adult population using CT scanning[73]
cIMT	Current evidence is insufficient to the balance of benefits and harms of using nontraditional risk factors to screen asymptomatic men and women with no history of CHD to prevent CHD events (I)[72]	cIMT is not recommended for routine measurement in clinical practice for risk assessment for first ASCVD event (B)[33]	ACPM: Does not recommend routine screening of the general adult population using cIMT[73]
Ultrasound of Abdominal Aorta	Recommends one-time screening for AAA by ultrasonography in men aged 65–75 y who have ever smoked (B) No recommendation for or against screening for AAA in men aged 65–75 y who have never smoked (C) Recommends against routine screening for AAA in women (D)[74]	Not addressed	ACPM: Recommends one-time AAA screening in men aged 65–75 y who have ever smoked Routine AAA screening in women is not recommended[73]

ECG		ACPM:
Stress	Recommends against routine screening with exercise treadmill test in adults with low risk for CHD events (D)[75]	Does not recommend routine screening of the general adult population using exercise stress testing[73]
	An exercise ECG may be considered for cardiovascular risk assessment in intermediate-risk asymptomatic adults (including sedentary adults considering starting a vigorous exercise program), predominantly when attention is paid to non-ECG markers, such as exercise capacity (B)[66]	
Resting	Insufficient evidence to recommend for or against routine ECG in adults at increased risk for CHD events (I)[75]	ACPM: Does not recommend routine screening of the general adult population using ECG[73]
	A resting ECG is reasonable for cardiovascular risk assessment in asymptomatic adults with HTN or diabetes (C)	
	A resting ECG may be considered for cardiovascular risk assessment in asymptomatic adults without HTN or diabetes (C)[66]	

Abbreviations: ACPM, American College of Preventive Medicine; FLP, fasting lipid panel.

[a] Strength of recommendation. Grade A: The USPSTF recommends the service. There is high certainty that the net benefit is substantial. Grade B: The USPSTF recommends the service. There is high certainty that the net benefit is moderate or there is moderate certainty that the net benefit is moderate to substantial. Grade C: The USPSTF recommends selectively offering or providing this service to individual patients based on professional judgment and patient preferences. There is at least moderate certainty that the net benefit is small. Grade D: The USPSTF recommends against the service. There is moderate or high certainty that the service has no net benefit or that the harms outweigh the benefits. Grade I: The USPSTF concludes that the current evidence is insufficient to assess the balance of benefits and harms of the service. Evidence is lacking, of poor quality, or conflicting; the balance of benefits and harms cannot be determined.[65]

[b] Evidence based on certainty of treatment effect. Level A: Multiple populations evaluated; data derived from multiple randomized clinical trials or meta-analyses. Level B: Limited populations evaluated; data derived from a single randomized trial or nonrandomized study. Level C: Very limited populations evaluated; only consensus opinion of experts, case studies, or standards of care.[66]

a source for information on blood pressure measurement, lipid screening, and use of ECGs in the primary care setting.

Studies report variable rates of blood pressure screening in the United States. One study of women in central Pennsylvania reported blood pressure measurement as the most commonly received preventive service, with 94.1% receiving screening in a 2-year period.[76] Another study demonstrated that blood pressure was measured in 56% of all adult visits and 93% of visits with hypertensive patients in office visits conducted in 2003 to 2004.[77] Seeing a specialist other than a cardiologist, older than 75 years, lack of insurance, absence of HTN-related comorbidities, and visits other than general medical examination visits were all associated with decreased odds of being screened for HTN.[77] Because blood pressure is one of the most important modifiable risk factors for CVD, this variability in blood pressure screening indicates that efforts are needed to improve the consistency of blood pressure screening in clinical practice.

Lipid screening is currently performed at highly variable rates throughout the United States. Among 6830 patients from 44 primary care practices in the Midwest, the rate of cholesterol screening every 5 years varied from 45% to 88%.[78] Similarly, cholesterol screening rates varied widely among 5071 patients at 60 non–university-based primary care practices in North Carolina. Although the median clinic screening rate of 40% every 2 years met the frequency recommended by the ATP-III's guidelines (once every 5 years), the rate of screening varied broadly from 26% to 54% among the different clinics.[79] Additionally, the 2-year screening rate differed significantly by specialty, with internal medicine providers screening at higher rates than family medicine providers (54% vs 38%) across the clinics.[79]

Lipid screening rates differ based on both patient and contextual factors. Patient factors associated with higher rates of lipid screening include older age, a diagnosis of diabetes, and higher body mass index.[76,79,80] Additionally, having a regular provider, having continuous health insurance coverage for the past year, and the presence of at least one chronic medical condition are associated with higher lipid screening rates.[76] At the contextual level, primary care provider density by county is positively associated with lipid screening.[76] Although some studies suggest no difference in lipid screening rates between men and women,[76,81] Rifas-Shiman and colleagues[80] found that women were screened at lower rates than men across all risk levels. Although there is clear evidence for racial and ethnic disparities in CVD prevalence,[6,7,82] outcomes,[6,7] and some treatment modalities,[6,83] evidence for such disparities in lipid screening rates is less consistent. Analysis of data from the Medical Expenditure Panel Survey, which constructs a nationally representative sample with oversampling of Hispanics and non-Hispanic blacks, from both 1996[84] and 2007[85] did not find significant racial or ethnic differences in cholesterol screening rates. In contrast, 2 independent studies using data from the National Health and Nutrition Examination Survey during the 1988–1994[86] and 1999–2006[87] periods conveyed that African Americans and Mexican Americans were less likely than whites to report serum cholesterol screening.

Given the lower absolute benefit from statin treatment in low-risk individuals,[41,49] variation in lipid screening rates based on some clinical factors may reflect appropriate risk stratification by providers. (Rates less than once every 5 years may very well be appropriate for low risk patients.) However, the widespread variation in lipid screening rates based on nonclinical factors suggests a nonsystematic approach to incorporating evidence-based preventive health services in primary care. Although differences between groups or clinics may seem inevitable, as some practices are more efficient in delivering preventive services than others, Solberg and colleagues[78] found significant variation between the delivery of different preventive services within individual clinics. This "marker of haphazard provision of clinical preventive services"[78(p124)] highlights the need for interventions aimed to systematically deliver evidence-based preventive measures, such as lipid screening. Complicating this task is the difficulty of implementing the ATP-III's guidelines in clinical practice as evident by data illustrating that higher-risk patients are more likely to be undertreated for dyslipidemia than those at lower risk. It is suggested that this is related to a lack of provider comfort with the complexity of ATP-III–based risk categorization.[81] Conversely, in a study of 24 primary care offices, higher global patient-centered medical home (PCMH) scores were associated with greater receipt of preventive health services, including lipid screening.[88] In particular, the relational principles of PCMH (such as identifying a personal physician, having continuity of care, and whole person–oriented care) were more strongly associated with lipid screening than the information technology capabilities of PCMH organizational structure.[88]

There are less available data on the current use of ECGs for screening in the primary care setting. In one study of 10 urban academic group internal medicine practices, ECGs were obtained in 4.4% of asymptomatic patients without known CVD.[89] There was significant variability among both group practices and providers, with the rate of ECG performance ranging from 0.8% to 8.6% among the 10 practices and from 0.0% to 24.0% among providers.[89] Clinical predictors of ECG use include older age, male sex, and clinical comorbidities. Additionally, older male providers, those who billed for ECG interpretation, and Medicare as a payment source were associated with obtaining ECGs.[89] Race and ethnicity were not analyzed as predictors of ECG screening.[89] Overall, variation in ECG screening was not well explained by patient characteristics and likely reflects the lack of sufficient evidence for the role of ECG screening in the primary care setting.[89]

IMPACT OF CHANGES WITHIN HEALTH CARE

The true impact of recent transformations within the health care system, such as widespread use of electronic health records (EHR), implementation of the Affordable Care Act (ACA), development of accountable care organization (ACOs), and expansion of PCMH principles, are yet to be seen.

EHR

Advocated for as a facilitator of quality health care delivery, EHRs are becoming increasingly prevalent. Reports of the effects of EHR implementation, however, are mixed.[90–95] Although proponents have pointed to increased use of clinical decision support within the EHR as a benefit, this has not consistently led to improvements in the quality of care[92]; however, EHRs have been used to successfully identify individuals at risk of developing CVD by readily identifying risk-factor clustering.[93]

ACA and ACOs

Although many provisions of the ACA have been implemented, the law will not be fully used until 2018; the effects of many of the recently implemented provisions have not yet been realized. There are several provisions, however, that will likely impact CVD screening and prevention in primary care. A Prevention and Public Health Fund was established by the ACA, which supports prevention and public health programs. Specifically, this fund will be used to increase the primary care workforce and develop programs to prevent tobacco use, obesity, heart disease, stroke and cancer, and to increase immunization rates.[96] Additionally, the ACA requires new health plans and

Medicare to provide coverage for preventive services rated A or B by the USPSTF (including AAA screening for men aged 65–75 years who have ever smoked and cholesterol screening in men older than 35 years or women older than 45 years or younger if at an increased risk for CHD).[96,97] There will also be federal matching payments for preventive services in Medicaid for states that offer A- and B-recommended services with no patient cost sharing.[96]

Through the ACA, the Centers for Medicare and Medicaid Services' Shared Savings Program promotes the growth of ACOs, the aims of which are to improve care for individuals, better the health of populations, and slow the growth of costs. Importantly, prevention is a key component of improving care, bettering health, and slowing growth of costs.[98,99] To accomplish these aims, ACOs must not only effectively manage patients' health care information but also use this information to inform patients about preventive care and increase patients' engagement in prevention through shared decision making.[98]

PCMH

The concept of the PCMH has been present for some time. In 2008, the American Academy of Family Physicians, American Academy of Pediatrics, American College of Physicians, and American Osteopathic Association developed joint principles describing the characteristics of the PCMH.[100] These principles describe a model in which patients have an ongoing relationship with a physician who provides continuous and comprehensive care. This physician leads a team of people who work together to provide care and arrange for care by other professionals when needed. Patients have enhanced access to care and increased options for communication with providers and staff. All of these principles are aligned to improve coordination of care, quality, and safety.[100] Research evaluating principles of the PCMH and the receipt of preventive services found a positive relationship with regard to lipid screening, suggesting that PCMH characteristics of practice organization may facilitate CVD screening best practice.[88]

SUMMARY

Any summary of scientific evidence is somewhat constrained as a particular snapshot in time, and lack of current evidence must not be equated with evidence against effectiveness. Many methods for CVD screening have insufficient evidence to currently recommend use in a general, asymptomatic adult population. This lack of evidence corresponds well with a 2012 Cochrane review evaluating the impact of general health checks (including screening measures) that found general health checks did not improve either overall health or cardiovascular morbidity and mortality.[101] Nonetheless, there is good evidence for some specific CVD screening modalities when used in the proper risk setting. Lipid measurement and abdominal aortic ultrasound, for example, are 2 screening techniques with strong data regarding who benefits from screening and the impact of screening on outcomes. Although current evidence does not support the use of other newer screening modalities for primary prevention of CVD, this may very well change as more high-quality trials are completed in the future.

Risk assessment is a vital first step in determining the appropriate approach to CVD screening. As discussed earlier, even with elevated LDL, younger adults without other risk factors, such as HTN, smoking, or diabetes, will not likely qualify for cholesterol-lowering medications according to the ATP-III's or ACC/AHA's guidelines. In this segment of the population, lipid screening may not be necessary. One study found that prescribed lipid management (ie, lifestyle counseling and medication initiation) was more closely related to pretreatment LDL than to calculated 10-year risk despite a body of research to the contrary, resulting in undertreatment of many intermediate- and high-risk individuals.[81] This finding highlights the importance of moving the assessment of CVD risk factors beyond the traditional focus on LDL and dyslipidemia to a more holistic and individualized approach as outlined by the ACC/AHA's 2013 risk assessment guidelines and championed by the PCMH movement.

Risk assessment tools, such as the Pooled Cohort Equations or Framingham calculator in a US population and SCORE cards or PROCAM calculator in a European population, can facilitate the estimation of risk and open the door for shared decision making regarding interventions to reduce cardiovascular risk. Shared decision-making tools are sometimes built into risk assessment tools (eg, QINTERVENTION tool for use in the United Kingdom: http://qintervention.org/; Mayo Clinic Shared Decision Making National Resource Center Statin/Aspirin Choice tool http://shareddecisions.mayoclinic.org/decision-aids-for-diabetes/cardiovascular-prevention/). These tools are designed to support patient-provider conversations regarding risk factor identification and the potential benefits and harms of screening for and/or treating a health condition. Including patients in the conversation regarding evidence, potential risks, and the various options for CVD screening will provide patients with the knowledge to make informed decisions regarding their health. Further research is needed on the facilitators of and barriers to efforts to implement global risk assessment strategies in a primary care setting.

The absolute benefit of treating risk factors to prevent CVD varies considerably as a function of baseline risk. In light of the current evidence, health organizations should be encouraged to reprioritize quality metrics by shifting the focus away from measuring individual biomarkers to performing global risk assessment to achieve CVD screening best practice.

ACKNOWLEDGMENTS

The authors would like to thank Mary Checovich, Senior Research Specialist with the University of Wisconsin Department of Family Medicine, for her organizational support in the development of this article.

REFERENCES

1. Kochanek KD, Xu J, Murphy SL, et al. Deaths: final data for 2009. Natl Vital Stat Rep 2011;60(3):1–17.
2. Centers for Disease Control and Prevention. Heart disease and stroke prevention addressing the nation's leading killers: at a glance 2011. Prev Chronic Dis 2011. Available at: http://www.cdc.gov/chronicdisease/resources/publications/aag/dhdsp.htm. Accessed May 16, 2013.
3. Cosford PA, Leng GC. Screening for abdominal aortic aneurysm [review]. Cochrane Database Syst Rev 2011;(2):CD002945.
4. Fleming C, Whitlock E, Beil T, et al. Screening for abdominal aortic aneurysm: a best-evidence systematic review for the US Preventive Service Task Force. Ann Intern Med 2005;142:203–11.
5. Khot UN, Khot MB, Bajzer CT, et al. Prevalence of conventional risk factors in patients with coronary heart disease. JAMA 2003;290(7):898–904.
6. Harold JG, Williams KA Sr. President's page: disparities in cardiovascular care: finding ways to narrow the gap. J Am Coll Cardiol 2013;62(6):563–5.

7. Ford ES. Trends in predicted 10-year risk of coronary heart disease and cardio-vascular disease among U.S. adults from 1999 to 2010. J Am Coll Cardiol 2013; 61(22):2249–52.

8. Drewnowski A. Obesity, diets, and social inequalities. Nutr Rev 2009;67(Suppl 1):S36–9.

9. Expert Panel on Detection Evaluation, Treatment of High Blood Cholesterol in Adults. Executive summary of the third report of the National Cholesterol Education Program (NCEP) Expert Panel on Detection, Evaluation, And Treatment of High Blood Cholesterol In Adults (Adult Treatment Panel III). JAMA 2001; 285(19):2486–97.

10. Wood D, De Backer G, Faergeman O, et al. Prevention of coronary heart disease in clinical practice: recommendations of the Second Joint Task Force of European and other Societies on Coronary Prevention. Atherosclerosis 1998; 140(2):199–270.

11. Califf RM, Armstrong PW, Carver JR, et al. 27th Bethesda Conference: matching the intensity of risk factor management with the hazard for coronary disease events. Task Force 5. Stratification of patients into high, medium and low risk subgroups for purposes of risk factor management. J Am Coll Cardiol 1996; 27(5):1007–19.

12. Matheny M, McPheeters M, Glasser A, et al. Systematic review of cardiovascular disease risk assessment tools. Evidence Synthesis No. 85. Rockville (MD): AHRQ Publication; 2011.

13. Barratt A, Wyer PC, Hatala R, et al. Tips for learners of evidence-based medicine: 1. Relative risk reduction, absolute risk reduction and number needed to treat. CMAJ 2004;171(4):353–8.

14. Goff DC Jr, Lloyd-Jones DM, Bennett G, et al. 2013 ACC/AHA guideline on the assessment of cardiovascular risk: a report of the American College of Cardiology/American Heart Association Task Force on Practice Guidelines. Circulation 2013. [Epub ahead of print].

15. James PA, Oparil S, Carter BL, et al. 2014 Evidence-based guideline for the management of high blood pressure in adults: report from the panel members appointed to the Eighth Joint National Committee (JNC 8). JAMA 2014;311(5): 507–20.

16. Sheridan S, Pignone M, Donahue K. Screening for high blood pressure: a review of the evidence for the U.S. Preventive Services Task Force. Am J Prev Med 2003;25(2):151–8.

17. US Preventive Services Task Force. Screening for high blood pressure: US Preventive Services Task Force reaffirmation recommendation statement. Ann Intern Med 2007;147(11):783–6.

18. Emerging Risk Factors Collaboration, Di Angelantonio E, Sarwar N, Perry P, et al. Major lipids, apolipoproteins, and risk of vascular disease. JAMA 2009;302(18): 1993–2000.

19. Akhabue E, Thiboutot J, Cheng JW, et al. New and emerging risk factors for coronary heart disease. Am J Med Sci 2014;347(2):151–8.

20. Humphrey LL, Fu R, Rogers K, et al. Homocysteine level and coronary heart disease incidence: a systematic review and meta-analysis. Mayo Clin Proc 2008; 83(11):1203–12.

21. O'Leary DH, Polak JF, Kronmal RA, et al. Carotid-artery intima and media thickness as a risk factor for myocardial infarction and stroke in older adults. Cardiovascular Health Study Collaborative Research Group. N Engl J Med 1999; 340(1):14–22.

22. Chambless LE, Heiss G, Folsom AR, et al. Association of coronary heart disease incidence with carotid arterial wall thickness and major risk factors: the Atherosclerosis Risk in Communities (ARIC) Study, 1987-1993. Am J Epidemiol 1997; 146(6):483–94.

23. Spence JD. Technology insight: ultrasound measurement of carotid plaque–patient management, genetic research, and therapy evaluation. Nat Clin Pract Neurol 2006;2(11):611–9.

24. Pletcher MJ, Tice JA, Pignone M, et al. Using the coronary artery calcium score to predict coronary heart disease events: a systematic review and meta-analysis. Arch Intern Med 2004;164(12):1285–92.

25. Kramer CK, Zinman B, Gross JL, et al. Coronary artery calcium score prediction of all cause mortality and cardiovascular events in people with type 2 diabetes: systematic review and meta-analysis. BMJ 2013;346:f1654.

26. Moyer VA, US Preventive Serivces Task Force. Screening for coronary heart disease with electrocardiography: US Preventive Services Task Force recommendation statement. Ann Intern Med 2012;157(7):512–8.

27. Ashley EA, Raxwal VK, Froelicher VF. The prevalence and prognostic significance of electrocardiographic abnormalities. Curr Probl Cardiol 2000;25(1): 1–72.

28. Cirino AL, Ho CY. Genetic testing for inherited heart disease. Circulation 2013; 128(1):e4–8.

29. Liao Y, McGee DL, Cooper RS, et al. How generalizable are coronary risk prediction models? Comparison of Framingham and two national cohorts. Am Heart J 1999;137(5):837–45.

30. Orford JL, Sesso HD, Stedman M, et al. A comparison of the Framingham and European Society of Cardiology coronary heart disease risk prediction models in the normative aging study. Am Heart J 2002;144(1):95–100.

31. Okwuosa TM, Greenland P, Ning H, et al. Yield of screening for coronary artery calcium in early middle-age adults based on the 10-year Framingham Risk Score: the CARDIA study. JACC Cardiovasc Imaging 2012;5(9):923–30.

32. Ridker PM, Cook NR. Statins: new American guidelines for prevention of cardiovascular disease. Lancet 2013;382(9907):1762–5.

33. Goff DC Jr, Lloyd-Jones DM, Bennett G, et al. 2013 ACC/AHA Guideline on the Assessment of Cardiovascular Risk: a Report of the American College of Cardiology/American Heart Association Task Force on Practice Guidelines. J Am Coll Cardiol 2013. [Epub ahead of print].

34. The Atherosclerosis Risk in Communities (ARIC) Study: design and objectives. The ARIC investigators. Am J Epidemiol 1989;129(4):687–702.

35. Fried LP, Borhani NO, Enright P, et al. The Cardiovascular Health Study: design and rationale. Ann Epidemiol 1991;1(3):263–76.

36. Friedman GD, Cutter GR, Donahue RP, et al. CARDIA: study design, recruitment, and some characteristics of the examined subjects. J Clin Epidemiol 1988;41(11):1105–16.

37. Govindaraju DR, Cupples LA, Kannel WB, et al. Genetics of the Framingham Heart Study population. Adv Genet 2008;62:33–65.

38. Wilson PW, D'Agostino RB, Levy D, et al. Prediction of coronary heart disease using risk factor categories. Circulation 1998;97(18):1837–47.

39. Assmann G, Cullen P, Schulte H. Simple scoring scheme for calculating the risk of acute coronary events based on the 10-year follow-up of the prospective cardiovascular Munster (PROCAM) study. Circulation 2002;105(3): 310–5.

40. Conroy RM, Pyorala K, Fitzgerald AP, et al. Estimation of ten-year risk of fatal cardiovascular disease in Europe: the SCORE project. Eur Heart J 2003; 24(11):987–1003.

41. Taylor F, Huffman MD, Macedo AF, et al. Statins for the primary prevention of cardiovascular disease. Cochrane Database Syst Rev 2013;(1):CD004816.

42. Pignone MP, Phillips CJ, Atkins D, et al. Screening and treating adults for lipid disorders. Am J Prev Med 2001;20(3 Suppl):77–89.

43. Helfand M, Carson S. Screening for lipid disorders in adults: selective update of 2001 US Preventive Services Task Force Review. Evidence synthesis no. 49. Rockville (MD): AHRQ Publication; 2008.

44. National Cholesterol Education Program Expert Panel on Detection Evaluation, Treatment of High Blood Cholesterol in Adults. Third report of the National Cholesterol Education Program (NCEP) Expert Panel on Detection, Evaluation, and Treatment of High Blood Cholesterol in Adults (Adult Treatment Panel III) final report. Circulation 2002;106(25):3143–421.

45. Stone NJ, Robinson J, Lichtenstein AH, et al. 2013 ACC/AHA guideline on the treatment of blood cholesterol to reduce atherosclerotic cardiovascular risk in adults: a report of the American College of Cardiology/American Heart Association Task Force on Practice Guidelines. Circulation 2013. [Epub ahead of print].

46. Mihaylova B, Emberson J, Blackwell L, et al. The effects of lowering LDL cholesterol with statin therapy in people at low risk of vascular disease: meta-analysis of individual data from 27 randomised trials. Lancet 2012;380(9841):581–90.

47. Taylor F, Ward K, Moore TH, et al. Statins for the primary prevention of cardiovascular disease. Cochrane Database Syst Rev 2011;(1):CD004816.

48. Cooper A, O'Flynn N. Risk assessment and lipid modification for primary and secondary prevention of cardiovascular disease: summary of NICE guidance. BMJ 2008;336(7655):1246–8.

49. Abramson JD, Rosenberg HG, Jewell N, et al. Should people at low risk of cardiovascular disease take a statin? BMJ 2013;347:f6123.

50. Mosca L, Benjamin EJ, Berra K, et al. Effectiveness-based guidelines for the prevention of cardiovascular disease in women–2011 update: a guideline from the American Heart Association. Circulation 2011;123(11):1243–62.

51. Helfand M, Buckley D, Freeman M, et al. Emerging risk factors for coronary heart disease: a summary of systematic reviews conducted for the US Preventive Services Task Force. Ann Intern Med 2009;151:496–507.

52. Helfand M, Buckley D, Fleming C, et al. Screening for intermediate risk factors for coronary heart disease: systematic evidence synthesis. Evidence synthesis No. 73. Rockville (MD): AHRQ Publication; 2009.

53. Buckley DI, Fu R, Freeman M, et al. C-reactive protein as a risk factor for coronary heart disease: a systematic review and meta-analyses for the US Preventive Services Task Force. Ann Intern Med 2009;151(7):483–95.

54. Homocysteine Studies Collaboration. Homocysteine and risk of ischemic heart disease and stroke: a meta-analysis. JAMA 2002;288(16):2015–22.

55. Bonaa KH, Njolstad I, Ueland PM, et al. Homocysteine lowering and cardiovascular events after acute myocardial infarction. N Engl J Med 2006;354(15):1578–88.

56. Lonn E, Yusuf S, Arnold MJ, et al. Homocysteine lowering with folic acid and B vitamins in vascular disease. N Engl J Med 2006;354(15):1567–77.

57. Schnyder G, Roffi M, Flammer Y, et al. Effect of homocysteine-lowering therapy with folic acid, vitamin B12, and vitamin B6 on clinical outcome after percutaneous coronary intervention: the Swiss Heart study: a randomized controlled trial. JAMA 2002;288(8):973–9.

58. Kavousi M, Elias-Smale S, Rutten JH, et al. Evaluation of newer risk markers for coronary heart disease risk classification: a cohort study. Ann Intern Med 2012; 156(6):438–44.
59. van Kempen BJ, Spronk S, Koller MT, et al. Comparative effectiveness and cost-effectiveness of computed tomography screening for coronary artery calcium in asymptomatic individuals. J Am Coll Cardiol 2011;58(16):1690–701.
60. Chou R, Arora B, Dana T, et al. Screening asymptomatic adults with resting or exercise electrocardiography: a review of the evidence for the US Preventive Services Task Force. Ann Intern Med 2011;155:375–85.
61. Austin MA, Hutter CM, Zimmern RL, et al. Genetic causes of monogenic heterozygous familial hypercholesterolemia: a HuGE prevalence review. Am J Epidemiol 2004;160(5):407–20.
62. Wonderling D, Umans-Eckenhausen MA, Marks D, et al. Cost-effectiveness analysis of the genetic screening program for familial hypercholesterolemia in The Netherlands. Semin Vasc Med 2004;4(1):97–104.
63. Nherera L, Marks D, Minhas R, et al. Probabilistic cost-effectiveness analysis of cascade screening for familial hypercholesterolaemia using alternative diagnostic and identification strategies. Heart 2011;97(14):1175–81.
64. United States Preventive Services Task Force. US Preventive Services Task Force. 2013. Available at: http://www.uspreventiveservicestaskforce.org/. Accessed October 21, 2013.
65. US Preventive Services Task Force. US Preventive Services Task Force grade definitions. 2012. Available at: http://www.uspreventiveservicestaskforce.org/uspstf/grades.htm. Accessed May 23, 2013.
66. Greenland P, Alpert JS, Beller GA, et al. 2010 ACCF/AHA guideline for assessment of cardiovascular risk in asymptomatic adults: a report of the American College of Cardiology Foundation/American Heart Association Task Force on Practice Guidelines. J Am Coll Cardiol 2010;56(25):e50–103.
67. Chobanian AV, Bakris GL, Black HR, et al. The seventh report of the Joint National Committee on Prevention, Detection, Evaluation, and Treatment of High Blood Pressure: the JNC 7 report. JAMA 2003;289(19):2560–72.
68. National Cholesterol Education Program-NHLBI, NIH. 2013. Available at: http://www.nhlbi.nih.gov/about/ncep/. Accessed October 21, 2013.
69. Minhas R, Humphries SE, Qureshi N, et al, NICE Guideline Development Group. Controversies in familial hypercholesterolaemia: recommendations of the NICE Guideline Development Group for the identification and management of familial hypercholesterolaemia. Heart 2009;95(7):584–7 [discussion: 587–91].
70. US Preventive Services Task Force. Screening for high blood pressure: US Preventive Services Task Force reaffirmation recommendation statement. 2007. Available at: http://www.uspreventiveservicestaskforce.org/uspstf07/hbp/hbprs.htm. Accessed January 2, 2014.
71. U.S Preventive Services Task Force. Recommendations and rationale: screening for lipid disorders in adults. 2008. Available at: http://www.uspreventiveservicestaskforce.org/uspstf08/lipid/lipidrs.htm. Accessed May 23, 2013.
72. US Preventive Services Task Force. Using nontraditional risk factors in coronary heart disease risk assessment: US Preventive Services Task Force recommendation statement. Ann Intern Med 2009;151:474–82.
73. Lim LS, Haq N, Mahmood S, et al. Atherosclerotic cardiovascular disease screening in adults: American College of Preventive Medicine position statement on preventive practice. Am J Prev Med 2011;40(3):381.e1–10.

74. US Preventive Services Task Force. Screening for abdominal aortic aneurysm: recommendation statement. Ann Intern Med 2005;142:198–202.
75. US Preventive Services Task Force. Screening for coronary heart disease: recommendation statement. 2004. Available at: http://www.uspreventiveservice staskforce.org/3rduspstf/chd/chdrs.htm. Accessed May 23, 2013.
76. McCall-Hosenfeld JS, Weisman CS, Camacho F, et al. Multilevel analysis of the determinants of receipt of clinical preventive services among reproductive-age women. Womens Health Issues 2012;22(3):e243–51.
77. Ma J, Stafford RS. Screening, treatment, and control of hypertension in US private physician offices, 2003-2004. Hypertension 2008;51(5):1275–81.
78. Solberg LI, Kottke TE, Brekke ML. Variation in clinical preventive services. Eff Clin Pract 2001;4(3):121–6.
79. Bertoni AG, Bonds DE, Steffes S, et al. Quality of cholesterol screening and management with respect to the National Cholesterol Education's Third Adult Treatment Panel (ATPIII) guideline in primary care practices in North Carolina. Am Heart J 2006;152(4):785–92.
80. Rifas-Shiman SL, Forman JP, Lane K, et al. Diabetes and lipid screening among patients in primary care: a cohort study. BMC Health Serv Res 2008;8:25.
81. Barham AH, Goff DC Jr, Chen H, et al. Appropriateness of cholesterol management in primary care by sex and level of cardiovascular risk. Prev Cardiol 2009; 12(2):95–101.
82. Allison MA, Ho E, Denenberg JO, et al. Ethnic-specific prevalence of peripheral arterial disease in the United States. Am J Prev Med 2007;32(4):328–33.
83. Rowe VL, Weaver FA, Lane JS, et al. Racial and ethnic differences in patterns of treatment for acute peripheral arterial disease in the United States, 1998-2006. J Vasc Surg 2010;51(4 Suppl):21S–6S.
84. Stewart SH, Silverstein MD. Racial and ethnic disparity in blood pressure and cholesterol measurement. J Gen Intern Med 2002;17(6):405–11.
85. Vaidya V, Partha G, Howe J. Utilization of preventive care services and their effect on cardiovascular outcomes in the United States. Risk Manag Healthc Policy 2011;4:1–7.
86. Nelson K, Norris K, Mangione CM. Disparities in the diagnosis and pharmacologic treatment of high serum cholesterol by race and ethnicity: data from the Third National Health and Nutrition Examination Survey. Arch Intern Med 2002;162(8):929–35.
87. Ford ES, Li C, Pearson WS, et al. Trends in hypercholesterolemia, treatment and control among United States adults. Int J Cardiol 2010;140(2):226–35.
88. Ferrante JM, Balasubramanian BA, Hudson SV, et al. Principles of the patient-centered medical home and preventive services delivery. Ann Fam Med 2010; 8(2):108–16.
89. Stafford RS, Misra B. Variation in routine electrocardiogram use in academic primary care practice. Arch Intern Med 2001;161(19):2351–5.
90. Rabinowitz I, Tamir A. The SaM (Screening and Monitoring) approach to cardiovascular risk-reduction in primary care–cyclic monitoring and individual treatment of patients at cardiovascular risk using the electronic medical record. Eur J Cardiovasc Prev Rehabil 2005;12(1):56–62.
91. Linder JA, Ma J, Bates DW, et al. Electronic health record use and the quality of ambulatory care in the United States. Arch Intern Med 2007;167(13):1400–5.
92. Romano MJ, Stafford RS. Electronic health records and clinical decision support systems: impact on national ambulatory care quality. Arch Intern Med 2011; 171(10):897–903.

93. Hivert MF, Grant RW, Shrader P, et al. Identifying primary care patients at risk for future diabetes and cardiovascular disease using electronic health records. BMC Health Serv Res 2009;9:170.

94. Walsh MN, Yancy CW, Albert NM, et al. Electronic health records and quality of care for heart failure. Am Heart J 2010;159(4):635–42.e1.

95. Zhou L, Soran CS, Jenter CA, et al. The relationship between electronic health record use and quality of care over time. J Am Med Inform Assoc 2009;16(4): 457–64.

96. Kaiser Family Foundation. Health reform implementation timeline. Health Reform 2013. Available at: http://kff.org/interactive/implementation-timeline/. Accessed August 7, 2013.

97. US Preventive Services Task Force. Affordable Care Act: A and B recommendations for preventive services. 2013. Available at: http://www.uspreventiveservices taskforce.org/uspstf/uspsabrecs.htm. Accessed January 2, 2014.

98. Berwick DM. Launching accountable care organizations–the proposed rule for the Medicare Shared Savings Program. N Engl J Med 2011;364(16):e32.

99. Quality Measurement & Health Assessment Group Center for Medicare and Medicaid Services. Quality performance standards narrative measure specifications. Accountable Care Organization 2013 Program Analysis. 2012. Available at: http://www.cms.gov/Medicare/Medicare-Fee-for-Service-Payment/shared savingsprogram/Downloads/ACO-NarrativeMeasures-Specs.pdf. Accessed August 8, 2013.

100. American Academy of Family Physicians. Joint principles of the Patient-Centered Medical Home. Del Med J 2008;80(1):21–2.

101. Krogsboll L, Jorgensen K, Gronhoj L, et al. General health checks in adults for reducing morbidity and mortality from disease [review]. Cochrane Database Syst Rev 2012;(10):CD009009.

Screening for Depression in the Primary Care Population

D. Edward Deneke, MD*, Heather Schultz, MD, MPH,
Thomas E. Fluent, MD

KEYWORDS

- Depression • Screening • Suicide • Primary care

KEY POINTS

- Depression is common in the primary care population, and imposes social, financial, and medical costs on patients on families.
- Screening for depression can be useful in the primary care setting if reliable systems of care are in place to ensure adequate treatment and follow-up.
- Use of collaborative care models for depression in the primary care setting have been shown to be a cost-effective means for providing depression-related care, but economic and cultural barriers continue to slow widespread adoption.
- Screening for suicide risk in the primary care population is generally not recommended. However, clinicians should familiarize themselves with the common risk factors for suicide and remain vigilant for patients at increased risk for self-harm.

INTRODUCTION

The *Diagnostic and Statistical Manual of Mental Disorders* (5th edition) defines major depressive disorder (MDD) as a mental health condition characterized by 5 or more of the following symptoms lasting for at least 2 weeks: depressed mood, diminished interest in activities (anhedonia), disordered sleep, fatigue, changes in appetite or changes in weight, persistent feelings of guilt or hopelessness, decreased concentration, psychomotor slowing, and thoughts of suicide; the 2 symptoms of depressed mood and anhedonia are cardinal, and at least 1 must be present for the diagnosis to be made (**Box 1**).[1] When assessing a patient for MDD, these symptoms need to represent a change from the patient's baseline, and must be accompanied by impairment in social or occupational functioning.

Conflicts of Interest: None.
Department of Psychiatry, University of Michigan Health System, University of Michigan, 4250 Plymouth Road, Ann Arbor, MI 48109-2700, USA
* Corresponding author.
E-mail address: edwardde@med.umich.edu

Prim Care Clin Office Pract 41 (2014) 399–420
http://dx.doi.org/10.1016/j.pop.2014.02.011
0095-4543/14/$ – see front matter © 2014 Elsevier Inc. All rights reserved.

Box 1
Diagnosing major depressive disorder

Five or more of the following symptoms are present during a 2-week period:

Note: Of the 5 symptoms, at least 1 must be depressed mood or anhedonia; symptoms need to represent a change from the patient's baseline, and be accompanied by an impairment in social or occupational functioning.

- Feeling depressed, sad, or hopeless most of the time (depressed mood)
- Decreased interest in pleasurable activities (anhedonia)
- Change in appetite (increase or decrease) and/or 5% or more change in weight
- Sleeping more or less often than usual
- Frequent feelings of worthlessness or excessive/inappropriate guilt
- Frequent fatigue
- Physical restlessness (psychomotor agitation) or slowed movements (psychomotor retardation)
- Indecisiveness or decreased concentration
- Recurrent thoughts of death or thoughts of suicide

From American Psychiatric Association, American Psychiatric Association DSM-5 Task Force. Diagnostic and statistical manual of mental disorders: DSM-5. 5th edition. Washington, DC: American Psychiatric Association; 2013.

Depressive disorders are highly prevalent in the general population and can be found across the age spectrum.[2] The estimated lifetime prevalence of MDD in the United States is approximately 13.2%,[3] with a 12-month prevalence of 6% to 7%.[2] Evidence suggests that upward of three-quarters of those who experience a major depressive episode will experience a subsequent episode,[4] with the mean number of episodes among adults with lifetime MDD being 4.7.[3] Approximately one-third of nonelderly patients[5] and two-thirds of elderly patients[6] are treated in the primary care setting.

Somatic symptoms (eg, headache, back pain, fatigue, and other physical complaints) are frequently found alongside symptoms of depression, often dominating the clinical picture and masking the underlying depressive disorder. This masking can sometimes make an accurate diagnosis more difficult. A 2005 literature review reported that approximately two-thirds of patients with depression present to primary care with primarily somatic complaints, and the presence of somatic complaints correlated with a decrease in the clinician's ability to recognize the depression.[7] Somatic symptoms comorbid with depression have been shown to be more prevalent in certain populations, including those who are pregnant, elderly, poor, incarcerated, and those suffering from other medical issues.[7]

Depression has a significant impact on the lives of the affected population. Given the symptoms of the disorder it should not be surprising that people suffering from depression often experience a decreased quality of life, as well as decreased productivity both at work and at home.[8,9] Depression can also have a negative impact on a person's self-reported global heath rating, whether taken alone or in combination with common chronic health conditions (**Table 1**).[10] In addition to depression's negative impact on health, people with depression have also been shown to have increased mortality rates.[11]

Table 1
Global mean health score by disease status

Chronic Condition	Mean Health Score[a]	
	Condition Alone	Condition Plus Depression
Baseline	90.6[b]	72.9[c]
Asthma	80.3	65.4
Angina	79.6	65.8
Arthritis	79.3	67.1
Diabetes	78.9	58.5
Two or more chronic conditions	71.8	56.1

[a] Derived from 16 self-reported health questions; scores range from 0 (worst health) to 100 (best health); sample includes more than 250,000 people representing 60 countries.
[b] Health score for those with neither depression nor a chronic health condition.
[c] Health score for those with depression alone (no chronic health condition).
Adapted from Moussavi S, Chatterji S, Verdes E, et al. Depression, chronic diseases, and decrements in health: results from the World Health Surveys. Lancet 2007;370:851–8.

Depression not only affects the person directly suffering from the disorder but also family members, employers, and others with whom the depressed person interacts. Spouses of people with depression have been shown to experience increased symptoms of depression and an increased emotional and financial burden.[12] Children of parents with depression have been shown to be at increased risk of mental illness,[13] and to demonstrate changes in health care use including decreased well-visit appointments, increased sick visits to primary care, and increased use of emergency, inpatient, and specialty care services.[14] The economic impact of depression on society is also significantly large, with estimates suggesting annual costs may exceed $80 billion in the United States alone.[15] Although lost productivity explains the bulk of this cost,[16,17] estimates suggest that roughly 30% can be attributed to direct medical expenditures.[15]

Multiple risk factors for depression have been demonstrated in the literature (**Box 2**). Gender is a major risk factor, with the lifetime prevalence of MDD about twice as high for women than for men.[5] Rates of depression have also been found to be higher in people with other psychiatric disorders, such as anxiety or substance-use disorders, and in people with comorbid medical issues or a family history of depression. Lower socioeconomic status and unemployment also appear to be risk factors for depression.[5] The average age of onset for depressive disorders is the mid-20s to 30s, with overall risk decreasing in the following decades.[5] Depression is less common in the community-living geriatric population, but clinicians should keep in mind that those who are elderly may be exposed to various age-specific risk factors, including loss of independence and increased medical burden.[13]

Depression has been found to be more common among whites than blacks, although depression in black populations has been found to be more severe and linked with greater functional impairment.[18] Racially linked disparities in severity and impairment are attributable, in part, to differences in securing necessary care.[19] Research suggests that treatment preferences and illness beliefs do not fully account for race-based differences in obtaining appropriate mental health care[20]; access-related factors such as the affordability, availability, accessibility, and acceptability of mental health care likely play a significant role.[21]

Depression is also associated with a variety of medical issues, and the relationship is particularly strong in diseases of the central nervous system such as traumatic brain

---

Box 2
Risk factors for depression

1. Family history of depression
2. Female gender
3. Poor social supports
4. Substance abuse
5. Prior depressive episode
6. Childhood trauma
7. Childbirth
8. Dementia
9. Stressful life events
10. Low socioeconomic status
11. Significant medical burden
12. Certain personality traits, such as low self-esteem or excessive pessimism

---

injury,[22] stroke,[23] and Parkinson disease.[24] Specific life experiences have also been identified as risk factors for depression, including childbirth,[25] childhood trauma,[26] and stressful life events.[27] Genetics seem to play a significant role in the pathophysiology of depression. The concordance rate for depression among monozygotic twins was found to be 37% in a large Swedish study involving more than 15,000 sets of twins.[28] Of note, this study also found a significant difference in the hereditability of depression between men (42%) and women (29%). As with most medical conditions, the precise role of genetics remains a mystery, with no single depression gene having been found; it is likely that the phenotype of depression is the product of a complex interplay between genetic vulnerability, conferred by small effects from a large number of genes, and environmental exposures.

CURRENT PRACTICE PATTERNS

The demand for depression-related care and the provision of that care in office-based settings in the United States is substantial; for example, the estimated number of visits for depression in office-based settings increased from 14.4 million in 1987 to 24.5 million in 2001.[29] Over this same period, the proportion of depression-related visits decreased for psychiatrists while it increased for primary care physicians: whereas psychiatrists accounted for 44% of visits in 1987 and 29% in 2001, primary care physicians accounted for 50% in 1987 and 64% in 2001.[29] Data from 1998 to 2007 suggest that the increase in outpatient treatment of depression has slowed, with the number of Americans receiving such care increasing from about 6.5 million in 1998 to 8.7 million in 2007.[30] These important data suggest that the growth in care grew more quickly for several groups that have been historically underserved, including blacks, Hispanics, and men.[30] Despite these improvements, evidence suggests that a substantial number of people in the United States remain untreated for their depression-related symptoms.[30]

Literature documenting screening rates for depression in primary care is not readily available; however, a 2009 review investigating the efficacy of depression screening among adults in primary care suggests that general mental health screening rates may be as high as 74%.[31] The specific disorders being screened were not delineated, but the investigators reasoned that screening programs for depression were likely among the most common, given the prevalence of depression within the primary care patient population. This review identified a large sample study investigating depression screening among outpatients within the Veterans Health Administration (VHA).[31] The study found that of the 85% of eligible patients screened, nearly 9% screened positive; among those screening positive, however, only 54% received follow-up evaluation, 24% of whom were subsequently diagnosed with a depressive disorder.[32]

While the rate of unidentified cases of depression presenting to United States primary care settings remains understudied, findings from the 2009 review suggest many adults with depression, perhaps as many as 40%, may not be properly identified by their primary care provider.[31] Researchers found that younger patients and those with less severe symptoms were among the most likely to be missed.[31] Another review identified somatization as one of the most important contributors to missing a diagnosis of depression in primary care.[33] This finding is particularly noteworthy, as up to two-thirds of depressed patients primarily present with somatic symptoms.[33] A review investigating the accuracy of depression diagnoses within primary care in North America, Europe, and Australia concluded that about half of the individuals with depression were not properly detected. Moreover, the investigators found that the risk of misidentification (false positives) was greater than the risk of missing cases, suggesting that primary care providers may need to exercise increased caution when making a definitive diagnosis in those screening positive.[34] One strategy that may help to improve depression screening and diagnosis is enhancing the structures and processes of care; that is, making the settings that carry out screening (and subsequent care) work better.

EVIDENCE FOR SCREENING

Evidence for the effectiveness of depression screening in the general population has been mixed. A 2005 review explored the utility of screening or case-finding instruments to improve the detection and management of depression in nonspecialist (ie, primary care) settings. Only minimal evidence linking routine administration of depression screening tools to rates of detection or treatment outcomes was found.[35] The investigators strongly discouraged the use of screening and case-finding instruments as stand-alone tools to identify those with depression. A subsequent meta-analysis revealed similar findings, concluding that screening settings themselves need to change to yield better results.[36] Of note, both reviews excluded studies involving enhanced systems of care, such as those that use care managers to support the primary care clinician in diagnosing and treating depression.

Two additional systematic reviews, completed in 2002 and 2009, reached similar conclusions[31,37]; however, when studies involving enhanced systems of care were included, investigators found that depression screening programs were effective in identifying and treating depression. Enhanced systems were those that included support staff, such as care managers, to augment the depression-related care provided by the clinician. Support staff assist clinicians with several functions, including patient education and follow-up, adjusting treatment plans, serving as a link between patients and the multiple components of the health care system (eg, mental health specialists and the primary care clinician), and (sometimes) proving limited mental health treatment. A meta-analysis investigating the efficacy of enhanced systems concluded that such models can effectively achieve improvements in depression outcomes in a wide range of settings.[38]

Although depression screening in usual care settings may not be cost-effective,[39] emerging evidence suggests that one-time screening for depression in settings with effective treatment programs (eg, enhanced settings with structured depression care) can make economic sense.[40] Structured collaborative care models (see later discussion) show promise in terms of both improving the quality of care and cost-effectiveness.[41,42]

SCREENING TOOLS FOR DEPRESSION

Several screening tools are available for use in the primary care setting. These tools vary in both their number and focus of questions. A meta-analysis comparing 19 screening tools with the number of questions varying from 1 to 30 found the median sensitivity and specificity to be 85% and 74%, respectively, with no significant difference found between measures.[43] In addition, brief screening tools have been shown to be as accurate as lengthier tools in detecting depression.[44] With many screening options and little evidence to differentiate the measures, primary care clinicians can easily become confused when trying to decide which tool to use with their patients. Decisions are likely often based on the availability of a given screening tool, as well as its ease of use for both patients and clinicians. To help minimize possible confusion, this article limits discussion to the following 6 commonly used tools: Patient Health Questionnaire–9 (PHQ-9), Patient Health Questionnaire–2 (PHQ-2), Beck Depression Inventory (BDI), Hospital Anxiety and Depression Scale (HADS), Geriatric Depression Scale (GDS), and Edinburgh Postnatal Depression Scale (EPDS) (**Table 2**).

Patient Health Questionnaire

The PHQ-9 (Appendix 1) is a popular choice for primary care clinicians, in part because of its brevity and ease of scoring. The PHQ-9 consists of 9 questions rating the severity of depressive symptoms over the past 2 weeks, with a tenth question used to assess impact of these symptoms on functioning. The first 9 questions are answered from 0 (not at all) to 3 (nearly every day). The sum of the first 9 questions gives the total score, with a total score of 10 marking the cutoff for likely depression. In addition to being a useful screening tool, the PHQ-9 has been demonstrated to be an effective tool in monitoring depression over time.[45] The PHQ-9 has been shown to be useful in a variety of populations, including blacks, non-Hispanic whites, Latinos, and Chinese Americans.[46] The PHQ-9 has also been validated in postpartum and geriatric populations.[47]

Table 2
Screening tools for depression

Screening Tool	No. of Items	Cutoff Score for Depression	Free for Clinical Use?
Patient Health Questionnaire–9	9	10 out of 21 possible points	Yes
Patient Health Questionnaire–2	2	3 out of 6 possible points	Yes
Hospital Anxiety and Depression Scale	14	8 out of 21 possible points	Yes
Beck Depression Inventory II	21	20 out of 63 possible points	No
Edinburgh Postnatal Depression Scale	10	10 out of 30 possible points	Yes
Geriatric Depression Scale–15	15	6 out of possible 15 points	Yes

The PHQ-2 is a brief variant of the PHQ-9, often used as an initial screen for depression. The PHQ-2 consists of the following 2 questions, reflecting the 2 cardinal symptoms of an MDD (depressed mood and anhedonia):

- During the last 2 weeks, how often have you been bothered by feeling down, depressed, or hopeless?
- During the last 2 weeks, how often have you often been bothered by having little interest or pleasure in doing things?

Each question is answered from 0 to 3, as in the PHQ-9, and the scores are added together for the total score. A total score greater than or equal to 3 is considered a positive screen. Using the cutoff score of 3, the PHQ-2 has been shown to have sensitivity of 83% and specificity of 92%.[47] Given the brevity of the screening tool, the PHQ-2 is a tempting choice for primary care clinicians struggling with a busy practice and ever-increasing screening recommendations. A common practice in primary care settings is to administer the PHQ-2 to patients and follow up with a more thorough PHQ-9 with those patients screening positive. Both screening tools are readily accessible for no fee from the manufacturer. Multiple translations are also available.

Beck Depression Inventory

The BDI-II is a 21-item self-report tool widely used in research for measuring the symptoms of depression. A shorter 7-item version designed for the primary care setting, the BDI for Primary Care (BDI-PC), is also available.[48] The BDI-II and BDI-PC are only available via license, thus limiting their use in the primary care setting.

Hospital Anxiety and Depression Scale

The HADS is a 14-item self-report scale, including two 7-item subscales for depression and anxiety, specifically designed for evaluation of psychiatric symptoms in patients with medical comorbidities.[49] The depression subscale focuses primarily on anhedonia and does not cover somatic symptoms. The HADS is copyrighted by the original authors and is available free of charge for clinical use.[50]

Geriatric Depression Scale

The GDS (Appendix 2) was specifically designed to screen for depression in the elderly population. Owing to the increased prevalence of medical comorbidities and somatic symptoms in this population, less focus is placed on somatic symptoms in comparison with other common screening tools. The tool comes in 3 versions consisting of 30, 15, or 5 simple yes/no questions. The 15-item version was found to have greater sensitivity and specificity than the 30-item scale.[51] The GDS is available free of charge from the designers, and is offered in multiple translations.

Edinburgh Postnatal Depression Scale

The EPDS has been well validated in pregnant and postpartum women.[52] The tool consists of 10 questions related to various symptoms of depression. The questions on the EPDS focus less on somatic symptoms (eg, weight change, sleep disturbances) and instead concentrate on depressed mood and anhedonia. Answers are graded in severity and scored on a range from 0 to 3. A total score of greater than 10 indicates possible depression. A study published in 2008 found the EPDS to have greater accuracy in depression screening among postpartum women when compared with the PHQ-9.[53] Like the PHQ-9 and GDS, the EPDS is available free for use from the publisher.

PROFESSIONAL GROUP RECOMMENDATIONS

Recommendations from the United States Preventive Services Task Force (USPSTF) and National Institute for Health and Care Excellence guidelines are summarized in **Table 3**.

United States Preventive Services Task Force

The most recent recommendations from the USPSTF suggest screening adults for depression in clinical settings with staff-assisted care supports in place to ensure accurate diagnosis, effective treatment, and follow-up.[54] The complexity of these staff-assisted care systems vary by site, but generally consist of either nurses or social workers providing assistance to the primary care clinician via care management, care coordination, or direct mental health treatment. The USPSTF review indicates that in primary care settings with such systems, treatment with antidepressants, psychotherapy, or a combination of both decreases comorbidity and improves outcomes in adults identified through screening; by contrast, screening in settings without these

Table 3
Professional group recommendations

US Preventive Services Task Force Guidelines[a]		National Institute for Health and Care Excellence Guidelines[b]
Screen adults for depression when staff-assisted depression care supports are in place to assure accurate diagnosis, effective treatment, and follow-up	Evidence Grade B[c]	Be alert to possible depression (particularly in people with a history of depression or a chronic physical health problem with associated functional impairment); for a person who may have depression, conduct a comprehensive assessment that does not rely simply on a symptom count
Do not routinely screen adults for depression when staff-assisted depression care supports are not in place. There may be considerations that support screening for depression in an individual patient	Evidence Grade C[d]	Routine depression screening is not recommended
Screen adolescents (12–18 y) for major depressive disorder when systems are in place to ensure accurate diagnosis, psychotherapy (cognitive-behavioral or interpersonal), and follow-up	Evidence Grade B[c]	—
Current evidence is insufficient to assess the balance of benefits and harms of screening of children (7–11 y)	Evidence Grade I[e]	—

[a] From the US Preventive Services Task Force (USPSTF).[54,55]
[b] From the National Institute for Health and Care Excellence Guidelines.[56]
[c] The USPSTF recommends the service. There is high certainty that the net benefit is moderate or there is moderate certainty that the net benefit is moderate to substantial.
[d] Clinicians may provide this service to selected patients depending on individual circumstances. However, for most individuals without signs or symptoms there is likely to be only a small benefit from this service.
[e] The USPSTF concludes that the current evidence is insufficient to assess the balance of benefits and harms of the service. Evidence is lacking, of poor quality, or conflicting, and the balance of benefits and harms cannot be determined.

systems shows minimal benefit. The USPSTF reported good evidence supporting the efficacy of both antidepressants and psychotherapy in treating adult patients with MDD. Reported risks of antidepressant use include a possible increase in suicidality, especially among younger adults (age 18–29 years), and upper gastrointestinal bleeding. The risk of such bleeding may be most elevated for older adults using selective serotonin reuptake inhibitors (SSRIs). The USPSTF found no studies including adverse events associated with screening.

The USPSTF also recommends screening adolescents aged 12 to 18 years for depression in clinical practices having systems (or referral systems) in place to ensure accurate diagnosis, psychotherapy (cognitive-behavioral or interpersonal therapy), and follow-up[55]; evidence was judged insufficient to balance the benefits and harms of depression screening in children aged 7 to 11 years. Although the USPSTF notes that SSRIs have been found to be helpful in treating some children and adolescents with MDD, SSRIs are also associated with an increased risk for suicidality and should therefore be used only under close clinical supervision. A variety of psychotherapies have also been shown to be beneficial for adolescents (eg, cognitive-behavioral, interpersonal), and potential harms of such therapies are judged to be small.

National Institute for Health and Clinical Excellence

The National Institute for Health and Clinical Excellence guidelines encourage a case-finding approach with at-risk groups, including patients with a history of depression, those with significant physical illness (particularly if associated with functional impairment and disability), and individuals with other mental health concerns such as dementia.[56,57] Patients with coronary heart disease and diabetes have been prioritized for screening. The following list outlines conditions or circumstances whereby screening should be strongly considered:

- Parkinson disease
- Dementia
- The puerperium
- Alcohol and drug abuse
- Abuse victims
- Physical disease such as cancer, cardiovascular disease, or diabetes
- Chronic pain
- Stressful home environments
- Elderly and socially isolated
- Multiple unexplained symptoms

CHANGES IN HEALTH CARE

The current consensus regarding depression screening in the primary care setting includes screening only if staff-assisted support systems are in place to provide accurate diagnosis, deliver effective treatment, and ensure follow-up. Providing access to comprehensive systems is not a minor feat, as access to mental health professionals is a large barrier to treatment.[58] Primary care is frequently the de facto provider for patients with depression but, despite strong efforts, a large number of cases of depression are missed or inadequately treated.[59]

Collaborative Care

Over the past several decades efforts have been made to develop effective systems of mental health care within the primary care setting. The evidence supports the use of staff-assisted support systems,[38,60] but substantial variation exists among these programs. The term collaborative care is often used to describe such programs, consisting of a multidisciplinary team tasked with providing quality depression care in the primary care setting (**Box 3**). A recent Cochrane review analyzed data from 79 randomized controlled trials of various collaborative care models, and concluded that "[c]ollaborative care is associated with significant improvement in depression and anxiety outcomes compared with usual care, and represents a useful addition to clinical pathways for adult patients with depression and anxiety."[60] Most care models detailed in this review consisted of a primary care clinician, a care manager (often a nurse or social worker), and a mental health specialist (MHS), usually a psychiatrist or psychologist embedded within the primary care setting. The roles of the primary care clinician are to refer the patient to the collaborative care program (usually through the help of screening tools), prescribe antidepressant medications as indicated, and consult regularly with the other team members. The care manager follows a panel of patients with a diagnosis of depression, providing disease education and self-management tools, motivating the patients for follow-up, and tracking outcome measurements such as PHQ-9 scores. The MHS meets regularly with the care manager to review cases, provides medication recommendations back to the primary care clinician for patients discussed with the care manager, and provides direct consultation with patients on an as-needed basis. Treatments offered to patients, including medications and psychotherapy, varied among systems. In most models, the MHS serves primarily a consultative role. The regularly scheduled (usually weekly) supervision between the MHS and the care manager allows the MHS to influence the care of a larger number of patients than would be possible the MHS were simply seeing all patients on his or her own.

Despite the significant evidence supporting the effectiveness of collaborative care models, dissemination has been slow. This lackluster performance is likely due, in part, to inflexible clinical care models, increased upfront costs of the model, and difficulty in developing a sustainable model in the traditional fee-for-service environments (eg, the collaborative care model could increase some nonbillable services, such as supervision between the MHS and the care manager).[61,62] However, upcoming changes to the United States health care system present significant opportunities for advancement of the collaborative care model for depression care.

Affordable Care Act and Accountable Care Organizations

The passage of the Patient Protection and Affordable Care Act (ACA) in 2010 will likely affect the United States health care system for the foreseeable future, influencing

---

Box 3
Key components of collaborative care

1. A multidisciplinary, multiprofessional approach, to include primary care physician and at least 1 other health professional, such as a care manager (nurse or social worker) and possibly a psychiatrist or psychologist

2. A management plan structured to include guidelines or protocols for evidence-based information, and pharmacologic and nonpharmacologic interventions

3. Organized, scheduled patient follow-ups, in person or by telephone

4. Enhanced interprofessional communication, to include team meetings, feedback, and so forth

From Gunn J, Diggens J, Hegarty K, et al. A systematic review of complex system interventions designed to increase recovery from depression in primary care. BMC Health Serv Res 2006;6:88.

depression care in several ways. For example, the ACA will expand the size of the insured population, thus increasing the number of patients seeking or needing care for depression from an already strained system. This influx of patients highlights the need for emphasis on population-based care models. Moreover, opportunities for alternative funding structures will likely arise through the formation of Accountable Care Organizations (ACOs).

ACOs consist of groups of coordinated health care providers tasked with providing medical care for a specific population, with reimbursements tied to cost savings and defined quality measures. Through utilization of ACOs established under the ACA, health systems have the option to participate in shared savings programs, allowing for funding of innovative models, such as collaborative care models, that struggle to thrive in traditional funding environments. As part of the shared savings programs, ACOs will be expected to meet specific quality measures established by Centers for Medicare and Medicaid Services. Among the 33 quality measures set for ACOs, one is intended for care of depression: screening for depression in all patients age 12 years and older and documentation of follow-up plans.[63]

Patient-Centered Medical Homes

The patient-centered medical home (PCMH) is a new model of primary care that emphasizes the delivery of comprehensive, accessible, and patient-centered care to patients within the primary care setting.[64] PCMHs focus on managing chronic diseases within the primary care setting, and coordination of care among providers is essential in achieving these goals. Given the high prevalence of depression within the primary care setting, depression care programs are a natural fit for PCMHs.[65] Specifically, collaborative care models share many common traits with PCMHs, including emphasizing multidisciplinary team-based approaches and effective communication between team members.[66] Successful implementations of collaborative care models with the PCMH can be found in the literature.[38,67–69]

Electronic Health Record

Electronic Health Records (EHRs) have the potential to significantly improve the quality of health care through ensuring accurate documentation of diagnosis and providing decision support for clinicians.[70,71] Use of EHRs in the primary care setting has been shown to benefit depression management; for example, EHRs can be used to trigger and help facilitate depression screening,[72,73] notify the primary care clinician of a depression diagnosis, and enable both accurate documentation and the provision of appropriate care.[74] However, EHRs frequently do not allow for the use of outcomes measures, such as tracking PHQ-9 scores over time, thus limiting their utility in assessing a given patient's progress in real time and on demand.[75] Of importance, the presence of EHRs in and of themselves does not guarantee improvement in depression care[76,77]: they need to be tailored to the particular demands (and resources) of a given setting, and structured to provide clinicians and patients with the information required to make informed decisions. As adoption of EHRs increase, studies will be needed to better understand their role in depression care programs and how they can best support collaborative models of care.

IMPLEMENTATION OF DEPRESSION CARE PROGRAMS

Implementation of depression programs, including screening, staff-assisted care support, and collaborative models of care, can be challenging. Recommendations from the literature are sparse, but consensus on key implementation strategies can be found.[62,78] For depression programs to be successful, buy-in from clinic leadership is essential; having a designated program champion to oversee the implementation is also valuable. In deciding the overall structure of the program, leaders, champions, clinicians, and other team members should not start from scratch, but instead rely on available evidence-based models on which to build their own program. A variety of models can be found in the literature.[38,60] Each clinical site is unique, and the chosen model should be used as a template to be molded to the site's particular needs. Barriers to changing clinical processes can emerge on multiple levels, from patients and providers to health systems and insurance providers. It is important that those involved in implementing a change process both acknowledge and seek to understand emergent barriers so that they can be dealt with appropriately.[62]

SPECIAL NOTE: SUICIDE SCREENING
What is Suicide?

When discussing suicide and self-injurious behaviors, consistent use of definitions is important for clear clinical communication as well as data collection and research. Suicide is defined as death caused by self-directed injurious behavior with intent to die. A suicide attempt is a nonfatal, self-directed, potentially injurious behavior with intent to die. Suicidal ideation involves thinking about, considering, or planning for suicide.[79]

By contrast, nonsuicidal self-injury (also known as deliberate self-harm) is the intentional, direct destruction of body tissue without conscious suicidal intent. The function of self-injury is complex. For instance, it is often associated with a need for relief/release of emotional pain, to provide a sense of control, to punish oneself, or to show distress to others.[80] Examples include cutting or hitting oneself, or ingesting toxic substances without the intent to die.

Epidemiology

Suicide was the 10th overall leading cause of death in the United States in 2010, with 38,364 total deaths.[81] Of note, in persons aged 25 to 34 years suicide was the second leading cause of death after unintentional injury. In 2010, suicide accounted for more than 1.4 million years of potential life lost before age 85 years.[82] Furthermore, for every person who dies by suicide, more than 30 others attempt suicide.[83] However, approximately two-thirds of suicides occur on the first attempt.[84] Men have a higher number of completed suicides (as they often use lethal means such as firearms), although women have a higher number of attempts.[85] Suicide is also closely related to psychiatric illness, and hopelessness and previous suicide attempts have been identified as strong prospective risk factors for suicide.[86] Although the prevalence of suicide is 0.01% in the general population, the risk increases 10-fold in depressed adults.[87] A summary of major risk and protective factors for suicide are shown in **Table 4**.

The Role of Primary Care Providers in Suicide Prevention

As per the 2012 National Strategy for Suicide Prevention, a report of the US Surgeon General, both primary care and emergency medicine providers are encouraged to screen for suicidality to improve the likelihood that the person will receive appropriate evaluation and treatment. These recommendations included screening, training to recognize risk, accurate diagnoses, implementation of trauma-informed policies and practices, easy access to mental health referrals, education of the warning signs of suicide risk, and continued care/improved aftercare.[83]

Of special importance, most individuals who complete suicide have presented to their primary care physician within a month of their death.[88] Furthermore, between

Table 4
Summary of major risk and protective factors for suicide

Risk Factors	Protective Factors
Male gender	Female gender (although females are more likely to attempt)
Previous attempt	Family/social support
Suicidal ideation	Hopeful
Mental illness	Access to mental health care
Caucasian	Prohibitive cultural or religious beliefs
Social isolation	Restricted access to lethal means
Recent loss (job, divorce)	
Alcohol/substance abuse	
Impulsivity	
Access to lethal means	
Hopelessness	
Family history of suicide	
History of childhood maltreatment	
Local epidemics of suicide	
Limited/no access to mental health care	
Physical illness/pain	

From Centers for Disease Control and Prevention. Suicide: risk and protective factors. Available at: http://www.cdc.gov/violenceprevention/suicide/riskprotectivefactors.html. Accessed December 27, 2013.

2% and 3% of primary care patients report suicidal ideation in the past month.[87] However, there are many ways to screen patients for suicidal ideation. For instance, the phrases in **Table 5** have been found to have different sensitivity, specificity, and positive predictive value for detecting patients with a plan to commit suicide.[87]

Table 5
Sensitivity, specificity, and predictive value for detecting patients with a plan to commit suicide

Phrase	Example Screening Question (To Provide a Clinical Example Only)	Sensitivity (%)	Specificity (%)	Positive Predictive Value (%)
"Thoughts of death"	Since your last visit have you had thoughts of death? What seems to trigger these thoughts?	100	81	5.9
"Wishing you were dead"	Do you ever find yourself wishing you were dead? If yes, explain how often this occurs? What makes this better/worse?	92	93	14
"Feeling suicidal"	Are you feeling suicidal? If yes, how often are you thinking of suicide? Do you have a plan? Do you have access to firearms or other lethal means?	83	98	30

Adapted from Gaynes BN, West SL, Ford CA, et al. Screening for suicide risk in adults: a summary of the evidence for the U.S. Preventive Services Task Force. Ann Intern Med 2004;140:822–35.

US Preventive Services Task Force

The USPSTF concluded in 2004 that the evidence is insufficient to recommend for or against routine screening by primary care clinicians to detect suicide risk in the general population. This situation was again reviewed in 2013, and the drafted recommendations indicated that: "There is insufficient evidence to conclude that screening adolescents, adults, and older adults in primary care adequately identifies patients at risk for suicide who would not otherwise be identified based on an existing mental health disorder, emotional distress, or previous suicide attempt."[89]

Practically speaking, the cost to clinicians of screening for suicide relates to the additional clinical time such screening requires. Among the trials reporting on potential negative effects of screening for patients, none found serious adverse effects.[89] For high-risk patients with a history of suicidal ideation or attempt, it is important that they do not have lethal means to harm themselves, such as firearms, poisons, or materials that could be used for hanging or suffocation.[90] Any patient who endorses active suicidal ideation should be specifically asked about access to lethal means and if they have a plan to harm themselves. Suicidal ideation with a plan and lethal means constitutes a psychiatric emergency warranting acute evaluation in the emergency department (by a psychiatrist, whenever possible).

Recommendations of Other Groups

- The American Academy of Child and Adolescent Psychiatry: Clinicians should be aware of patients at high risk for suicide.[91]
- The American Academy of Pediatrics: Pediatricians should ask questions about mood disorders, sexual orientation, suicidal thoughts, and other risk factors associated with suicide during routine health care visits.[92]
- The American Medical Association: All adolescents should be asked annually about behaviors or emotions that indicate recurrent or severe depression or risk of suicide. Physicians should screen for depression or suicidal risk in those with risk factors such as family dysfunction, declining school grades, and history of abuse.[93]

Confidentiality and Patient Safety

Although there are few exceptions to maintaining confidentiality within the doctor-patient relationship, most states have "duty to warn" and "duty to protect" laws. These laws often address potential harm not only to others but also to self. Physicians should be mindful of their state laws regarding special circumstances when confidentiality may be breached, and to whom the information can be given. Clinicians can refer to the National Conference of State Legislators for more information regarding the laws in their state: http://www.ncsl.org/issues-research/health/mental-health-professionals-duty-to-warn.aspx.

Resources for Suicidal Patients

Primary care physicians should be aware of local resources, such as crisis centers and psychiatric emergency departments, to which a suicidal patient might be referred. Any patient who screens positive for active suicidal ideation with a plan and access to lethal means should be treated emergently. If a patient is not currently suicidal, but has a history of suicide attempts or suicidal ideation, it is important to provide the number for the national suicide prevention lifeline.

- National Suicide Prevention Lifeline: 1-800-273-TALK (8255). This confidential service is available 24 hours per day, 7 days per week to those who are in emotional distress or suicidal crisis.

SUMMARY

Depression is common in the primary care setting, and can significantly affect patients and families in several ways. Somatic symptoms frequently mask the underlying depression, leading to challenges in accurate diagnoses. Most depressed patients receive care solely in primary care, making this setting the optimal place for the use of targeted interventions. Screening for depression is the first step in treating depression, but is insufficient in providing quality care if subsequent support is not in place. Several effective screening measures exist, many of which are widely available for clinical use. In addition to screening, systems should be in place to help ensure that the patients follow through with the treatment plan. Various models of care have been discussed in the literature, but further changes to current clinical culture and funding structures are needed before widespread adoption of these innovative systems can take place.

Thoughts of suicide are not uncommon in the depressed population. The current evidence is inadequate to describe risks/benefits of suicide screening in the asymptomatic adult population. However, primary care providers might identify patients with multiple risk factors or who are in high levels of emotional distress, and refer them for further mental health evaluation (acutely if suicide risk is deemed imminent). Most effective treatments of suicidal patients involve psychotherapy, and the primary care provider can provide support, referrals, and coordination of care. It remains important to recognize warning signs for suicide, such as a patient who talks about death or threatens self-harm.

REFERENCES

1. American Psychiatric Association, American Psychiatric Association DSM-5 Task Force. Diagnostic and statistical manual of mental disorders: DSM-5. 5th edition. Washington, DC: American Psychiatric Association; 2013.
2. Kessler RC, Chiu WT, Demler O, et al. Prevalence, severity, and comorbidity of 12-month DSM-IV disorders in the National Comorbidity Survey Replication. Arch Gen Psychiatry 2005;62:617–27.
3. Hasin DS, Goodwin RD, Stinson FS, et al. Epidemiology of major depressive disorder: results from the National Epidemiologic Survey on Alcoholism and Related Conditions. Arch Gen Psychiatry 2005;62:1097–106.
4. Kessler RC, Zhao S, Blazer DG, et al. Prevalence, correlates, and course of minor depression and major depression in the National Comorbidity Survey. J Affect Disord 1997;45:19–30.
5. Kessler RC, Berglund P, Demler O, et al. The epidemiology of major depressive disorder: results from the National Comorbidity Survey Replication (NCS-R). JAMA 2003;289:3095–105.
6. Harman JS, Veazie PJ, Lyness JM. Primary care physician office visits for depression by older Americans. J Gen Intern Med 2006;21:926–30.
7. Tylee A, Gandhi P. The importance of somatic symptoms in depression in primary care. Prim Care Companion J Clin Psychiatry 2005;7:167–76.
8. Daly EJ, Trivedi MH, Wisniewski SR, et al. Health-related quality of life in depression: a STAR*D report. Ann Clin Psychiatry 2010;22:43–55.
9. Simon GE. Social and economic burden of mood disorders. Biol Psychiatry 2003;54:208–15.
10. Moussavi S, Chatterji S, Verdes E, et al. Depression, chronic diseases, and decrements in health: results from the World Health Surveys. Lancet 2007;370: 851–8.

11. Cuijpers P, Smit F. Excess mortality in depression: a meta-analysis of community studies. J Affect Disord 2002;72:227–36.

12. Benazon NR, Coyne JC. Living with a depressed spouse. J Fam Psychol 2000; 14:71–9.

13. Olfson M, Marcus SC, Druss B, et al. Parental depression, child mental health problems, and health care utilization. Med Care 2003;41:716–21.

14. Sills MR, Shetterly S, Xu S, et al. Association between parental depression and children's health care use. Pediatrics 2007;119:e829–36.

15. Donohue JM, Pincus HA. Reducing the societal burden of depression: a review of economic costs, quality of care and effects of treatment. Pharmacoeconomics 2007;25:7–24.

16. Wang PS, Simon G, Kessler RC. The economic burden of depression and the cost-effectiveness of treatment. Int J Methods Psychiatr Res 2003;12:22–33.

17. Stewart WF, Ricci JA, Chee E, et al. Cost of lost productive work time among US workers with depression. JAMA 2003;289:3135–44.

18. Williams DR, Gonzalez HM, Neighbors H, et al. Prevalence and distribution of major depressive disorder in African Americans, Caribbean blacks, and non-Hispanic whites: results from the National Survey of American Life. Arch Gen Psychiatry 2007;64:305–15.

19. Miranda J, Cooper LA. Disparities in care for depression among primary care patients. J Gen Intern Med 2004;19:120–6.

20. Hunt J, Sullivan G, Chavira DA, et al. Race and beliefs about mental health treatment among anxious primary care patients. J Nerv Ment Dis 2013;201:188–95.

21. Cook BL, Doksum T, Chen CN, et al. The role of provider supply and organization in reducing racial/ethnic disparities in mental health care in the U.S. Soc Sci Med 2013;84:102–9.

22. Jorge RE, Robinson RG, Moser D, et al. Major depression following traumatic brain injury. Arch Gen Psychiatry 2004;61:42–50.

23. Robinson RG. Poststroke depression: prevalence, diagnosis, treatment, and disease progression. Biol Psychiatry 2003;54:376–87.

24. McDonald WM, Richard IH, DeLong MR. Prevalence, etiology, and treatment of depression in Parkinson's disease. Biol Psychiatry 2003;54:363–75.

25. Marcus SM, Flynn HA, Blow FC, et al. Depressive symptoms among pregnant women screened in obstetrics settings. J Womens Health (Larchmt) 2003;12: 373–80.

26. Green JG, McLaughlin KA, Berglund PA, et al. Childhood adversities and adult psychiatric disorders in the national comorbidity survey replication I: associations with first onset of DSM-IV disorders. Arch Gen Psychiatry 2010;67:113–23.

27. Kendler KS, Karkowski LM, Prescott CA. Causal relationship between stressful life events and the onset of major depression. Am J Psychiatry 1999;156: 837–41.

28. Kendler KS, Gatz M, Gardner CO, et al. Swedish national twin study of lifetime major depression. Am J Psychiatry 2006;163:109–14.

29. Stafford RS, MacDonald EA, Finkelstein SN. National patterns of medication treatment for depression, 1987 to 2001. Prim Care Companion J Clin Psychiatry 2001;3:232–5.

30. Marcus SC, Olfson M. National trends in the treatment for depression from 1998 to 2007. Arch Gen Psychiatry 2010;67:1265–73.

31. O'Connor EA, Whitlock EP, Gaynes B, et al. Screening for depression in adults and older adults in primary care: an updated systematic review. Rockville (MD): 2009.

32. Desai MM, Rosenheck RA, Craig TJ. Case-finding for depression among medical outpatients in the Veterans Health Administration. Med Care 2006;44: 175–81.
33. Timonen M, Liukkonen T. Management of depression in adults. BMJ 2008;336: 435–9.
34. Mitchell AJ, Vaze A, Rao S. Clinical diagnosis of depression in primary care: a meta-analysis. Lancet 2009;374:609–19.
35. Gilbody S, House AO, Sheldon TA. Screening and case finding instruments for depression. Cochrane Database Syst Rev 2005;(4):CD002792.
36. Gilbody S, Sheldon T, House A. Screening and case-finding instruments for depression: a meta-analysis. CMAJ 2008;178:997–1003.
37. Pignone M, Gaynes BN, Rushton JL, et al. Screening for depression. Rockville (MD): 2002.
38. Thota AB, Sipe TA, Byard GJ, et al. Collaborative care to improve the management of depressive disorders: a community guide systematic review and meta-analysis. Am J Prev Med 2012;42:525–38.
39. Paulden M, Palmer S, Hewitt C, et al. Screening for postnatal depression in primary care: cost effectiveness analysis. BMJ 2009;339:b5203.
40. Valenstein M, Vijan S, Zeber JE, et al. The cost-utility of screening for depression in primary care. Ann Intern Med 2001;134:345–60.
41. Unutzer J, Katon WJ, Fan MY, et al. Long-term cost effects of collaborative care for late-life depression. Am J Manag Care 2008;14:95–100.
42. Katon W, Russo J, Lin EH, et al. Cost-effectiveness of a multicondition collaborative care intervention: a randomized controlled trial. Arch Gen Psychiatry 2012;69:506–14.
43. Williams JW Jr, Pignone M, Ramirez G, et al. Identifying depression in primary care: a literature synthesis of case-finding instruments. Gen Hosp Psychiatry 2002;24:225–37.
44. Akena D, Joska J, Obuku EA, et al. Comparing the accuracy of brief versus long depression screening instruments which have been validated in low and middle income countries: a systematic review. BMC Psychiatry 2012;12:187.
45. Kroenke K, Spitzer RL, Williams JB, et al. The patient health questionnaire somatic, anxiety, and depressive symptom scales: a systematic review. Gen Hosp Psychiatry 2010;32:345–59.
46. Huang FY, Chung H, Kroenke K, et al. Using the Patient Health Questionnaire-9 to measure depression among racially and ethnically diverse primary care patients. J Gen Intern Med 2006;21:547–52.
47. Kroenke K, Spitzer RL, Williams JB. The Patient Health Questionnaire-2: validity of a two-item depression screener. Med Care 2003;41:1284–92.
48. Steer RA, Cavalieri TA, Leonard DM, et al. Use of the Beck Depression Inventory for Primary Care to screen for major depression disorders. Gen Hosp Psychiatry 1999;21:106–11.
49. Herrmann C. International experiences with the Hospital Anxiety and Depression Scale—a review of validation data and clinical results. J Psychosom Res 1997;42:17–41.
50. Mapi Research Trust. HADS (Hospital Anxiety and Depression Scale). Available at: http://www.mapi-trust.org/services/questionnairelicensing/catalog-questionnaires/240-hads. Accessed October 25, 2013.
51. Mitchell AJ, Bird V, Rizzo M, et al. Diagnostic validity and added value of the Geriatric Depression Scale for depression in primary care: a meta-analysis of GDS30 and GDS15. J Affect Disord 2010;125:10–7.

52. Hewitt C, Gilbody S, Brealey S, et al. Methods to identify postnatal depression in primary care: an integrated evidence synthesis and value of information analysis. Health Technol Assess 2009;13:1–145, 147–230.

53. Hanusa BH, Scholle SH, Haskett RF, et al. Screening for depression in the post-partum period: a comparison of three instruments. J Womens Health (Larchmt) 2008;17:585–96.

54. U.S. Preventive Services Task Force. Screening for depression in adults: recommendation statement. 2009. Available at: http://www.uspreventiveservicestaskforce.org/uspstf09/adultdepression/addeprrs.htm. Accessed October 10, 2013.

55. U.S. Preventive Services Task Force. Screening and treatment for major depressive disorder in children and adolescents: recommendation statement. 2009. Available at: http://www.uspreventiveservicestaskforce.org/uspstf09/depression/chdeprrs.htm. Accessed October 10, 2013.

56. National Institute for Health and Clinical Excellence. Treatment and management of depression in adults, including adults with a chronic physical health problem. 2009. Available at: http://www.nice.org.uk/nicemedia/live/12329/45890/45890.pdf. Accessed December 27, 2013.

57. Pilling S, Anderson I, Goldberg D, et al. Depression in adults, including those with a chronic physical health problem: summary of NICE guidance. BMJ 2009;339:b4108.

58. Cunningham PJ. Beyond parity: primary care physicians' perspectives on access to mental health care. Health Aff (Millwood) 2009;28:w490–501.

59. Olfson M, Marcus SC, Tedeschi M, et al. Continuity of antidepressant treatment for adults with depression in the United States. Am J Psychiatry 2006;163:101–8.

60. Archer J, Bower P, Gilbody S, et al. Collaborative care for depression and anxiety problems. Cochrane Database Syst Rev 2012;(10):CD006525.

61. Bachman J, Pincus HA, Houtsinger JK, et al. Funding mechanisms for depression care management: opportunities and challenges. Gen Hosp Psychiatry 2006;28:278–88.

62. Pincus HA, Pechura CM, Elinson L, et al. Depression in primary care: linking clinical and systems strategies. Gen Hosp Psychiatry 2001;23:311–8.

63. RTI International, Telligen. Accountable Care Organization 2013 program analysis: quality performance standards narrative measure specifications. Research Triangle Park (NC): 2012.

64. Agency for Healthcare Research and Quality. Defining the PCMH. Available at: http://pcmh.ahrq.gov/page/defining-pcmh. Accessed December 8, 2013.

65. Croghan TW, Brown JD. Integrating mental health treatment into the patient centered medical home. Rockville (MD): Agency for Healthcare Research and Quality; 2010. AHRQ Publication No. 10-0084-EF.

66. Gunn J, Diggens J, Hegarty K, et al. A systematic review of complex system interventions designed to increase recovery from depression in primary care. BMC Health Serv Res 2006;6:88.

67. Baik SY, Crabtree BF, Gonzales JJ. Primary care clinicians' recognition and management of depression: a model of depression care in real-world primary care practice. J Gen Intern Med 2013;28:1430–9.

68. Crabtree BF, Nutting PA, Miller WL, et al. Summary of the National Demonstration Project and recommendations for the patient-centered medical home. Ann Fam Med 2010;8(Suppl 1):S80–90 S92.

69. Chung H, Kim A, Neighbors CJ, et al. Early experience of a pilot intervention for patients with depression and chronic medical illness in an urban ACO. Gen Hosp Psychiatry 2013;35:468–71.

70. Institute of Medicine. Crossing the quality chasm: a new health system for the 21st century. Washington, DC: 2001.
71. Blumenthal D, Tavenner M. The "meaningful use" regulation for electronic health records. N Engl J Med 2010;363:501–4.
72. Klein EW, Hunt JS, Leblanc BH. Depression screening interfaced with an electronic health record: a feasibility study in a primary care clinic using optical mark reader technology. Prim Care Companion J Clin Psychiatry 2006;8:324–8.
73. Gill JM, Dansky BS. Use of an electronic medical record to facilitate screening for depression in primary care. Prim Care Companion J Clin Psychiatry 2003;5: 125–8.
74. Rollman BL, Hanusa BH, Gilbert T, et al. The electronic medical record. A randomized trial of its impact on primary care physicians' initial management of major depression [corrected]. Arch Intern Med 2001;161:189–97.
75. Kobus AM, Harman JS, Do HD, et al. Challenges to depression care documentation in an EHR. Fam Med 2013;45:268–71.
76. Harman JS, Rost KM, Harle CA, et al. Electronic medical record availability and primary care depression treatment. J Gen Intern Med 2012;27:962–7.
77. Rollman BL, Hanusa BH, Lowe HJ, et al. A randomized trial using computerized decision support to improve treatment of major depression in primary care. J Gen Intern Med 2002;17:493–503.
78. Rollman BL, Weinreb L, Korsen N, et al. Implementation of guideline-based care for depression in primary care. Adm Policy Ment Health 2006;33:43–53.
79. Centers for Disease Control and Prevention. Definitions: self-inflicted violence. 2012. Available at: http://www.cdc.gov/violenceprevention/suicide/definitions.html. Accessed October 10, 2013.
80. Lloyd-Richardson EE, Perrine N, Dierker L, et al. Characteristics and functions of non-suicidal self-injury in a community sample of adolescents. Psychol Med 2007;37:1183–92.
81. Centers for Disease Control and Prevention. 10 leading causes of death by age group—2010. Available at: http://www.cdc.gov/injury/wisqars/pdf/10LCID_All_Deaths_By_Age_Group_2010-a.pdf. Accessed October 10, 2013.
82. Centers for Disease Control and Prevention. Years of potential life lost (YLL) reports, 1999-2010. Available at: http://webappa.cdc.gov/sasweb/ncipc/ypll10.html. Accessed October 10, 2013.
83. U.S. Department of Health and Human Services (HHS) Office of the Surgeon General and National Action Alliance for Suicide Prevention. 2012 national strategy for suicide prevention: goals and objectives for action: a report of the U.S. Surgeon General and of the National Action Alliance for Suicide Prevention. Washington, DC: HHS; 2012.
84. Mann JJ. A current perspective of suicide and attempted suicide. Ann Intern Med 2002;136:302–11.
85. Nock MK, Borges G, Bromet EJ, et al. Suicide and suicidal behavior. Epidemiol Rev 2008;30:133–54.
86. Brown GK, Beck AT, Steer RA, et al. Risk factors for suicide in psychiatric outpatients: a 20-year prospective study. J Consult Clin Psychol 2000;68:371–7.
87. Gaynes BN, West SL, Ford CA, et al. Screening for suicide risk in adults: a summary of the evidence for the U.S. Preventive Services Task Force. Ann Intern Med 2004;140:822–35.
88. Luoma JB, Martin CE, Pearson JL. Contact with mental health and primary care providers before suicide: a review of the evidence. Am J Psychiatry 2002;159: 909–16.

89. U.S. Preventive Services Task Force. Screening for suicide risk in adolescents, adults, and older adults: draft recommendation statement. 2013. Available at: http://www.uspreventiveservicestaskforce.org/uspstf13/suicide/suicidedraftrec. htm. Accessed October 10, 2013.

90. Mann JJ, Apter A, Bertolote J, et al. Suicide prevention strategies: a systematic review. JAMA 2005;294:2064–74.

91. Suicide and suicide attempts in adolescents. Committee on Adolescents. American Academy of Pediatrics. Pediatrics 2000;105:871–4.

92. American Academy of Child and Adolescent Psychiatry. Practice parameter for the assessment and treatment of children and adolescents with suicidal behavior. American Academy of Child and Adolescent Psychiatry. J Am Acad Child Adolesc Psychiatry 2001;40:24S–51S.

93. American Medical Association, Department of Adolescent Health. Guidelines for adolescent preventive services (GAPS): recommendations monograph. 2nd edition. Chicago: American Medical Association, Dept. of Adolescent Health; 1995.

APPENDIX 1: PATIENT HEALTH QUESTIONNAIRE–9

PATIENT HEALTH QUESTIONNAIRE-9 (PHQ-9)				
Over the <u>last 2 weeks</u>, how often have you been bothered by any of the following problems? *(Use "✔" to indicate your answer)*	Not at all	Several days	More than half the days	Nearly every day
1. Little interest or pleasure in doing things	0	1	2	3
2. Feeling down, depressed, or hopeless	0	1	2	3
3. Trouble falling or staying asleep, or sleeping too much	0	1	2	3
4. Feeling tired or having little energy	0	1	2	3
5. Poor appetite or overeating	0	1	2	3
6. Feeling bad about yourself — or that you are a failure or have let yourself or your family down	0	1	2	3
7. Trouble concentrating on things, such as reading the newspaper or watching television	0	1	2	3
8. Moving or speaking so slowly that other people could have noticed? Or the opposite — being so fidgety or restless that you have been moving around a lot more than usual	0	1	2	3
9. Thoughts that you would be better off dead or of hurting yourself in some way	0	1	2	3

FOR OFFICE CODING ___0___ + _____ + _____ + _____

=Total Score: _____

If you checked off <u>any</u> problems, how <u>difficult</u> have these problems made it for you to do your work, take care of things at home, or get along with other people?

Not difficult at all	Somewhat difficult	Very difficult	Extremely difficult
☐	☐	☐	☐

Developed by Drs. Robert L. Spitzer, Janet B.W. Williams, Kurt Kroenke and colleagues, with an educational grant from Pfizer Inc. No permission required to reproduce, translate, display or distribute.

From Patient Health Questionnaire Screeners. Available at: http://www.phqscreeners. com/overview.aspx?Screener=02_PHQ-9.

APPENDIX 2: GERIATRIC DEPRESSION SCALE, SHORT FORM

MOOD SCALE (short form)

Choose the best answer for how you have felt over the past week:

1. Are you basically satisfied with your life? YES/NO

2. Have you dropped many of your activities and interests? YES/NO
3. Do you feel that your life is empty? YES/NO
4. Do you often get bored? YES/NO
5. Are you in good spirits most of the time? YES/NO
6. Are you afraid that something bad is going to happen to you? YES/NO
7. Do you feel happy most of the time? YES/NO
8. Do you often feel helpless? YES/NO
9. Do you prefer to stay at home, rather than going out and doing new things? YES/NO
10. Do you feel you have more problems with memory than most? YES/NO
11. Do you think it is wonderful to be alive now? YES/NO
12. Do you feel pretty worthless the way you are now? YES/NO
13. Do you feel full of energy? YES/NO
14. Do you feel that your situation is hopeless? YES/NO
15. Do you think that most people are better off than you are? YES/NO

From Geriatric Depression Scale. Available at: http://www.stanford.edu/~yesavage/GDS.english.short.html.

Genomics in Primary Care Practice

Kathryn Teng, MD[a],*, Louise S. Acheson, MD, MS[b]

KEYWORDS

- Primary care • Preventive care • Family health history • Ancestry • Genomic • Value

KEY POINTS

- Family health history is a proxy for genomic testing, and can inform and guide preventive care plans.
- Family health history can be a useful tool to discuss risk and engage patients in preventive care plans.
- Both family health history and DNA analysis provide probabilistic risk, not deterministic risk.
- Both bloodline ancestry and shared environmental factors are important predictors for many disease states.
- Education at all levels is needed to stay current and to provide efficient genomically informed, value-based care.
- Genetic counselors can be valuable partners and resources to interpret and educate patients regarding genomic risk and risk associated with family health history.

INTRODUCTION

Since the completion of the Human Genome Project in 2003, clinicians and patients alike have anticipated the promise of genomics. We have hoped that genomic information would provide answers to several age-old questions: What causes disease? Why are some people afflicted over others? Why do some people respond to certain therapies over others? Particularly for primary care clinicians, it was hoped that genomics would provide additional information that would allow us to more precisely predict and prevent disease. Instead, we have observed that progress has been slow in the realm of disease prediction. While new discoveries linking genomics and disease are published almost weekly, the use of genomics in standard clinical practice, in most fields other than oncology, has lagged behind. For various reasons including

The authors do not have any conflicts of interest.

[a] Internal Medicine, Center for Personalized Healthcare (Cleveland Clinic), 9500 Euclid Avenue, NE5-203, Cleveland, OH 44195, USA; [b] Departments of Family Medicine, Oncology, and Reproductive Biology, University Hospitals Case Medical Center, Case Western Reserve University, 11100 Euclid Avenue, Cleveland, OH 44106-5036, USA

* Corresponding author.

E-mail address: tengk@ccf.org

http://dx.doi.org/10.1016/j.pop.2014.02.012
0095-4543/14/$ – see front matter © 2014 Elsevier Inc. All rights reserved.
primarycare.theclinics.com

outstanding questions of disease association versus prediction, unproven clinical utility, cost of clinical trials, genomic testing and analytics, limited reimbursement, and a lag in clinician education, genomics has been slow to reach its potential promise in primary care medicine.

Compounding the questions surrounding the fundamental clinical utility of genomic information for risk prediction is the change we are currently facing with health care reform (eg, the Patient Protection and Affordable Care Act). We have reached a new era in health care: one in which costs will be heavily scrutinized, quality and impact on clinical outcomes will need to be proved, and value has become the new buzzword. The specific problem we are facing is that in the United States, health care spending continues to increase and is expected to reach 18.4% of the gross domestic product by 2017.[1] Yet despite our high levels of health care spending, when compared with other developed nations, the United States consistently performs poorly in measures of access, outcomes, and quality of care. We have reached an era in which we are increasingly being held accountable for following evidence-based standards of care and for which care coordination will be critical. How does genomics fit into this model, and what will its role be?

This article aims to discuss the current role of genomics for risk assessment in primary care practice and how it might interface with value-based health care initiatives. The US Preventive Services Task Force (USPSTF) has issued some evidence-based recommendations for personalized prevention based on family history or genetic testing.[2] In the United States, the Evaluating Genomic Applications in Practice and Prevention Working Group, an independent expert group similar to the USPSTF, makes recommendations about clinical applications of genomic tests, based on systematic reviews of evidence.[3] Through use of a case example, these recommendations are critically explored with the goal of highlighting their applicability and utility within the primary care setting.

Case discussion: the effects of gene variants on disease risk are complex, so the predictive value of genomic profiles for individuals is limited

Mrs Jones is a 50-year-old woman with no significant medical history, who has just moved from another state and presents for a new patient annual preventive care/physical examination visit with Dr Brown, a primary care physician. She brings with her the results of a personal genomic test that she received as a 50th birthday gift. Of most interest to her, these results indicate that she is at increased risk for coronary heart disease and decreased risk for colon cancer. Mrs Jones has been dreading her screening colonoscopy, which she knows is recommended at age 50. She asks Dr Brown what she should do about the elevated risk for coronary heart disease and whether she can forgo screening colonoscopy based on the personal genomic test results (**Box 1**).

This case highlights 2 important features: first, the use of genomics in the adult primary care setting is sometimes driven by patients; second, clinicians need to understand and be able to educate patients about the limitations of genomic testing. The cost of personal genomic testing has fallen dramatically in the last 5 years, and is now as low as US$99. As a result, it is reasonable to assume that with a push in consumer advertising[4] the uptake and interest in such tests will increase. Although the medical community has considered that such information might be psychologically harmful to patients, harm has not been shown in several studies.[5,6] In fact, studies have shown that consumers have properly understood their results,[6,7] but it is unclear as to whether such information has influenced long-term change in behavior. Regardless, it is clear that there is interest among laypeople to have access to genomic

---

Box 1
Genomics in the primary care setting

- Genomics investigates the interaction of genes with the rest of the genome and with the environment

- The use of genomics in the adult primary care setting is sometimes driven by patients

- Clinicians need to understand and be able to educate patients about the limitations of genomic testing

- Genetic markers or single-nucleotide polymorphisms identified through genome-wide association studies research are associated with disease, but not necessarily causative of disease

---

information, and they are looking to their clinicians to help interpret this information and use it in their preventive care plans.[8]

For clinicians to appropriately assess genomic testing results, there are a few concepts that are essential to understand. First is the complexity of genomics (**Table 1**); second is the multifactorial origin of most diseases and personal characteristics; and third is the imperfect ability of DNA analysis to predict disease risk.

The study of genomics holds great promise because it investigates the interaction of genes with the rest of the genome and with the environment, to determine what might cause multifactorial disorders commonly seen in primary care practice. Many genomic studies attempt to understand how variations in a single base pair on a DNA molecule, called single-nucleotide polymorphisms (SNPs), correlate with disease, drug response, or other phenotypes. The SNPs and other genetic markers are often found by a type of genomic research called genome-wide association studies (GWAS). GWAS scan the genomes of many people looking for genetic markers that can be used to predict risk for a disease. Once these markers are identified, they might be used to better understand the role these genes play in development of disease and how disease might be prevented or treated.

In addition to seeking variations in a panel of SNPs found in population studies to be associated with diseases, other types of genomic studies reveal many rare variants, rearrangements of DNA, copy-number variations, and inactivation of DNA sequences by epigenetic changes such as methylation. Most of these findings are used more for genetic diagnosis than for risk prediction. Sequencing of a person's whole genome or whole exome (the 1% of the genome that codes for proteins) is currently on the frontier of clinical application, but is hindered by the sheer volume of results whose significance is unknown.[9]

A very important concept must be emphasized: the genetic markers or SNPs that are identified using GWAS research are associated with disease but are not

---

Table 1
The complexity of genomics

Gene	A unit of DNA that carries the instructions for making a specific protein or set of proteins
Genetics	The study of a particular gene
Genome	An organism's complete set of DNA
Genomics	The study of the function and interactions of the DNA in a genome

necessarily causative of disease. Fundamentally this means that genomic information identified from GWAS is usually probabilistic, not deterministic. Furthermore, the ethnicity of the populations studied matters because certain genetic markers may be more prevalent in certain ethnic populations than in others (population stratification). Associations of genetic alterations with disease are applicable when the association has been found in multiple ethnic groups or in populations similar to those that want to use the information. Even when a single genetic alteration is associated with a very high susceptibility to disease (as in hereditary cancer syndromes), not everyone with the genetic change will get the disease (many adult-onset conditions have less than 100% penetrance). Furthermore, manifestations of an inherited disease may vary from mild to severe, as in cystic fibrosis (variable expressivity).

Case discussion continued: gene variants associated with disease in one population may not be informative for individuals from another population

Dr Brown reviewed the genomic report that Mrs Jones had brought in. He notes that her increased risk for coronary heart disease (CHD) is based on a customized panel of 15 to 20 SNPs that have been reported in the literature to be associated with CHD. These markers have been identified in subjects of European ethnicity only. Dr Brown inquires about Mrs Jones' ethnicity, and she tells him that her mother and father are from Africa. She does not have any known European ancestry. As such, this result may not be applicable to her. Her risk for CHD cannot be accurately determined by this panel of markers, because CHD is multifactorial and these genetic markers have been found to be applicable only in people of European ancestry.

Likewise, when Dr Brown examines Mrs Jones' results for colorectal cancer risk, he notes that the risk level is based on presence of an SNP that is associated with cancer in populations with European and Asian ancestry. There are inadequate data to extrapolate risk to African ethnicities. He explains to Mrs Jones that the risk score for colorectal cancer may not apply to her and does not truly reduce her estimated risk for colorectal cancer. He recommends that she proceed with screening for colorectal cancer according to age-appropriate screening guidelines for colorectal cancer in the general population.

He emphasizes to Mrs Jones the nature of genomic testing—that in the case of multifactorial diseases such as CHD and colorectal cancer, it is usually probabilistic and not deterministic. Gene variants associated with disease risk in populations leave much uncertainty regarding individual risk prediction (Box 2).

Case discussion continued: family health history is a "genomic test" that shows combined effects of many genes, behavior, and environment

As part of her annual preventive care visit, Mrs Jones completed a family health history questionnaire sent to her from Dr Brown's office. Dr Brown reviews the family health history and notes that both of Mrs Jones' parents had adult-onset diabetes. There is no family health history of premature CHD or stroke, nor is there a family health history of colon cancer. He tells Mrs Jones that this family health history remarkably increases her lifetime risk of developing diabetes (to 75%). He screens for glucose intolerance, and reinforces the need for preventive measures (Box 3).

Family health history has long been used as a proxy for genomic risk and to guide clinical care. Family health history can be used to inform risk stratification and to guide appropriate screening and preventive care in circumstances whereby it is safer or more cost-effective to apply certain preventive measures to a high-risk subset rather than universally.[10–12] Individuals with a family health history of disease have been

---

Box 2
Genomic testing, screening, and prevention

- Many diseases are multifactorial
- For multifactorial diseases, genomic testing results are usually probabilistic, not deterministic
- Genomic test results are not always applicable to the individual patient
- Clinicians should adhere to recommended guidelines for screening and prevention

---

found to be more knowledgable about risk factors for disease,[13] and discussion of family health history has been shown in some, but not all studies to motivate these patients to greater compliance with disease screening and adherence to medical recommendations.[14–17] However, some studies have shown, for example, that even people with a family health history of colon cancer are not following the recommended guidelines for colon cancer screening.[18,19] Interviews with patients in general practice suggest that laypeople variably interpret their own family health histories, including behavioral and environmental risk factors as well as genetics.[20]

Unfortunately, collection of family health history is inconsistent, and not much time is devoted to it in primary care practice.[21] Only recently are electronic health records becoming capable of organizing family history as structured data, so that eventually risk assessment based on family health history can be systematic[22–24]; consequently, the evidence basis for clinical utility of family health history–based risk assessment is not yet well developed.[25,26] Recent and ongoing research to simplify and deploy computerized tools for collection of family health history and risk assessment in primary care offers promising results.[16,27–31]

Family health history confers an overall higher predictive value than does SNP analysis.[32] Unlike traditional genetic testing, which looks for uncommon genetic changes with exceedingly high predictive and/or diagnostic value, most SNPs have a very modest effect size. The median odds ratio given is 1.33[33]; this translates to a relative risk (RR) of approximately 1.3 for a condition with a prevalence of 8%.[34] In other words, given that the general population risk of breast cancer is 8%, if a patient had the disease-associated SNP with an RR of 1.3 her lifetime risk for breast cancer would increase from 8% to approximately 10%. By contrast, family health history is the most consistent risk factor for nearly every disease.[35] Unlike a personal genomic test that conveys only information about several genes, a family health history captures information about combined effects of multiple genes and environmental exposures, because families (unless separated at birth) share tens of thousands of similar genes, similar learned behavior patterns, and similar environments. Close family members presumably are also exposed to the same environmental stressors that increase risk (a risk that may be further elevated when certain genetic markers are also present). In many cases, having a single affected first-degree (parent, sibling, child) relative

---

Box 3
Family health history and disease-risk assessment

- Family health history can be used to personalize disease-risk assessment
- Reviewing family health history and recognizing patterns of disease is important, especially in the primary care setting
- Collection of family health history is inconsistent

---

doubles the risk of disease (ie, RR ~2).[36] Returning to the earlier example of breast cancer, this translates to an increase from an 8% to approximately 16% lifetime risk of breast cancer for a woman whose mother had breast cancer in middle age, with no additional family health history of cancer. For this reason, most experts recommend continuing to use family health history rather than SNPs for personalizing risk-assessment analysis at present (**Box 4**).

Case discussion continued: patterns of familial and inherited susceptibility to cancer and other diseases

Dr Brown also sees that Mrs Jones has reported a history of ovarian cancer in her mother at age 60 and, to his surprise, a history of breast cancer in her maternal grandfather at an unknown age. Based on this family history, particularly the uncommon occurrence of breast cancer in a male relative, along with ovarian cancer in the same lineage, Dr Brown is concerned that Mrs Jones might carry a BRCA gene mutation that has been shown to dramatically increase the risk for hereditary breast-ovarian cancer.[45–47] Hereditary breast-ovarian cancer syndrome is an autosomal dominant condition, which means that offspring of an affected individual have a 50% chance of inheriting the BRCA mutation, putting Mrs Jones potentially at high risk for developing breast and ovarian cancer.

Dr Brown expresses his concern to Mrs Jones regarding her elevated risk for breast cancer based on family health history, and she reassures him that she had a screening mammogram done earlier this year. Dr Brown can refer to special recommendations for cancer surveillance and prevention in women with known deleterious BRCA gene mutations (see the related article in this issue by de la Cruz and colleagues addressing the topic of breast cancer screening); these take into account both the elevated lifetime risk and the fact that inherited cancers tend to develop at earlier ages than in the general population.

*Dr Brown is perplexed that Mrs Jones' personal genomic test did not identify her as being at high risk for breast cancer. On closer review of the report, however, he notes that the genomic test does not include specific testing for BRCA1 gene mutations (testing for BRCA mutations involves sequencing the gene, rather than SNP analysis) and does not consider family health history. This report includes SNPs associated with familial (multifactorial) breast cancer but not for the genes that cause hereditary breast cancer. Nevertheless, Dr Brown recognizes that not all women who inherit these mutations will get cancer (**Box 5, Table 2**).*

Box 4
Family health history resources

- Family health history questionnaires can be completed by patients, outside of a clinical encounter[37,38]

- Those that generate structured data with enough detail for use in risk assessment for common adult diseases generally take about 20 minutes for patients to complete, depending on family size and medical conditions included[39,40]

- Some have been validated in comparison with family health histories obtained by genetic counselors[23,29,40]

- The US Surgeon General makes available an online tool for recording family health history: My Family Health Portrait[41]

- Links to family history resources are on the National Human Genome Institute Web site[42]

- Resources from the Genetic Alliance take a narrative approach to family health history[43]

- The American Medical Association also has a pamphlet about family health histories[44]

Box 5
Interpreting risk: familial history, genomic testing, and ethnicity

- It is important to understand the differences between sporadic, familial (multifactorial), and hereditary diseases

- Accurate interpretation of genomic test results is critical

- Ethnicity can be a risk factor for certain diseases. Ethnicity is complex and not always obvious

---

For the primary care clinician, even in the genomic era, the use of family health history to predict disease risk is still the mainstay of preventive care. Moreover, because of the growing emphasis toward value-based care, whereby clinicians are being asked to do more, to do better, and to do so in less time, primary care clinicians must ensure they effectively interpret a well-conducted family health history so as to readily identify patterns of disease. The first step toward doing this is to understand that disease can be grouped into 3 categories (**Table 3**).

As such, when asking about family health history it is prudent to first ask about hereditary diseases. Most such diseases, such as cystic fibrosis or sickle cell anemia, present in childhood. However, a handful usually present in adulthood, and these include hereditary breast-ovarian cancer syndrome and Lynch syndrome (hereditary nonpolyposis colorectal cancer), neurofibromatosis, multiple endocrine neoplasias, Charcot-Marie-Tooth disease, and other late-onset neurologic conditions. Next, clinicians should look for patterns of familial inheritance: diseases for which family history is a known risk factor and for which early screening can improve outcomes. Most of the conditions that are seen and managed in primary care medicine (such as diabetes and CHD) would fall into this category of familial or multifactorial disease.

Although there are commonalities in the patterns of family health history between hereditary and familial conditions, there are also some differences. For both hereditary and familial conditions it is common to find multiple family members with the same condition, early onset of disease, and disease in the sex less often affected. Clues to hereditary disease would also include the following: family members with different but related conditions (such as breast cancer and ovarian cancer or prostate cancer), a discernible pattern of inheritance (such as autosomal dominant with successive generations affected), and high-risk ethnicity.[10]

Early age at onset of the disease increases predicted familial risk, and also the chance of a hereditary susceptibility. For example, risk modeling estimates that a

---

Table 2
Lifetime risks for developing breast or ovarian cancer in women with and without a cancer-associated BRCA mutation

Gene	Condition	Lifetime Incidence WITHOUT a Cancer-Associated Mutation (%)	Lifetime Incidence WITH a Cancer-Associated Mutation (%)
BRCA1	Breast cancer	12	55–65
	Ovarian cancer	1.4	39
BRCA2	Breast cancer	12	45
	Ovarian cancer	1.4	11–17

Data from Refs.[48–50]

Table 3	
Categories of disease	
Sporadic	With no apparent inheritance pattern
Familial or multifactorial	Greater preponderance of disease in a family than would be expected by chance, but no identifiable hereditary syndrome or known genetic etiology
Hereditary	Part of a known hereditary syndrome/disease with known or suspected genetic origin

non-Ashkenazi Jewish woman diagnosed with breast cancer at age 30 years has an approximately 10% chance of having a *BRCA* mutation, compared with an approximately 1% chance for a woman diagnosed at age 70 years.[51] In individuals without a personal history of breast cancer, a family history of early-onset breast cancer is also predictive of genetic etiology. For example, based on the genetic testing results of more than 185,000 individuals, the prevalence of *BRCA* mutations among individuals with no cancer diagnosis and no risk factors (ie, no family health history of early breast cancer or of ovarian cancer in any relative, not of Ashkenazi Jewish heritage) is 1.5%.[52] By contrast, individuals with no personal history of cancer who have more than 1 first-degree or second-degree relative with breast cancer before age 50 years have a 5.6% a priori risk of *BRCA* mutation. If they are of Ashkenazi Jewish ancestry, the probability of a mutation increases to 16.4%.[52]

RACE, ETHNICITY, AND ANCESTRY

The relationship between race and ethnicity, morbidity and mortality, and health care utilization and outcomes is a hot topic in today's health care environment. Despite significant progress in recent decades, a patient's racial or ethnic identity continues to be associated with access to health care and the quality of such care.[53–57] Like access to health care proper, there are also well-articulated concerns about disparate access to genomic medicine and its priority relative to well-proven primary care and preventive measures,[58] as well as well-developed literature on the influence of the environment and social factors (poverty, environmental hazards, institutional and individual forms of discriminatory treatment) on health outcomes.[54,56] Taken as a whole, evidence suggests that many factors contribute to the nation's racially linked disparities in health status, health care quality, and health care outcomes. In light of this evidence, a person's racial and ethnic identity can play an important role in identification of risk for disease, and can sometimes allow clinicians to appropriately customize preventive care for those at highest risk.

Following the Human Genome Project, genomic research has found that genetic variations among individuals are much greater than genetic differences among racial groups. Physical appearance is not a reliable way to predict genetic characteristics. Through genomics, the concepts of race, ethnicity, and ancestry have been redefined as imprecise, primarily social categories. Nonetheless, these imprecise categories are sometimes helpful for directing the use and interpretation of family health history and genetic tests (**Table 4**).

One definition of ancestry corresponds to the "inherited properties shared with others of your bloodline," hereafter referred to as bloodline ancestry.[60] Because

Table 4	
Definitions of race, ethnicity, and ancestry	
Race	A "socioeconomic concept wherein groups of people sharing certain physical characteristics are treated differently[59]"
Ethnicity	Refers to "a shared culture and way of life, especially reflected in language, religion, and material culture[59]"
Ancestry	*Bloodline ancestry*: "Inherited properties shared with others of your bloodline,"[60] tracing back paternal and maternal lineages. For example, some genetics professionals ask, "what is the ancestry/national origin of each of your grandparents?"
	Biogeographic ancestry: Based on migration of human populations throughout history[61]
	Continental ancestry: Some genomic profiles compare the individual's genetic markers with those that distinguish populations now living in various continents[61]
	Founder effect: Some population groups that have been geographically or socially isolated, and whose modern representatives descended from relatively few individuals, have an unusual prevalence of certain genetic traits[61]

bloodline ancestry refers to blood traits, it is important to remember that ancestry, from this perspective, is not physically obvious. Bloodline ancestry plays a role in risk prediction for several adult conditions; for example, hereditary breast cancer is more prevalent in people of Ashkenazi Jewish descent.

Another pattern highlighting the importance of bloodline ancestry is the preponderance of recessively inherited diseases in individuals of certain populations because of their shared genetic heritage. For example, individuals descended from equatorial Africa have an increased risk for sickle cell anemia[62,63]; individuals of Mediterranean, Middle Eastern, and Asian descent have an increased risk for thalassemia[64]; and individuals of northern European descent have an increased risk for hereditary hemochromatosis.[65] One of the most common reasons for this high rate of disease within a particular population is genetic isolation, which occurs when populations are distanced from other populations in terms of geography or cultural barriers,[66] and selective advantage conferred by the disease/carrier state occurring when the genetic variant persists because it offers some type of protection or survival advantage.[62] In the case of sickle cell anemia and thalassemia, there may be a selective advantage of having these carrier states: they are known to be protective against malaria infection.[62,64]

It is important that although some disease aggregates to particular bloodline groups, sometimes the concentration of disease within a given population is attributable to shared environmental factors rather than genetic factors. An example of this is adult-onset diabetes, whereby shared socioeconomic and cultural factors are responsible for higher rates of disease in certain groups than in others.[67]

In summary, both bloodline ancestry and shared environmental factors are important predictors for many disease states. Because bloodline ancestry is not easily identifiable, race and ethnicity (which encompass a broad range of social, religious, and cultural attributes[68,69]) may sometimes be used as rough proxies for genetic risk (eg, equatorial African lineage and sickle cell disease; Ashkenazim lineage and hereditary breast cancer; Celtic or Northern European lineage and hemochromatosis). In an era of value-based health care, appropriate identification of a patient's lineage can be a critical step toward risk identification and appropriate utilization of screening and preventive care.

Case discussion continued: personalized preventive recommendations

Dr Brown screens and counsels Mrs Jones on risk factors for CHD, and encourages her to engage in at least 150 minutes of moderate aerobic exercise or 75 minutes of vigorous aerobic activity per week, along with muscle training at least 2 days per week.[70] He orders age-appropriate screening for colorectal cancer. In regard of family health history of breast cancer, he requests confirmatory records of Mrs Jones' mammograms, and offers her a consultation with a genetic counselor and a breast specialist to further discuss her risk for breast cancer and to determine the optimal strategy for breast cancer prevention. He informs her that genetic tests for hereditary cancer susceptibility may involve sequencing whole genes such as BRCA1 and BRCA2 (not the same as the SNP profile that she received), and are most informative if a person who has already been diagnosed with the cancer, in this case, Mrs Jones' mother, can be tested initially. If a genetic alteration is identified in a relative with cancer, then testing Mrs Jones or other family members can determine whether each individual inherited the genetic alteration that confers higher risk for cancer, and therefore needs special preventive care, or did not inherit the known mutation, and therefore has the same risk for cancer as the general population and can follow usual preventive recommendations (**Box 6**).

With a focus on value-based health care, greater emphasis is being placed on maximizing limited face time with patients, with the goal to not only provide higher-quality care, but to do so in less time and at a lower cost. One of the ways that clinicians can meet this goal is through health care teams. In this era of genomic medicine, medical geneticists and genetic counselors are important consultants or collaborators for primary care clinicians. Genetic counselors are master's-trained allied health care professionals with specific expertise in identifying and educating patients at risk for inherited conditions. With increasing demands and limited time, it can often be difficult for primary care clinicians to provide comprehensive risk assessment and genetic counseling.[71] Genetic counselors, often working in close collaboration or under the supervision of a physician medical geneticist, can serve as partners to clinicians, helping to determine what additional testing is needed based on initial risk assessment with family history, helping patients to decide whether to obtain a genetic test, clarifying insurance coverage, and facilitating pretest and posttest counseling with patients and their families. Patients who may benefit from a referral to a genetic counselor include those with a personal or family history of a hereditary condition, those in whom a primary care clinician suspects increased risk based on personal or family health history, or patients with other mitigating factors such as a family history that is not known or unclear. There are various resources for finding genetic services and genetic counselors.[72–74]

Box 6
Specialists and genetic counselors

- Primary care physicians should refer to medical specialists when appropriate
- Genetic counselors educate patients and facilitate genetic testing when necessary

SUMMARY

Primary care clinicians face many challenges in the current health care environment. Clinicians are being asked to provide better quality, better safety, and better access, with fewer resources and less time. The hope for genomics is that it will enable primary care clinicians to better predict and prevent illness, while at the same time improving efficiencies and reducing costs by driving appropriate utilization of resources and enabling better health. The good news is that, at present, the most important and least expensive tool for prediction of most diseases seen in adult medicine is still the family health history. As a proxy for genomic testing, family health history can inform and guide preventive care plans; moreover, family health history can be used as a tool to discuss environmental, social, or cultural risk factors, and health care team members (including social workers, nurse educators, community health workers, health educators, and dieticians/nutritionists) can be employed to help meet identified needs.

Of importance, both family health history and DNA analysis provide probabilistic information and are not deterministic, and clinicians must remember that environmental exposures and patient behavioral choices can play a large role in causing disease. Knowing this, clinicians are better positioned to assess patient risks and are better informed to engage patients as partners in achieving better health. The challenges going forward for primary care clinicians will be to stay up to date on genomic risk, educate patients about the magnitude of inherited risk in relation to other factors, and help patients and communities influence modifiable risk factors. To stay current and provide efficient genomically informed, value-based care, clinicians will need to target efforts toward education at all levels (including medical training), partner with medical geneticists and genetic counselors, create electronic decision-support tools that can integrate family history and evidence-based risk prediction at the point of care, and generate evidence for the clinical utility and cost-benefit of applying genomic medicine. If these challenges are met successfully in the future, the United States health care system will be well on its way toward providing both genomically informed and value-based health care.

ACKNOWLEDGMENTS

The authors would like to thank Jennifer DiPiero for her assistance in preparing this article for publication.

REFERENCES

1. National health expenditures and selected economic indicators, levels and annual percent change: calendar years 2006-2021 table 1. 2012. Available at: http://www.cms.gov/Research-Statistics-Data-and-Systems/Statistics-Trends-and-Reports/NationalHealthExpendData/Downloads/Proj2011PDF.pdf. Accessed August 8, 2013.
2. US Preventive Services Task Force. Genetic risk assessment and BRCA mutation testing for breast and ovarian cancer susceptibility: recommendation statement. Ann Intern Med 2005;143(5):355–61.
3. Berg AO. The CDC's EGAPP initiative: evaluating the clinical evidence for genetic tests. Am Fam Physician 2009;80(11):1218.
4. 23andMe launches first national TV campaign. 2013. Available at: http://mediacenter.23andme.com/press-releases/poh_ad_campaign/. Accessed August 14, 2013.

5. Bloss CS, Schork NJ, Topol EJ. Effect of direct-to-consumer genomewide profiling to assess disease risk. N Engl J Med 2011;364:524–34.

6. Bloss CS, Wineinger NE, Darst BF, et al. Impact of direct-to-consumer genomic testing at long term follow-up. J Med Genet 2013;50(6):393–400.

7. Kaphingst KA, McBride CM, Wade C, et al. Patients' understanding of and responses to multiplex genetic susceptibility test results. Genet Med 2012; 14(7):681–7.

8. Powell KP, Christianson CA, Cogswell WA, et al. Educational needs of primary care physicians regarding direct-to-consumer genetic testing. J Genet Couns 2012;21(3):469–78.

9. Veenstra DL, Piper M, Haddow JE, et al. Improving the efficiency and relevance of evidence-based recommendations in the era of whole-genome sequencing: an EGAPP methods update. Genet Med 2013;15(1):14–24.

10. Doerr M, Teng K. Family history: still relevant in the genomics era. Cleve Clin J Med 2012;79(5):331–6.

11. Dunlop K, Barlow-Stewart K, Giffin M. Family health history: a role in prevention. Aust Fam Physician 2010;39(10):793–4.

12. Martin AJ, Lord SJ, Verry HE, et al. Risk assessment to guide prostate cancer screening decisions: a cost-effectiveness analysis. Med J Aust 2013;198(10): 546–50.

13. Sud R, Roy B, Emerson J, et al. Associations between family history of cardiovascular disease, knowledge of cardiovascular disease risk factors and health behaviours. Aust J Prim Health 2013;19(2):119–23.

14. Zlot AI, Valdez R, Han Y, et al. Influence of family history of cardiovascular disease on clinicians' preventive recommendations and subsequent adherence of patients without cardiovascular disease. Public Health Genomics 2010;13(7–8): 457–66.

15. Zlot AI, Bland MP, Silvey K, et al. Influence of family history of diabetes on health care provider practice and patient behavior among nondiabetic Oregonians. Prev Chronic Dis 2009;6(1):A27.

16. Ruffin MT 4th, Nease DE Jr, Sen A, et al. Effect of preventive messages tailored to family history on health behaviors: the Family Healthware Impact Trial. Ann Fam Med 2011;9(1):3–11.

17. Wijdenes M, Henneman L, Qureshi N, et al. Using web-based familial risk information for diabetes prevention: a randomized controlled trial. BMC Public Health 2013;13:485.

18. Bronner K, Mesters I, Weiss-Meilnik A, et al. Do individuals with a family history of colorectal cancer adhere to medical recommendations for the prevention of colorectal cancer? Fam Cancer 2013;12:629–37.

19. Lin OS, Gluck M, Nguyen M, et al. Screening patterns in patients with a family history of colorectal cancer often do not adhere to national guidelines. Dig Dis Sci 2013;58(7):1841–8.

20. Walter FM, Emery J. 'Coming down the line'—patients' understanding of their family history of common chronic disease. Ann Fam Med 2005;3(5): 405–14.

21. Acheson LS, Wiesner GL, Zyzanski SJ, et al. Family history-taking in community family practice: implications for genetic screening. Genet Med 2000;2(3):180–5.

22. Scheuner MT, de Vries H, Kim B, et al. Are electronic health records ready for genomic medicine? Genet Med 2009;11(7):510–7.

23. Qureshi N, Wilson B, Santaguida P, et al. Collection and use of cancer family history in primary care. Evid Rep Technol Assess (Full Rep) 2007;(159):1–84.

24. Kannry J, Williams MS. The undiscovered country: the future of integrating genomic information into the EHR. Genet Med 2013;15(10):842–5.

25. Berg AO, Baird MA, Botkin JR, et al. National Institutes of Health State-of-the-Science Conference Statement: family history and improving health. Ann Intern Med 2009;151(12):872–7.

26. Qureshi N, Wilson B, Santaguida P, et al. Family history and improving health. Evid Rep Technol Assess (Full Rep) 2009;(186):1–135.

27. Emery J, Morris H, Goodchild R, et al. The GRAIDS Trial: a cluster randomised controlled trial of computer decision support for the management of familial cancer risk in primary care. Br J Cancer 2007;97(4):486–93.

28. Qureshi N, Armstrong S, Dhiman P, et al. Effect of adding systematic family history enquiry to cardiovascular disease risk assessment in primary care: a matched-pair, cluster randomized trial. Ann Intern Med 2012;156(4): 253–62.

29. Walter FM, Prevost AT, Birt L, et al. Development and evaluation of a brief self-completed family history screening tool for common chronic disease prevention in primary care. Br J Gen Pract 2013;63(611):e393–400.

30. Scheuner MT, Hamilton AB, Peredo J, et al. A cancer genetics toolkit improves access to genetic services through documentation and use of the family history by primary-care clinicians. Genet Med 2014;16:60–9.

31. Biswas S, Atienza P, Chipman J, et al. Simplifying clinical use of the genetic risk prediction model BRCAPRO. Breast Cancer Res Treat 2013;139(2):571–9.

32. Do CB, Hinds DA, Francke U, et al. Comparison of family history and SNPs for predicting risk of complex disease. PLoS Genet 2012;8(10):e1002973.

33. Hindorff LA, Sethupathy P, Junkins HA, et al. Potential etiologic and functional implications of genome-wide association loci for human diseases and traits. Proc Natl Acad Sci U S A 2009;106(23):9362–7.

34. Viera AJ. Odds ratios and risk ratios: what's the difference and why does it matter? South Med J 2008;101(7):730–4.

35. Yoon PW, Scheuner MT, Khoury MJ. Research priorities for evaluating family history in the prevention of common chronic diseases. Am J Prev Med 2003;24(2): 128–35.

36. Hemminki K, Sundquist J, Bermejo JL. How common is familial cancer? Ann Oncol 2008;19(1):163–7.

37. Wilson BJ, Carroll JC, Allanson J, et al. Family history tools in primary care: does one size fit all? Public Health Genomics 2012;15(3–4):181–8.

38. Reid GT, Walter FM, Brisbane JM, et al. Family history questionnaires designed for clinical use: a systematic review. Public Health Genomics 2009; 12(2):73–83.

39. O'Neill SM, Rubinstein WS, Wang C, et al. Familial risk for common diseases in primary care: the Family Healthware Impact Trial. Am J Prev Med 2009;36(6): 506–14.

40. Acheson LS, Zyzanski SJ, Stange KC, et al. Validation of a self-administered, computerized tool for collecting and displaying the family history of cancer. J Clin Oncol 2006;24(34):5395–402.

41. My family health portrait tool. US Surgeon General. Available at: https:// familyhistory.hhs.gov/fhh-web/home.action. Accessed November 4, 2013.

42. Family history. Bethesda (MD): National Human Genome Research Institute; 2013. Available at: http://www.genome.gov/27527640. Accessed November 4, 2013.

43. Family health history. Genetic Alliance. Available at: http://www.geneticalliance. org/fhh. Accessed November 4, 2013.

44. Family medical history in disease prevention. American Medical Association. Available at: http://www.ama-assn.org/resources/doc/genetics/family_history02.pdf. Accessed November 4, 2013.

45. Ford D, Easton DF, Bishop DT, et al. Risks of cancer in BRCA1-mutation carriers. Breast Cancer Linkage Consortium. Lancet 1994;343(8899):692–5.

46. Ford D, Easton DF, Stratton M, et al. Genetic heterogeneity and penetrance analysis of the BRCA1 and BRCA2 genes in breast cancer families. The Breast Cancer Linkage Consortium. Am J Hum Genet 1998;62(3):676–89.

47. Struewing JP, Hartge P, Wacholder S, et al. The risk of cancer associated with specific mutations of BRCA1 and BRCA2 among Ashkenazi Jews. N Engl J Med 1997;336(20):1401–8.

48. Antoniou A, Pharoah PD, Narod S, et al. Average risks of breast and ovarian cancer associated with BRCA1 or BRCA2 mutations detected in case series unselected for family history: a combined analysis of 22 studies. Am J Hum Genet 2003;72(5):1117–30.

49. Chen S, Parmigiani G. Meta-analysis of BRCA1 and BRCA2 penetrance. J Clin Oncol 2007;25(11):1329–33.

50. Howlader N, Noone AM, Krapcho M, et al, editors. SEER cancer statistics review, 1975-2010. Bethesda (MD): National Cancer Institute; 2013. Based on November 2012 SEER data submission, posted to the SEER website. Available at: http://seer.cancer.gov/csr/1975_2010/. Accessed November 4, 2013.

51. Antoniou AC, Pharoah PP, Smith P, et al. The BOADICEA model of genetic susceptibility to breast and ovarian cancer. Br J Cancer 2004;91(8):1580–90.

52. Myriad Genetic Laboratories, Inc. Mutation prevalence tables. 2010. Available at: http://www.myriad.com/lib/brac/brca-prevalence-tables.pdf. Accessed August 8, 2013.

53. Hunt LM, Kreiner MJ. Pharmacogenetics in primary care: the promise of personalized medicine and the reality of racial profiling. Cult Med Psychiatry 2013;37(1):226–35.

54. Williams DR. Miles to go before we sleep: racial inequities in health. J Health Soc Behav 2012;53(3):279–95.

55. Sorkin DH, Ngo-Metzger Q, De Alba I. Racial/ethnic discrimination in health care: impact on perceived quality of care. J Gen Intern Med 2010;25(5):390–6.

56. Richardson LD, Norris M. Access to health and health care: how race and ethnicity matter. Mt Sinai J Med 2010;77:166–77.

57. National healthcare disparities report 2012. US Department of Health and Human Services. Available at: http://www.ahrq.gov/research/findings/nhqrdr/nhdr12/nhdr12_prov.pdf. Accessed November 4, 2013.

58. Burke W, Edwards KA, Goering S, et al, editors. Achieving justice in genomic translation: re-thinking the pathway to benefit. New York: Oxford University Press; 2011.

59. Ulmer C, McFadden B, Nerenz DR, Institute of Medicine (US), Subcommittee on Standardized Collection of Race/Ethnicity Data for Healthcare Quality Improvement, editors. Race, ethnicity, and language data: standardization for health care quality improvement. Washington, DC: The National Academies Press; 2009.

60. Webster's online dictionary: definition: ancestry. Available at: http://www.websters-online-dictionary.org/definitions/Ancestry. Accessed August 12, 2013.

61. Royal CD, Novembre J, Fullerton SM, et al. Inferring genetic ancestry: opportunities, challenges, and implications. Am J Hum Genet 2010;86(5):661–73.

62. McCavit TL. Sickle cell disease. Pediatr Rev 2012;33(5):195–204.

63. Sickle-cell anaemia: report by the secretariat. World Health Organization; 2005. Available at: http://apps.who.int/iris/bitstream/10665/20659/1/B117_34-en.pdf. Accessed November 4, 2013.
64. Vallance H, Ford J. Carrier testing for autosomal-recessive disorders. Crit Rev Clin Lab Sci 2003;40(4):473–97.
65. McCarthy GM, Crowe J, McCarthy CJ, et al. Hereditary hemochromatosis: a common, often unrecognized, genetic disease. Cleve Clin J Med 2002;69(3): 224–6, 229–30, 232–3.
66. Arcos-Burgos M, Muenke M. Genetics of population isolates. Clin Genet 2002; 61:233–47.
67. Link CL, McKinlay JB. Disparities in the prevalence of diabetes: is it race/ethnicity or socioeconomic status? Results from the Boston Area Community Health (BACH) survey. Ethn Dis 2009;19(3):288–92.
68. O'Loughlin J. Understanding the role of ethnicity in chronic disease: a challenge for the new millennium. CMAJ 1999;161(2):152–3.
69. Pearce N, Foliaki S, Sporle A, et al. Genetics, race, ethnicity, and health. BMJ 2004;328(7447):1070–2.
70. American Heart Association recommendations for physical activity in adults. Available at: http://www.heart.org/HEARTORG/GettingHealthy/PhysicalActivity/StartWalking/American-Heart-Association-Recommendations-for-Physical-Activity-in-Adults_UCM_307976_Article.jsp. Accessed August 12, 2013.
71. Mester JL, Schreiber AH, Moran RT. Genetic counselors: your partners in clinical practice. Cleve Clin J Med 2012;79(8):560–8.
72. Find a genetic counselor. National Society of Genetic Counselors. Available at: http://nsgc.org/p/cm/ld/fid=164. Accessed November 4, 2013.
73. American College of Medical Genetics and Genomics. Available at: https://www.acmg.net/ACMG/Terms_and_Conditions/ACMG/Terms_and_Conditions.aspx?redirect=https://www.acmg.net/ACMG/Find_Genetic_Services/ACMG/ISGweb/FindaGeneticService/aspx?hkey=720856ab-a827-42fb-a788-b618b15079f9. Accessed November 4, 2013.
74. Genetic testing registry. Available at: http://www.ncbi.nlm.nih.gov/gtr/. Accessed November 4, 2013.

Index

Note: Page numbers of article titles are in **boldface** type.

A

Abdominal aorta, ultrasonography of, 381–382, 386
Abuse Assessment Screen, 269–271
Accountable Care Organizations, 164, 166–170, 177
    cardiovascular disease and, 389–390
    colorectal cancer and, 347
    depression and, 408–409
    lung cancer and, 323
    prostate cancer and, 366
    sexually transmitted infections and, 232
Adenomatous polyps, colorectal, 332, 341–343
Affordable Care Act, 166–167
    breast cancer and, 298
    cardiovascular disease and, 389–390
    colorectal cancer and, 346
    contraception and, 247–248
    depression and, 408–409
    genomic testing and, 422
    intimate partner violence and, 273
    lung cancer and, 321–322
    prostate cancer and, 365
    sexually transmitted infections and, 232
    substance abuse and, 205
Age, as breast cancer risk factor, 284
AIDS. *See* HIV infection.
Air pollution, lung cancer due to, 311
Al-Anon, 202
Alcohol abuse. *See also* Substance abuse.
    breast cancer risk and, 290
Alcohol Use Disorders Identification Test–Consumption (AUDIT-C), 195, 198
Alcoholics Anonymous, 201–202
American Academy of Child and Adolescent Psychiatry Clinicians, 412
American Academy of Family Physicians
    breast cancer screening recommendations of, 292, 297
    intimate partner violence screening guidelines of, 272
    on substance abuse, 194
American Academy of Pediatrics
    intimate partner violence screening guidelines of, 272
    on substance abuse, 194
    suicide screening recommendations of, 412
American Association for Thoracic Surgery, lung cancer screening recommendations
    of, 315

Prim Care Clin Office Pract 41 (2014) 437–449
http://dx.doi.org/10.1016/S0095-4543(14)00026-8
0095-4543/14/$ – see front matter © 2014 Elsevier Inc. All rights reserved.
primarycare.theclinics.com

Moving?

Make sure your subscription moves with you!

To notify us of your new address, find your **Clinics Account Number** (located on your mailing label above your name), and contact customer service at:

Email: **journalscustomerservice-usa@elsevier.com**

800-654-2452 (subscribers in the U.S. & Canada)
314-447-8871 (subscribers outside of the U.S. & Canada)

Fax number: **314-447-8029**

Elsevier Health Sciences Division
Subscription Customer Service
3251 Riverport Lane
Maryland Heights, MO 63043

*To ensure uninterrupted delivery of your subscription, please notify us at least 4 weeks in advance of move.

Printed and bound by CPI Group (UK) Ltd, Croydon, CR0 4YY

03/10/2024

01040495-0008